Fatigue in Sport and Exercise

Fatigue is an important concern for all athletes, sportspeople and coaches, and in clinical exercise science. There remains considerable debate about the definition of fatigue, what causes it, what its impact is during different forms of exercise, and what the best methods are to combat fatigue and improve performance. This is the first student-focused book to survey the contemporary research evidence into exercise-induced fatigue and to discuss how knowledge of fatigue can be applied in sport and exercise contexts.

The book examines the different 'types' of fatigue and the difficulties of identifying which types are prevalent during different types of exercise. It introduces the fundamental science of fatigue, focusing predominantly on physiological and neuromuscular aspects, and explores key topics in detail, such as energy depletion, lactic acid, dehydration, electrolytes and minerals, and the perception of fatigue. Every chapter includes real case studies from sport and exercise, as well as useful features to aid learning and understanding, such as definitions of key terms, guides to further reading, discussion questions, and principles for training and applied practice. *Fatigue in Sport and Exercise* is an invaluable companion for any degree-level course in sport and exercise physiology, fitness and training, or strength and conditioning.

Shaun Phillips is Lecturer in Sport, Physical Education, and Health Sciences (Sports Physiology) at the University of Edinburgh, Scotland. His research interests include perceptual and self-regulation of exercise performance, fatigue mechanisms in short-duration and endurance exercise, and the impact of novel exercise interventions for improving mental health. Shaun is an invited reviewer for a number of international peer-reviewed journals, and has provided research and consultancy services for numerous elite and professional sport and health organizations.

Fatigue in Sport and Exercise

Shaun Phillips

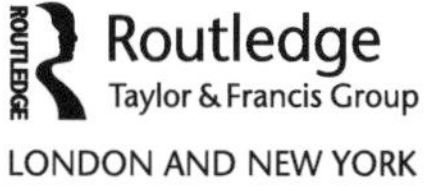

LONDON AND NEW YORK

First published 2015
by Routledge
2 Park Square, Milton Park, Abingdon, Oxon OX14 4RN

and by Routledge
711 Third Avenue, New York, NY 10017

Routledge is an imprint of the Taylor & Francis Group, an informa business

British Library Cataloguing in Publication Data
A catalogue record for this book is available from the British Library

Library of Congress Cataloging in Publication Data
Phillips, Shaun (Shaun Martyn)
Fatigue in sport and exercise / Shaun Phillips.
pages cm
Includes bibliographical references and index.
1. Exercise – Physiological aspects. 2. Sports – Physiological aspects.
3. Fatigue. I. Title.
QP321.P477 2015
612.7′6 – dc23
2014037639

ISBN: 978-0-415-74222-1 (hbk)
ISBN: 978-1-315-81485-8 (ebk)

Typeset in Goudy
by Florence Production Limited, Stoodleigh, Devon, UK

To Jody, for her patience and support.
To my parents, for everything.

Contents

Illustrations

Figures

Tables

Preface

Since I began my studies as a sport and exercise science undergraduate, I have been intrigued by the difficulty and complexity behind answering some of the fundamental questions in the discipline. This interest developed as I specialised in physiology and became fascinated with the processes regulating human exercise performance. Over time, these interests merged my focus to the difficulties of answering one of the enduring questions: why do we fatigue during exercise?

At face value, this seems like a relatively simple question to answer. After all, anyone who has taken part in sport or exercise will probably be aware of some of the common sensations that we associate with fatigue, such as breathlessness, sore muscles, heavy tired limbs, and an overwhelming desire to stop and rest. Surely then, all we have to do is trace the physical causes of these sensations, and we will arrive at our answer? Well, in one way or another this is what fatigue research has been doing for over a century, and in doing so, this research has served to open our eyes to the incredibly complex and multi-faceted probable causes behind fatigue in sport and exercise. The number of variables that can influence fatigue processes during exercise (some of which are discussed in this book), along with the intricate and integrated functioning of the human body, are partly responsible for this complexity. As a result, the reasons behind why we fatigue during exercise are probably more keenly debated now than they have ever been, with a body of research supporting one particular fatigue mechanism often accompanied by an equally relevant body of research rejecting the same mechanism.

It is important that students of the sport, exercise, and health sciences understand the theories and hypotheses behind what causes fatigue during exercise. However, the teaching of fatigue is often overlooked, or limited to a superficial overview of the 'classical' theories. Unfortunately, these theories often are outdated, significantly challenged by contemporary research, or simply wrong. As a human physiology lecturer, I appreciate the difficulties that lecturers can face when trying to teach such a wide-ranging and complex area as fatigue. I believe that one of the reasons sport and exercise fatigue is not more substantially taught is that the body of literature is so large and diverse that it is difficult for the lecturer to condense the knowledge base into an appropriate form. I also believe lecturers appreciate the difficulty that students may have when trying to study sport and exercise fatigue, for the same reason. This was the inspiration behind this book: to address in one volume some of the key hypotheses and current thinking behind how and why humans fatigue during sport and exercise.

So what is the aim of the book? That is two-fold. First: to bring together current thinking on some of the key hypotheses behind fatigue in sport and exercise in order to help students understand and appreciate this fascinating area of investigation. Second: to encourage students to widen their thinking and challenge their existing beliefs behind what causes fatigue in sport and exercise. Some ideas regarding the how and why of sport and exercise fatigue have entered general consciousness (at the expense of other equally valid ideas) despite significant evidence against them. Both the well-known and the not so well-known ideas will be discussed critically and fairly. I have no agenda behind this book other than to inspire a greater level of teaching and understanding of an important topic.

Unfortunately, the full scope of this enormous area of research cannot be included in a single undergraduate volume. To devote as much space as possible to the topic at hand, the book is focused exclusively on sport and exercise fatigue, and will not include detailed discussions of common biochemical or physiological principles. I invite the reader to consult any of the excellent existing undergraduate texts in exercise physiology to support their reading of this book as required. The book focuses on prevalent hypotheses of sport and exercise fatigue that have generated significant research interest (and sometimes have entered the consciousness of the sport and exercise public), as well as more contemporary ideas that are helping to shed new light on the topic. It is hoped that the topics addressed will allow old concepts to be clarified and corrected where necessary, and new thinking to be showcased.

The discussions in the book are based on fatigue from a physiological perspective. The reader is reminded that the influence of other factors not exclusively related to physiology on the fatigue process should be considered. I encourage any interested readers to contact me for further discussion of any information included in the book, or indeed of any information not included. The topics discussed in the book are intricate and often subject to intense debate. To fully appreciate this, the reader is encouraged to use the chapters as a foundation for further study by accessing some of the references cited in each chapter.

A final important point: please do not read this book expecting that come the end you will know precisely what causes fatigue in an exercising human. I do not promise concrete answers, because in the majority of cases they do not yet exist. Instead, I offer an insight into a fascinating, frustrating, and ever changing world of sport and exercise science research. I hope your time with this book is informative, intriguing, challenging, and enjoyable.

Shaun Phillips

Part I

What is fatigue?

Chapter 1

Defining and measuring fatigue in sport and exercise

Part 1 – Defining fatigue

1.1 Introduction

The study of fatigue in humans has been a source of interest for over a century. Since the early work of Mosso[1] and Hill[2], the how and why of human fatigue has been subjected to debate and speculation. Despite huge forward strides in technology that provide us with a much clearer and in-depth observation of the function of the body, many of the observations made by these early pioneers still provide the foundation on which we study fatigue today:

> The first [phenomenon characterising fatigue] is the diminution of the muscle force. The second is fatigue as a sensation. That is to say, we have a physical fact which can be measured and compared and a psychic fact that eludes measurement.[1]

> With young athletic people one may be sure that they really have gone 'all-out', moderately certain of not killing them, and practically certain that their stoppage is due to oxygen want and to lactic acid in their muscles. Quantitatively the phenomena of exhaustion may be widely different; qualitatively they are the same, in our athlete, in your normal man, in your dyspnoeic patient.[2]

> [The limit of exercise] has often been associated with the heart alone, but the facts as a whole indicate that the sum of the changes taking place throughout the body brings about the final cessation of effort.[3]

> Fatigue of brain reduces the strength of the muscles.[1]

> Strength is kept in bounds by the inability of the higher centres to activate the muscles to the full.[4]

> It is not will, not the nerves, but it is the muscle that finds itself worn out after the intense work of the brain.[1]

It is outside the scope of this book to provide a detailed history of all aspects of fatigue research. However, before progressing it is important to appreciate the historical nature of research into human fatigue.

Given its long history, it could be assumed that an unambiguous, universally accepted definition of fatigue has been developed, which all researchers and students of fatigue can use as a benchmark for understanding and applying knowledge. Unfortunately, this is far from true. The long history of research has only served to extend the number of available 'definitions' of fatigue (a non-exhaustive sample of these is in Table 1.1).

The definitions in Table 1.1 highlight one of the main issues in sport and exercise fatigue research: the inability to agree on a single definition of fatigue. This inability hinders and clouds the scientific investigation of fatigue, as there is no single meter on which to gauge and compare study results.[5] In addition, the exercise intensity, amount of muscle mass involved, and the type and duration of exercise can all influence fatigue mechanisms (discussed in Chapter 7).[6] Therefore, experimental data will take on different applications and meanings depending on the type of exercise studied and which definition of fatigue is prevalent in the minds of the researchers and the consumers of that research.

Another source of confusion is that researchers often use the terms 'fatigue' and 'exhaustion' interchangeably. A participant who is no longer able to maintain a given power output during a time to exhaustion test will often be classified as having reached 'exhaustion'. However, they may still be fully capable of continuing exercise at a lower intensity. The definition of exhaustion as: 'a total loss of strength; to consume or use up the whole of'[7] implies that attaining a state of exhaustion results in a complete inability to continue functioning, not simply an inability to continue at a given work

Table 1.1 Different definitions of fatigue, emphasising the variation in the quantification and interpretation of fatigue

1	The moment when a participant is unable to maintain the required muscle contraction or performed workload.
2	Extreme tiredness after exertion; reduction in efficiency of a muscle, organ etc. after prolonged activity.
3	The failure to maintain the required or expected force.
4	Fatigue produced by failure to generate output from the motor cortex.
5	A loss of maximal force generating capacity.
6	A reversible state of force depression, including a lower rate of rise of force and a slower relaxation.
7	Any exercise-induced reduction in the ability of a muscle to generate force or power; it has peripheral and central causes.
8	Failure to continue working at a given exercise intensity.
9	Any exercise-induced reduction in the ability to exert muscle force or power, regardless of whether or not the task can be sustained.
10	A progressive reduction in voluntary activation of muscle during exercise.

rate. Therefore, the concepts of fatigue and exhaustion are different constructs that should not be confused. This becomes more difficult when there are examples in the scientific literature of researchers using different criteria to define and discuss the concept of exhaustion.[5–6] It is important to remember that in this book fatigue is the focus of discussion, not exhaustion.

Key point

The term 'fatigue' has many definitions, and this makes the consistent interpretation and comparison of research findings into fatigue difficult.

Look again at the definitions of fatigue given in Table 1.1. In particular, focus on definitions 2, 4, and 9. Do you think these definitions adequately define and describe the complex, multifaceted phenomenon of exercise-induced fatigue? For example, definition 2 specifically refers to a 'reduction in efficiency of a muscle, organ etc. after prolonged activity' – should we interpret this to mean that there is no such thing as fatigue during short-duration activity? Ask an 800-metre runner what they think of that! Definition 4 states fatigue is due to 'failure to generate output from the motor cortex'. This definition appears to discount the potential influence of peripheral factors in the development of fatigue (Section 1.1.1). Definition 9 defines fatigue as occurring 'whether or not the task can be sustained'. Does this definition clarify or cloud the differences between fatigue and exhaustion discussed above? As you can see, not only might the multitude of fatigue definitions cause misunderstanding, but also the available definitions are open to challenge and debate regarding their veracity for actually defining sport and exercise fatigue in all of its potential states. Clearly, it would be useful if a single, 'unified' definition of fatigue could be achieved. However, care is needed here, for, as Marino *et al.*[5] state, 'to prematurely arrive at a definition [of fatigue] that is only accepted because no better one exists may only confirm our own biases and misrepresent the reality of fatigue'.

1.2 Prevalent fatigue theories: peripheral and central fatigue

Fatigue can be broadly categorised into two types: peripheral fatigue and central fatigue. A basic understanding of these two types of fatigue is fundamental to successfully understanding the information provided in Part II of this book. A description of the key peripheral and central sites that may contribute to fatigue is in Table 1.2.

Table 1.2 Possible sites involved in the development of peripheral and central exercise-induced fatigue

I Peripheral fatigue

A Exercise-related changes in the internal environment

1 Accumulation of lactate and H^+. H^+ is partly buffered, increasing carbon dioxide production from bicarbonate.
2 Accumulation of heat, leading to increased sweat secretion. The loss of water may lead to dehydration.

B Exercise-related changes within muscle fibres

1 Accumulation of P_i in the sarcoplasm, decreasing contractile force due to cross-bridge inhibition.
2 Accumulation of H^+ in the sarcoplasm, decreasing contractile force due to cross-bridge inhibition. Accumulation of H^+ may also depress Ca^{2+} re-uptake in the sarcoplasmic reticulum.
3 Accumulation of sarcoplasmic Mg^{2+}. Mg^{2+} counteracts Ca^{2+} release from the sarcoplasmic reticulum.
4 Inhibition of Ca^{2+} release from the sarcoplasmic reticulum by accumulation of P_i (see point 1). Ca^{2+} release is inhibited by precipitation of calcium phosphate in the sarcoplasmic reticulum and phosphorylation of Ca^{2+} release channels.
5 Decline of glycogen stores and (in extreme cases) decline of blood glucose levels.
6 Decreased conduction velocity of action potentials along the sarcolemma, probably as a result of biochemical changes in and around the muscle fibres. This has no known immediate effect on muscle force production.
7 Increased efflux of K^+ from muscle. Increased K^+ in the lumen of the t-tubuli may block the tubular action potential and lessen force due to a depression of excitation-contraction coupling.

II Central fatigue

1 The conduction of axonal action potentials may become blocked at axonal branching sites, leading to a loss of muscle fibre activation.
2 Motor neuronal drive may be influenced by reflex effects from muscle afferents.
3 Stimulation of type III and IV nerves decreasing motor neuron firing rate and inhibiting motor cortex output.
4 The excitability of cells within the cerebral motor cortex may change during the course of maintained motor tasks, as suggested by measurements using transcranial magnetic stimulation.
5 Synaptic effects of serotoninergic neurons may become enhanced, causing increased tiredness and fatigue. This may occur from increased brain influx of the serotonin precursor tryptophan, via exercise-induced decreases in the blood concentration of BCAAs.
6 Exercise-induced release of cytokines; IL-6 induces sensations of fatigue and IL-1 induces sickness behaviour.

BCAAs = branched-chain amino acids; Ca^{2+} = calcium; H^+ = hydrogen; IL = interleukin; K^+ = potassium; Mg^{2+} = magnesium; P_i = inorganic phosphate.

Source: adapted from Ament and Verkerke.[6]

1.2.1 Peripheral fatigue

Peripheral fatigue states that the sites of fatigue sit outside of the central nervous system (CNS). More specifically, peripheral fatigue is associated with an attenuation of muscle force production caused by a process or processes distal to the neuromuscular junction.[6] The concept of peripheral fatigue originates from the early work of AV Hill and colleagues in the 1920s.[8–11] This work, some of which Hill conducted using himself as the participant, led to the conclusion that immediately before termination of exercise, the oxygen requirements of the exercising muscles exceed the capacity of the heart to supply that oxygen. This develops an anaerobiosis within the working muscles, causing lactic acid accumulation. Because of this change in the intramuscular environment, continued contraction becomes impossible and the muscle reaches a state of failure. Hill interpreted these findings to mean that lactic acid is only produced in the body under anaerobic conditions, and that fatigue is caused by increased intramuscular lactic acid concentrations.[12] Coupled with study findings that appeared to demonstrate improved exercise performance when oxygen was inhaled,[13] Hill and colleagues concluded that the primary limiting factor in exercise tolerance was the heart's capacity to pump blood to the active muscles. This theory, termed the cardiovascular/anaerobic/catastrophic model of human exercise performance ('catastrophic' due to the predicted failure of homeostatic cardiac function), became the dominant theory within exercise science teaching and research.[12] A schematic of the theory is in Figure 1.1.

Despite its dominance in the minds of sport and exercise physiologists, there are issues with the cardiovascular/anaerobic/catastrophic model of exercise performance. First, consider the way in which many of the studies underpinning this model were conducted, namely with Hill himself acting as researcher and participant. This is clearly not the most objective or reliable research approach. Hill's background as a muscle physiologist may also have influenced his focus on the muscle as the loci of fatigue and pre-empted his interpretation of his findings,[12] although this is somewhat speculative. Second, Hill and colleagues stated that the maximal cardiac output of the heart is attained due to the development of myocardial ischaemia. Simply put, the heart cannot pump any more blood as it can no longer consume oxygen at a greater rate. However, the development of sophisticated monitoring equipment has allowed us to confirm that, while a ceiling of cardiac output is attained during maximal intensity exercise, a healthy human heart does not develop ischaemia even during maximal exercise.[14] Third, the model depicted in Figure 1.1 clearly shows that the attainment of a 'maximal' cardiac output limits the flow of blood to the working muscles, causing an 'anaerobiosis' that prevents oxidative removal of lactic acid. This results in lactic acid accumulation within the muscle that directly interferes with the contractile ability of the muscle fibres, causing muscle fatigue. The role of lactic acid in exercise-induced fatigue will be discussed in detail in Chapter 3. It is

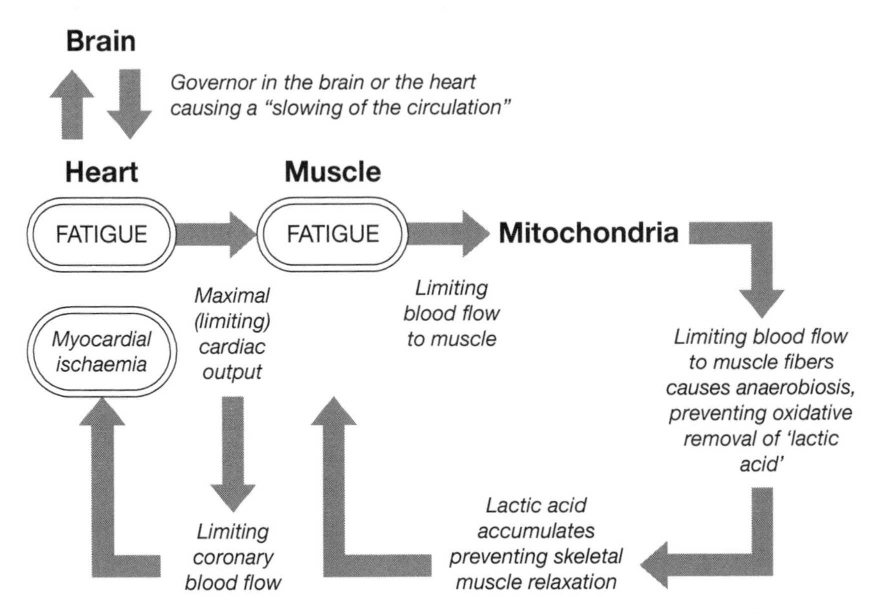

Figure 1.1 A schematic of the cardiovascular/anaerobic/catastrophic model of exercise performance. This theory became, and arguably remains, the dominant paradigm on which the vast majority of exercise physiology teaching and research is conducted. Adapted from Noakes.[12]

sufficient to say at this stage that there is an increasing body of evidence which seriously challenges the concept that lactic acid is the cause of altered contractile function in exercising skeletal muscle.[15–17] Furthermore, there is a lack of evidence to demonstrate that muscles actually become anaerobic during exercise or that oxygen consumption or cardiac output consistently reach a maximal point (defined by a plateau in values with increasing exercise intensity), which would be a requirement for their implication in fatigue during maximal exercise.[12] Fourth, Hill's model suggests that the development of fatigue in the periphery would result in the brain recruiting additional muscle fibres in an attempt to help out those fatiguing fibres and thereby maintain exercise intensity, with this response continuing until all available muscle fibres had been maximally recruited. Only at this point would 'fatigue' begin to develop. However, this prediction is contradictory to other aspects of the model, as continued recruitment of muscle would exacerbate the metabolic crisis (i.e. developing anaerobiosis) that the model predicts causes exercise termination.[18] We now know that regardless of the exercise duration or intensity, fatigue develops before full recruitment of all available muscle fibres. Approximately 35–50% of muscle mass is recruited during prolonged exercise,[19] rising to only ~60% during maximal exercise.[20] Finally, refer again to the schematic of the model in Figure 1.1. Near the top left of the figure is a picture of the brain with the phrase 'governor in the brain or the heart causing a "slowing" of the circulation'. Hill and colleagues proposed myocardial ischaemia as the cause of attainment of the 'exercise limiting' maximal cardiac output. If myocardial ischaemia was allowed to develop and persist during intense exercise a clear threat to the integrity of the cardiac tissue, and hence the athletes themselves, would occur. Hill and colleagues explained the absence of this life-threatening condition by proposing the existence of a governor, located in either the brain or heart, which reduces activity of the heart at the onset of myocardial ischaemia, thereby protecting it from damage.[9] However, we have already mentioned that myocardial ischaemia does not occur in a healthy heart during even the most severe exercise. Therefore, different components of this model of exercise fatigue do not appear to marry up. However, the theory remained, and arguably still stands as the most quoted explanation of exercise-induced fatigue.

Key point

Peripheral fatigue is the term for fatigue caused by factors that reside outside of the central nervous system, distal to the neuromuscular junction.

Further issues occur when the model is tested against some of the definitions of fatigue highlighted in Table 1.1. Many individuals, from recreational exercisers to elite athletes, will identify with a progressive inability to maintain a given running speed or cycling cadence despite best efforts; a form of fatigue defined in example 8 in Table 1.1. Many have also felt the reluctance of their muscles to provide them with a maximal effort when required to break away from the pack in the middle of a race, as defined in example 5 in Table 1.1. These are both definitions of fatigue where the athlete is more than capable of continuing exercise, just at a slightly lower intensity. Indeed, so are fatigue definitions 2, 3, 6, 7, 9, and 10. These definitions of fatigue, that have been both subjectively experienced and experimentally demonstrated, cannot exist based on Hill's catastrophe model of fatigue. This is because the model states that fatigue is indeed a catastrophic, 'all or nothing' event that results in complete failure of the working muscles to continue producing force. However, with extremely rare exceptions, catastrophic muscle or organ failure does not occur at exhaustion in healthy individuals during any form of exercise.[21] In this vein, the model also does not account for the observation that athletes begin exercise of different durations at different paces: a harder initial pace for shorter duration events, and a reduced initial pace for longer events (Section 6.4.3), and that they are generally able to exercise at a higher intensity during competition compared to training. This suggests two things: that physiological mechanisms are not solely responsible for the regulation of exercise intensity (if they were, the athlete would surely maximise their physiological capability regardless of the duration of exercise), and that humans display an anticipatory aspect of exercise regulation, possibly related to factors including perception of task effort and motivation.[12] Clearly, this aspect of exercise regulation cannot be attributed purely to peripheral components, i.e. the skeletal muscles (see the 'To think about' example at the end of the chapter). Indeed, if exercise is limited purely by attainment of a maximal cardiac output, as Hill suggested, then psychological aspects such as motivation, focus, and confidence have no role to play in exercise performance. This is clearly not the case. It therefore appears that the long-standing model of 'catastrophic' exercise-induced fatigue does not hold all the answers, and is likely too simplistic to adequately explain the complex phenomena of human muscle fatigue (Table 1.2).

Key point

The cardiovascular/anaerobic/catastrophic model of exercise performance does not satisfactorily explain many of the definitions of fatigue stated in this chapter, or many of the real-world observations and sensations experienced when a person reaches 'fatigue'.

1.2.2 Central fatigue

Whereas peripheral fatigue occurs via processes outside of the CNS, unsurprisingly central fatigue proposes that the origin of fatigue is located within the CNS, with a loss of muscle force occurring through processes proximal to the neuromuscular junction. Specifically, this refers to locations within the brain, spinal nerves and motor neurons. Just as there are multiple definitions for fatigue, there are several definitions of central fatigue, although these definitions have similarities:

> A negative central influence that exists despite the subject's full motivation.

> A force generated by voluntary muscular effort that is less than that produced by electrical stimulation.

> A subset of fatigue associated with specific alterations in central nervous system function that cannot reasonably be explained by dysfunction within the muscle itself.

> The loss of contractile force or power caused by processes proximal to the neuromuscular junction.[22]

Some of these definitions are questionable; for example, assessing a person's motivation to continue exercise, or whether someone has the 'full motivation' to perform is very difficult. However, the definitions are all similar in that they provide only vague definitions of central fatigue, with no specific information about locations or mechanisms of impairment.

> On an examination of what takes place in fatigue, two series of phenomena demand our attention. The first is the diminution of the muscle force. The second is fatigue as a sensation.[1]

> There appear, however, to be two types of fatigue, one arising entirely within the central nervous system, the other in which fatigue of the muscles themselves is superadded to that of the nervous system.[3]

The two quotes above were made in 1915 and 1931, respectively, indicating that an awareness of the potential for both peripheral and central fatigue process has existed for at least a century. However, the idea of a central component to the fatigue process did not immediately become popular from a research perspective, perhaps because it was superseded by the work of Hill and others about a decade later that focused on the periphery as the loci of fatigue during exercise (Section 1.1.1).[12]

In fact, comparatively little research effort was spent on the role of the CNS in fatigue until the last few decades.[22] This seems strange, considering for how long the possibility of a central component of fatigue has been known. It is also interesting to note that the second quote above, which acknowledges both a central and peripheral fatigue, was added into the Bainbridge text at the request of AV Hill, the 'father' of the peripheral catastrophe fatigue model.[12] However, the central component quickly vanished from the teaching of exercise fatigue, as the perceived importance of peripheral fatigue became more engrained.[12]

Central fatigue as a hypothesis may not have gained traction due to the publication of research findings that appeared to support the theory of peripheral muscle fatigue (Section 1.1.1). However, it may also have been due to limitations in the ability to measure central fatigue because of a lack of objective, clearly defined measurement tools (this is discussed further in the next section of the chapter). In fact, difficulties remain to the present day when trying to test central fatigue theories accurately (Chapter 6), although technological advances are making this more possible (Part II, Chapter 6).[23–4] A common research approach for studying central fatigue is the comparison of maximal voluntary contraction (MVC) force with the force generated by supramaximal electrical stimulation of the muscle itself (Section

1.2.1). Studies applying this technique have reported a parallel reduction in MVC and electrically stimulated (i.e. non-CNS mediated) force during repeated muscle contractions, leading to the suggestion that central processes do not play a role in muscle fatigue.[25–6] However, as Davis and Bailey[22] summarise, this may not be the case for the following reasons:

- Maintaining a maximal CNS 'drive' is difficult and even unpleasant, and requires a well-familiarised and motivated participant to achieve it.
- Even if a participant is well motivated, it is not always possible to maintain maximal CNS drive to some muscles.
- It is more difficult to maximally recruit all motor units during repeated maximal concentric contractions compared with eccentric contractions. Therefore, the reported impact of central fatigue on exercise performance may be influenced by the specific exercise protocols used in different research studies.

These issues help to highlight some of the problems associated with measuring central fatigue. However, the objectivity of central fatigue measurement tools is important, as it helps to remove some of the potential subjectivity involved in the assessment of a person's 'willingness' to continue exercise. The issues with objectively measuring central fatigue may be part of the reason why central fatigue is sometimes only accepted when experimental findings do not support any peripheral causes for fatigue,[22] making central fatigue almost a 'condition of exclusion'. Furthermore, quantification of the presence of central fatigue, for example by observation of reduced maximal voluntary contraction force, does not offer insights into the causes behind the development of central fatigue (potential causes of central fatigue are discussed in Chapter 6). An unwillingness and/or inability to generate sufficient drive from the CNS to the muscles is a likely cause of exercise-induced fatigue in the majority of people.[22] It is therefore important for the advancement of knowledge into fatigue processes during exercise that research attempts to overcome the challenges associated with investigating central fatigue.

Key point

Central fatigue is the term for fatigue caused by factors that reside within the central nervous system (brain, spinal cord, and motor neurons).

1.2.3 Peripheral and central fatigue: summary

Sections 1.2.1 and 1.2.2 have introduced the two overriding theories of fatigue in sport and exercise. It may already be apparent that both theories have limitations in terms of the research that has investigated them, and in their ability to explain sport and exercise fatigue. In fact, the ability of either theory to independently, consistently, and effectively explain fatigue in all sport and exercise scenarios is highly questionable. However, it must be remembered that peripheral and central fatigue are simply umbrella terms used to classify multiple specific processes that are thought to contribute to fatigue. It is some of these processes that will be discussed in Part II of the book, and in so doing, the relative merits of peripheral and central fatigue will be evaluated. It is also easy to consider peripheral and central fatigue as two opposing theories that have no common ground or influence over one another. As will be mentioned throughout the book, the body responds to exercise in an integrated fashion. Therefore, it is likely that peripheral and central fatigue processes overlap and influence one another. Such potential links of influence will be highlighted as relevant in Part II.

Part 2 – Measuring fatigue

To understand sport and exercise fatigue research, it is important to appreciate how fatigue is measured and assessed. The following is a brief introduction to some of the common methods of measuring fatigue. This will provide context for the more detailed discussions in Part II.

1.3 Direct methods of fatigue assessment

1.3.1 Maximal voluntary force generation/electrical stimulation

Accurate measurement of the force generating capacity of muscle is crucial for the reliable assessment of muscle fatigue.[27] The maximal isometric force production (MVC for maximal voluntary contraction) is often used for this purpose. Participants are instructed to exert what they believe to be their maximum force against a piece of apparatus that does not enable dynamic contraction of the muscle (hence the term isometric force production; Figure 1.2). Strong verbal encouragement is provided by the investigator in an effort to assist the participant in reaching a true maximal contraction. There are numerous examples in the literature of the use of MVC force as an indication of fatigue. For example, Nybo and Nielsen[28] investigated the influence of hyperthermia on fatigue following exercise at 60% VO_{2max} until exhaustion in temperatures of 40°C and 18°C. Following exercise, participants undertook a two-minute MVC of the knee extensor muscles with force output continually monitored. The authors found that while force output decreased over the two minutes in both trials, the drop was significantly greater in the hot trial, indicating a negative effect of hyperthermia on force production and, hence, greater central fatigue. However, there are concerns with the use of MVC for assessing fatigue. Force production can be limited by the voluntary effort/motivation of the participant. Not even strong encouragement and feedback may be sufficient to enable someone to achieve a true maximal contraction.[27] In addition, MVC can be limited by factors present within the CNS or in the periphery. Therefore, it is not possible to clearly determine potential mechanisms for reduced MVC.

How, therefore, were Nybo and Nielsen[28] able to conclude that reduced force output in the hot exercise trial was due to greater levels of central fatigue? The answer is they also utilised a technique called electrical stimulation. Here, an electrical signal is externally applied to the motor neuron of the muscle, or directly to the muscle itself, which causes it to contract (Figure 1.2). This is usually done in short, repeated bursts, or twitches, to prevent over-stimulation of the muscle that can attenuate force production and lead to an incorrect interpretation of muscle fatigue.[29] The important concept behind electrical stimulation is that it removes the CNS from the equation as the electrical stimulation to contract the muscle is externally and directly applied. Therefore, potential limitations to muscle contraction present in the CNS can be discounted, and the ability of the muscle itself to contract is isolated. Voluntary contractile ability can be interpreted using the simple formula:

$$MVC / MVC + ES$$

where MVC is the maximal voluntary contraction force and ES is the force generated by electrical stimulation, superimposed onto the MVC (referred to as total muscle force). Solving this equation provides the voluntary

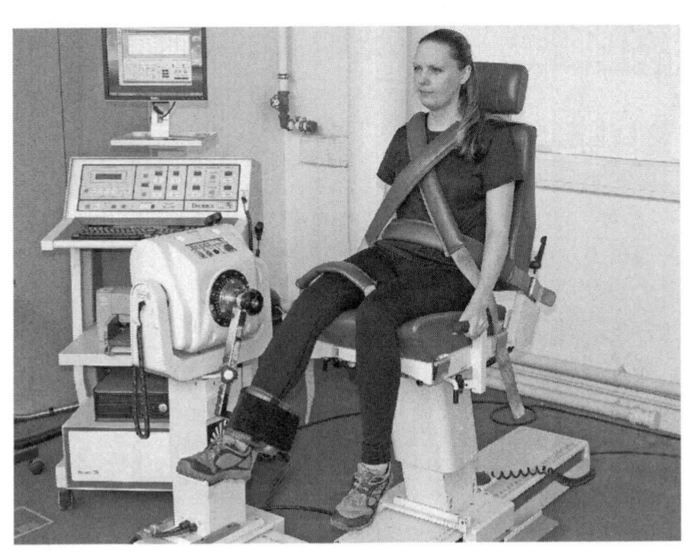

Figure 1.2 A person preparing to undertake a maximal voluntary contraction of the quadriceps muscles.

activation percentage, which is the percentage of the total possible muscle force that can be achieved by a voluntary contraction. As the right side of the equation includes the muscle force produced by isolated, non-CNS mediated contractile force, the voluntary activation percentage provides an estimate of the degree of central activation present in any given muscle contraction. Currently, MVC and ES are the most direct methods of assessing muscle fatigue.

1.3.2 Low-frequency fatigue

Low-frequency fatigue (LFF) is characterised by a proportionately greater loss of force during low-frequency compared with high-frequency muscle stimulation.[30] This form of fatigue can take hours or even days to dissipate, and may play a key role in the decline in muscle force production.[30] Low-frequency fatigue is typically interpreted by measuring torque responses to different frequencies of electrical stimulation and examining changes in the ratio of force production at a given frequency (usually 20 Hz) to that at a standardised frequency (usually 50 or 80 Hz). Decreases in this ratio are interpreted as LFF. Low-frequency fatigue may increase the requirement for greater CNS activation to elicit a given muscle force.[30] Consequently, this could cause an increase in effort perception for a given force production, potentially contributing to the development of central fatigue.

Low-frequency fatigue has been reported during high-intensity and submaximal exercise,[31] and therefore has the potential to be used as a fatigue measure during a variety of exercise scenarios. The use of ES to quantify LFF may be subject to limitations including preferential recruitment of fast-twitch motor units near the sites of ES, potentially overestimating fatigue due to the greater fatigability of fast twitch units,[32] varied recruitment thresholds of motor neuron axons so that different motor units may be recruited by ES in different trials,[33] and the inability of ES to accurately account for the influence of muscle damage on LFF, as ES only stimulates a fraction of the muscle mass and damage is not uniform throughout a muscle.[34] However, Martin *et al.*[35] reported that LFF can be accurately assessed by ES via large surface electrodes (termed transcutaneous stimulation). Assessment of LFF is of course limited in its applicability by the requirement to use laboratory-based ES on a small amount of muscle mass during exercise that is not representative of most sporting situations.

Key point

Many of the techniques commonly used to measure fatigue during exercise are limited in their ability to measure fatigue during real-world sport-specific activities.

1.4 Indirect methods of fatigue assessment

1.4.1 Endurance time ('time to exhaustion')

Many research studies have utilised an endurance test, commonly known as a time to exhaustion test, to assess and/or quantify fatigue, particularly the influence of an intervention on the development of fatigue. Use of these tests is partly based on the assumption that there is a relationship between the force generating capacity of muscles and the time to exhaustion.[27] However, this assumed relationship has been demonstrated to vary considerably during repeated isometric contractions.[36] Also, gross time to exhaustion tests (e.g. a cycle to exhaustion at 80% VO_{2max}) exhibit large coefficients of variation (up to ~35%),[37] suggesting that time to exhaustion tests should not be the only measure used to determine the influence of a treatment on performance/fatigue.[38] Conversely, more recent research has shown that treadmill based time to exhaustion tests are inherently reliable when time to exhaustion is transformed using statistical modelling based on the speed-duration relationship.[39] However, the runs in the Hinckson and Hopkins[39] study only lasted between ~2 and 8 minutes. Most other research into the reliability of time to exhaustion tests has used longer duration exercise, which may be less reliable than shorter exercise due to the multitude of factors that can influence a person's decision of whether or not to continue, such as motivation and boredom. In addition, the variability in time to exhaustion of the shorter runs before statistical modelling (9–16%) was still quite large. Finally, Hinckson and Hopkins[39] acknowledge that the conversion of changes in time to exhaustion via the statistical models used in their study is specific to the particular statistical model used and to the individual participant. As a result, the conversions are only approximate. Therefore, the ability of converted time to exhaustion scores to detect small changes in performance or fatigue is unknown.

1.4.2 Electromyography

Electromyography (EMG) is the analysis of the electrical activity of muscle tissue. The two common forms of EMG are surface EMG (non-invasive) and needle EMG (invasive). For ethical reasons, surface EMG is most prevalent in the sports science literature. Here, surface electrodes are attached to specific locations on the muscle (Figure 1.3). These electrodes detect the electrical signal transmitted through the superficial muscle tissue, allowing the amplitude of the electrical activity to be determined. The amplitude of the signal is related to the number and size of action potentials (electrical signals transmitted down motor neurons into the muscle). Changes in the frequency of these action potentials or in the number of muscle fibres activated can be detected, however EMG cannot distinguish between these two occurrences.[27]

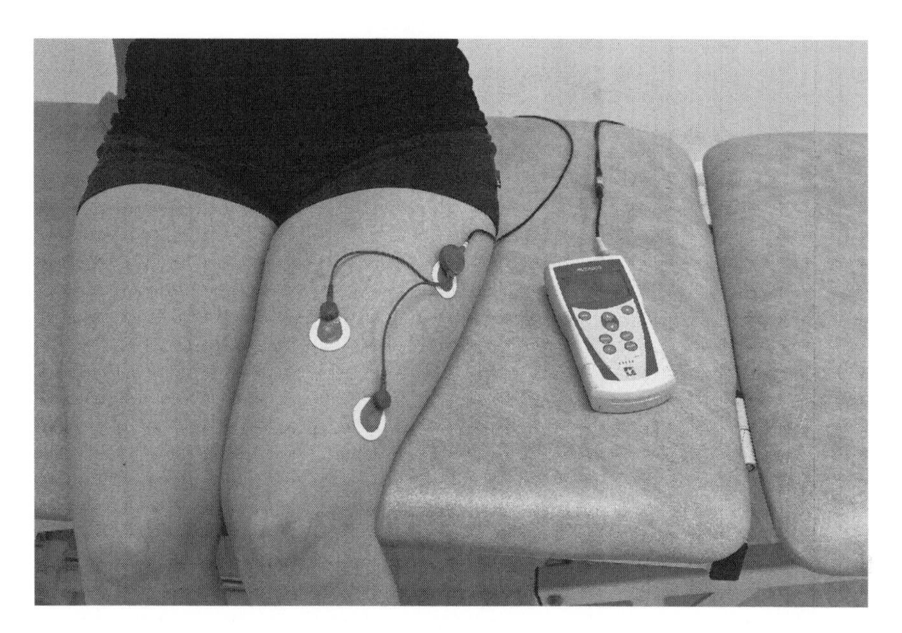

Figure 1.3 Surface electromyography of the quadriceps muscles.

Electromyography amplitude falls progressively during repeated maximal isometric contractions, likely due to a reduction in the activity of motor units and, hence, a reduction in muscle force production.[40] However, this does not automatically mean that EMG is a good indicator of muscle fatigue, as the cause and effect relationship between EMG amplitude and fatigue is still under debate. During repeated or sustained submaximal contractions a rise in EMG activity is seen in the presence of a reduction in muscle force production (i.e. muscle electrical activity is increasing yet force is reducing). This is probably due to the progressive requirement for more muscle fibre recruitment as contractions progress and existing muscle fibres begin to fatigue.[27] However, during repeated submaximal contractions there is a large inter-participant variability in EMG response. This is shown in Figure 1.4, where two participants recorded an increase in EMG activity as MVC force declined, but the other two participants recorded almost no change in EMG activity with MVC force decline. Furthermore, EMG principally records the neural component of muscle contraction; if causes of reduced muscle force production were occurring inside the muscle, independent of neural input, EMG would not detect this.[27] Finally, EMG can only be used with any form of validity during isometric contractions, as changes in muscle length alter the relationship between EMG and neuromuscular activation.[27] This indicates that EMG may not be a particularly useful or appropriate index of fatigue during many sport-specific muscle actions.

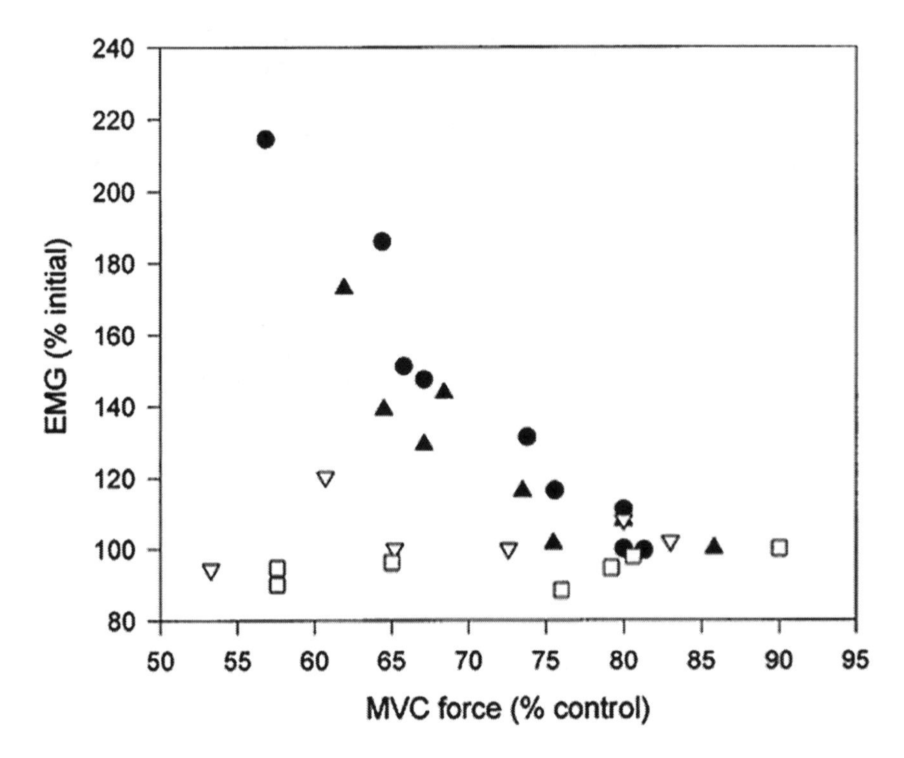

Figure 1.4 Electromyography activity during repeated quadriceps contractions at 30% of initial maximal voluntary contraction in relation to the maximal voluntary contraction force. Notice how two participants (black circles and triangles) show an increase in electromyography activity as maximal voluntary contraction force decreases, yet two participants (white triangles and squares) show a stable electromyography activity in the face of declining maximal voluntary contraction force. Data from Mengshoel *et al.*[41]

1.4.3 Muscle biopsies

In a muscle biopsy, a small piece of muscle tissue is removed from an intact human muscle for examination. In sport and exercise science research, the needle biopsy is most common. Here, local anaesthetic is applied to the area after which a needle is inserted into the muscle (commonly the vastus lateralis of the quadriceps). Muscle biopsies can be used for quantifying muscle fibre composition, muscle energy content, and the concentration and activity of a multitude of enzymes involved in energy production that can provide an insight into the functional capacity of the muscle and changes in this capacity following an intervention, such as a training period.

The actual process of conducting a biopsy, if done correctly, can provide a sample of muscle tissue that can be used in a variety of analyses for determination of the variables described above and more. A potential limitation is that a biopsy sample may not be representative of the entire muscle from which it is drawn. In this situation, results extrapolated from a biopsy sample to the full muscle would be inaccurate. In addition, if repeated biopsy samples are required, variations in the sampling site may affect the validity and/or reliability of the data. However, the main concern with the use of muscle biopsies in fatigue research is whether the measurements made on the muscle sample are actually indicative of fatigue. For example, muscle biopsies are often taken to assess the rate and extent of muscle glycogen degradation during and after exercise, with differences in the rate of degradation and end-exercise concentration often cited as a causative mechanism of fatigue. However, a closer analysis of the literature appears to indicate that carbohydrate ingestion during exercise does not attenuate muscle glycogen depletion[42] (discussed further in Part II). Of course, one of the primary limitations of the muscle biopsy technique is gaining the necessary ethical approval and, perhaps even more of a challenge, informed consent to actually conduct the procedure.

1.4.4 Blood sampling

Blood sampling is a staple tool in sports science research. Methods of sampling vary, from simple fingertip or earlobe capillary sampling (Figure 1.5) to arterial and venous sampling and cannulation. The frequency and method of blood sampling will depend on the aims of the research, the aims of the sampling (what blood variables will be measured and what they will be used for), and ethical and consensual restrictions. These same factors will, in part, determine the blood-borne variables that a researcher measures. Common measurements include blood glucose and lactate contractions and basic haematological variables, which can be accurately measured using capillary blood sampling with very small volumes of blood. Other measurements include the concentration of blood-borne substances such as hormones, free-fatty acids, antioxidants, and intra-muscular substances such as creatine kinase and myoglobin.

Blood sampling conducted by a trained person in an appropriate environment, and adhering to appropriate codes of conduct and safety, carries minimal risk to the participant or the person taking the sample. However, as with muscle biopsies, the fatigue researcher needs to consider how representative, and therefore useful, their blood-borne analyses are in helping to quantify or explain fatigue. A classic example is the testing of blood lactate. Observation of high blood lactate concentrations at the point of fatigue led to the often-repeated conclusion that high blood lactate concentrations *cause* fatigue (see part 1 of this chapter). However, ample evidence now exists to debate, or even refute, this claim (Chapter 3). Similarly, blood lactate concentration has been, and frequently still is, taken

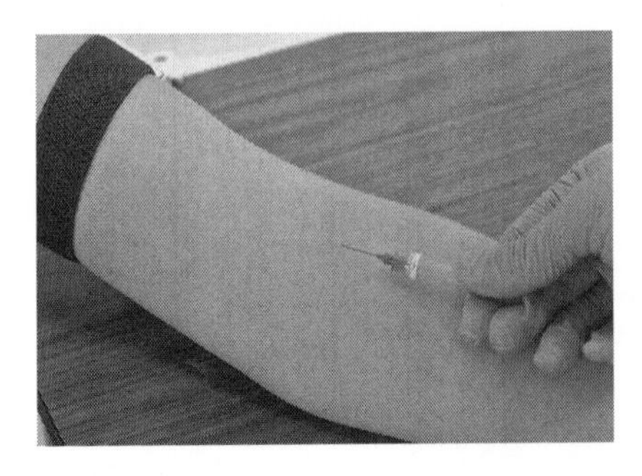
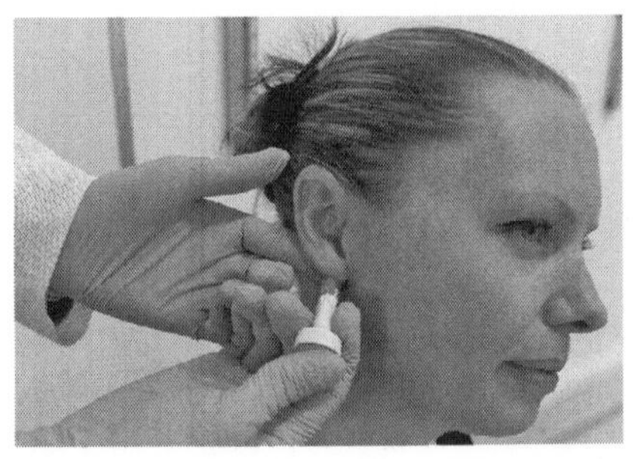

Figure 1.5 Antecubital venous blood sampling (left) and capillary earlobe sampling (right).

as a surrogate measure of intramuscular lactate concentration and, therefore, a measure of the biochemical status of the muscle. However, blood lactate concentration is not a valid measure of muscle lactate concentration during exercise as it only reflects activities undertaken a few minutes prior to sampling, and the balance between lactate movement into and out of the blood.[43–4] This will be discussed further in Chapter 3, and blood-based indicators of fatigue will be discussed throughout Part II.

Key point

Blood sampling and, in particular, muscle biopsies require strong justifications before ethical approval will be granted to use these techniques in sports science research.

1.4.5 Perceptual measurements

Numerous rating scales have been developed which attempt to quantify an individual's psychological, perceptual, and motivational responses to exercise. This is a hugely complex task, and specific scales have been produced that measure varied aspects such as sensation of effort, motivation, pain, enjoyment, concentration, attention, lethargy, and many more. It is impractical to highlight all of these scales. To provide an overview of this aspect of fatigue assessment discussion will focus on the most commonly used of these scales, and a contemporary addition to the repertoire.

1.4.5.1 Ratings of perceived exertion

The most commonly used perceptual scale is the Borg rating of perceived exertion (RPE) scale (also referred to as the Borg 6–20 scale). Developed in

1970 by Gunnar Borg,[45] the scale provides a quantifiable representation of an individual's level of exertion during exercise. The scale is generally used to provide a holistic measure of exertion (determined by the combined sensation of exertion from breathing, muscle soreness and strain, cardiovascular load, body temperature etc). As a result, perceived exertion during exercise is classed as having peripheral, respiratory-metabolic, or non-specific origins.[46] The seemingly arbitrary 6–20 range of the original Borg scale was developed due to the observed correlation between heart rate and RPE ratings, such that the given score on the scale can be multiplied by 10 and provide a close approximation of the exercising person's heart rate (e.g. an RPE of 12 approximates a heart rate of 120 bpm). However, this calculation is at best an approximation due to the multitude of factors that can influence the heart rate response to exercise.

Many studies have demonstrated that the RPE scale can be used to accurately establish intensity during exercise.[47–9] The scale is fairly simple to use provided appropriate instructions are given, however its use in young children is inappropriate or limited due to inabilities to cognitively rate perceived exertion (0–3 years of age) or provide a cohesive RPE score (4–7 years); little is known about the ability of adolescents to provide accurate RPE scores.[50]

It is important to look a little deeper at what information is actually being provided when a person gives their 'rating of perceived exertion'. This is highlighted by the fact that the origins of how we sense and then 'perceive' exertion during exercise are still not fully understood.[51–2] Furthermore, interventions can be made that alter the relationship between exercise intensity (usually measured by heart rate) and RPE, such as the use of music,[53] altered sensory perception strategies,[54] and the provision of accurate and inaccurate feedback regarding exercise intensity and the duration of the exercise bout that remains to be completed (Chapter 6).[55]

1.4.5.2 Task effort awareness scale

The task effort awareness (TEA) scale was developed and first used by Swart *et al.*[56] The scale is designed to quantify the magnitude of the psychological/psychic sensations of effort and the extent to which a person is consciously aware of this effort.[56] The scale attempts to identify the psychological and mental effort required to perform a given bout of exercise at a chosen intensity based on the degree of attention and mental effort experienced during exercise. Importantly, participants are instructed to disregard the physical sensations they may be feeling when giving a TEA rating. Therefore, the scale attempts to separate the psychological sensations of effort from the physical sensations.

Swart *et al.*[56] reported that during prolonged cycling interspersed with high-intensity efforts, the physical and psychological sensations of exertion did not increase linearly with one another. This suggests that physical and psychological sensations of effort are distinct but related 'cues' that may combine to regulate exercise intensity.[57] This is interesting data, and the TEA scale appears to provide an additional dimension from which to study the regulation of exercise. However, at the time of writing Swart *et al.*[56] are the only authors to have published a study using the TEA scale. Therefore, more research is required to further understand the role that the TEA scale may play in exercise fatigue research.

1.4.6 Magnetic resonance imaging

One of the challenges in understanding the complex function of the body during exercise, and therefore determining fatigue mechanisms, is being able to 'see' exactly what is happening in various body systems and tissues while exercise is taking place, or in the post-exercise period. Without this ability, determining the exact mechanisms of fatigue will remain a process of indirect deductions and educated guesses.

The development of magnetic resonance imaging (MRI) techniques in medical and health settings has opened a new window into the workings of the body during exercise. An MRI machine produces a strong magnetic field around a person. This magnetic field acts on protons within the body. Protons are very sensitive to magnetisation and get 'pulled' in the direction of the magnet, where they essentially 'line-up' in the direction of the magnetic field. A radio frequency pulse is then directed to the part of the body to be examined. This pulse causes the protons to spin at a particular frequency and in a particular direction. When the pulse is turned off, the protons return to their natural alignment within the magnetic field and release the energy absorbed from the radio frequency pulse. This energy is detected and converted into an image, allowing the body part in question to be 'seen'.

Magnetic resonance imaging has been applied in exercise research to investigate the energetics and intracellular environment of intact skeletal muscle,[58–60] skeletal muscle fibre orientation and architecture,[61] and the cardiac responses to exercise.[62] In addition, functional MRI (*f*MRI) has been employed to investigate the activity of brain regions in response to specific stimuli that are associated with performance during exercise, such as carbohydrate mouth rinses.[63] The use of MRI has the potential to significantly improve our understanding of the processes involved in enhancing, and limiting, performance from a metabolic, anatomical, functional, and regulatory perspective. Unfortunately, there are obvious limitations to the application of MRI technology, not least of which is the prohibitive cost of purchasing the equipment and the requirement for trained practitioners to run it. In addition, techniques such as *f*MRI are still limited in their application to sport and exercise as they require a participant to lie still within the machine in order to provide accurate results. This rules out using *f*MRI to investigate most real-time or real-world sporting activities.

1.4.7 Transcranial magnetic stimulation

Transcranial magnetic stimulation is another non-invasive medical technique that is being increasingly used in sport and exercise research. Transcranial magnetic stimulation involves placing an electromagnetic coil in contact with the head. The coil emits short electromagnetic pulses that pass through the skull and cause small electrical currents to penetrate a few inches into the brain. These currents cause activity of neurons in the areas of the brain to which they are directed. This stimulated brain activity results in an action; for example, if transcranial magnetic stimulation is used on the primary motor cortex, muscle activity is produced (this is referred to as a motor evoked potential). These motor evoked potentials can be used to examine the ability of the motor cortex to activate skeletal muscles. For example, research investigating the use of carbohydrate mouth rinses (which are thought to influence central drive to muscles) used transcranial magnetic stimulation to demonstrate significant increases in motor evoked potentials when carbohydrate mouth rinses were used.[64] This is another example of how technology can provide fascinating new insights into the complexity behind our responses to exercise. Unfortunately, much like MRI techniques, the requirement for expensive equipment and well trained practitioners limits the employment of transcranial magnetic stimulation in the study of sport and exercise fatigue.

Key point

Researchers must consider whether the measurements they intend to make will actually provide relevant information about the fatigue process before deciding whether or not to employ them.

1.5 Summary

- Human fatigue has been researched for over a century, and many of the findings and questions stimulated by this early research are still relevant today.
- Fatigue research is hampered by the multiple definitions of fatigue that exist, meaning there is no single meter on which to compare study findings. This may slow the rate of progress of fatigue research.
- The two most prevalent fatigue theories are peripheral and central fatigue. Peripheral fatigue was originally modelled by Hill and colleagues in the

1920s, while the concept of a central component to fatigue was also being discussed around this time.

- Peripheral fatigue is characterised by processes occurring outside of the central nervous system, distal to the neuromuscular junction. The absence of a consistent link between any single physiological variable and the development of fatigue during exercise, as well as the contemporary refuting of many components of the peripheral fatigue model of Hill and colleagues, suggests additional explanations for exercise-induced fatigue are required.
- Central fatigue is the term for fatigue that resides within the central nervous system. A central component to fatigue has been speculated for over a century, but comparatively little research effort was spent investigating this suggestion until the last few decades. This may be due to the prevalent support for peripheral fatigue, and limitations in the ability to measure central fatigue because of a lack of objective, clearly defined measurement tools. As a result, central fatigue is sometimes only accepted when experimental findings do not support any peripheral causes for fatigue.
- Both peripheral and central fatigue theories have limitations in terms of the research that has investigated them, and in their ability to explain sport and exercise fatigue, and the ability of either to independently, consistently, and effectively explain fatigue is questionable.
- Peripheral and central fatigue are umbrella terms used to classify multiple specific processes that are thought to contribute to fatigue.
- Peripheral and central fatigue should not be considered as opposing theories that have no common ground or influence over one another.
- The two primary direct methods of fatigue assessment are the quantification of voluntary and electrically stimulated muscle force production and the assessment of low-frequency fatigue. Both methods are laboratory-based and require carefully controlled procedures to produce accurate results. Assessment of force production cannot detect limitations from central regions or the periphery, therefore cannot determine mechanisms for fatigue development. Low-frequency fatigue assessment takes place on a small amount of muscle mass, therefore its applicability to real-world sport and exercise situations is limited.
- Indirect methods of fatigue assessment include time to exhaustion tests, electromyography, muscle biopsies, blood sampling, perceptual measurements, and magnetic resonance imaging. All these measures have positives and negatives associated with their ability to shed light on fatigue development during exercise. Choice of which to use will depend on factors including the specific research design, availability of equipment, ethical and consensual restrictions, and the informed decision by the researcher of which methods will provide information that can actually

help to quantify potential causes of fatigue development during the exercise protocol or research scenario employed.

To think about . . .

In 2005 the great Ethiopian distance runner Kenenisa Bekele set a new world record for the 10,000 metres of 26 minutes 17 seconds; a record that as of publication of this book still stands. During that race, Bekele ran the first 9 kilometres at an average pace of 2 minutes 38 seconds per kilometre. However, he ran the final kilometre in 2 minutes 32 seconds, 6 seconds faster than his average speed for the first 90% of a world-record setting race! This is by no means a 'fluke' performance; in fact, it is commonplace in endurance sports to see a significant increase in exercise intensity near the end of a race, regardless of how hard the athlete was pushing throughout the event.

As you read the coming chapters of this book, keep this scenario in your mind. As we discuss each theory of fatigue, ask yourself: does that theory help to explain what Kenenisa Bekele did in his world record run? After all, if a theory does not explain what we see in the real world, perhaps it's time to have a re-think . . .

Test yourself

Answer the following questions to the best of your ability. This will reinforce the key knowledge that you require before progressing with the rest of the book. Try to understand the information gained from answering these questions before you progress with the book.

1. Define the term exercise-induced fatigue.
2. Write a short paragraph highlighting why the study of fatigue is complex and subject to so much debate and indecision.
3. Briefly describe the two most prevalent fatigue theories.
4. What are the key contemporary research findings that cast doubt on the veracity of the peripheral catastrophe model of exercise performance?
5. What are the main direct and indirect methods of exercise-induced fatigue assessment?
6. What considerations does a researcher need to make before deciding which of the above measurements to employ in a research study?

References

1 Mosso A (1915) *Fatigue*. London: Allen and Unwin Ltd.
2 Hill AV (1926) *Muscular Activity*. Baltimore, MD: Williams & Wilkins.
3 Bainbridge FA (1931) *The Physiology of Muscular Exercise* (3rd ed). New York: Longmans, Green and Co.
4 Merton PA, Pampiglione G (1950) Strength and fatigue. *Nature:* 166.
5 Marino FE, Gard M, Drinkwater EJ (2011) The limits to exercise performance and the future of fatigue research. *Br J Sports Med* 45: 65–7.
6 Ament W, Verkerke GJ (2009) Exercise and fatigue. *Sports Med* 39 (5): 389–422.
7 Moore B, ed. (2004) *The Australian Concise Oxford Dictionary* (4th edn). South Melbourne: Oxford University Press.
8 Hill AV, Lupton H (1923) Muscular exercise, lactic acid, and the supply and utilization of oxygen. *QJ Med* 16: 135–71.
9 Hill AV, Long CHN, Lupton H (1924) Muscular exercise, lactic acid and the supply and utilisation of oxygen: parts VII–VIII. *Proc Royal Soc* 97: 155–76.
10 Hill AV, Long CHN, Lupton H (1924) Muscular exercise, lactic acid, and the supply utilization of oxygen: parts I–III. *Proc Royal Soc* 96: 438–75.
11 Hill AV, Long CHN, Lupton H (1924) Muscular exercise, lactic acid, and the utilization of oxygen: parts IV–VI. *Proc Royal Soc* 97: 84–138.
12 Noakes TD (2012) Fatigue is a brain-derived emotion that regulates the exercise behaviour to ensure the protection of whole-body homeostasis. *Front Physiol* 3: 1–13.
13 Hill L, Flack M (1910) The influence of oxygen inhalations on muscular work. *J Physiol* 5.
14 Raskoff WJ, Goldman S, Cohn K (1976) The 'athletic heart': prevalence and physiological significance of left ventricular enlargement in distance runners. *J Am Med Assoc* 236: 158–62.
15 Bandschapp O, Soule CL, Iaizzo PA (2012) Lactic acid restores skeletal muscle force in an in vitro fatigue model: are voltage-gated chloride channels involved? *Am J Physiol* 302: C1019–25.
16 Kristensen M, Albertsen J, Rentsch M, *et al.* (2005) Lactate and force production in skeletal muscle. *J Physiol* 562: 521–6.
17 Nielsen OB, de Paoli F, Overgaard K (2001) Protective effects of lactic acid on force production in rat skeletal muscle. *J Physiol* 536: 161–6.
18 St Clair Gibson A, Noakes TD (2004) Evidence for complex systems integration and dynamic neural regulation of skeletal muscle recruitment during exercise in humans. *Br J Sports Med* 38: 797–806.
19 Amann, M, Eldridge MW, Lovering AT, *et al.* (2006) Arterial oxygenation influences central motor output and exercise performance via effects on peripheral locomotor muscle fatigue in humans. *J Physiol* 575 (3): 937–52.
20 Albertus Y (2008) *Critical Analysis of Techniques for Normalising Electromyographic Data*. PhD thesis, University of Cape Town, Cape Town: 1–219.
21 Noakes TD, St Clair Gibson A (2004) Logical limitations to the 'catastrophe' models of fatigue during exercise in humans. *Br J Sports Med* 38: 648–9.
22 Davis JM, Bailey SP (1997) Possible mechanisms of central nervous system fatigue during exercise. *Med Sci Sports Exerc* 29 (1): 45–57.
23 Graham TE, Rush JWE, MacLean DA (1995) Skeletal muscle amino acid metabolism and ammonia production during exercise. In: Hargreaves M (ed.) *Exercise Metabolism*. Champaign, IL: Human Kinetics: 131–75.
24 Gandevia SC, Allen GM, Butler JE, *et al.* (1996) Supra-spinal factors in human muscle fatigue: evidence for sub-optimal output from the motor cortex. *J Physiol* 490: 529–36.

25 Bigland-Ritchie B, Thomas CK, Rice CL, *et al.* (1992) Muscle temperature, contractile speed, and motor neuron firing rates during human voluntary contractions. *J Appl Physiol* 73: 2457–61.
26 Enoka RM, Stuart DG (1992) Neurobiology of muscle fatigue. *J Appl Physiol* 72: 1631–48.
27 Vøllestad NK (1997) Measurement of human muscle fatigue. *J Neurosci Meth* 74: 219–27.
28 Nybo L, Nielsen B (2001) Hyperthermia and central fatigue during prolonged exercise in humans. *J Appl Physiol* 91 (3): 1055–60.
29 Jones DA (1996) High- and low-frequency fatigue revisited. *Acta Physiol Scand* 156: 265–70.
30 Keeton RB, Binder-Macleod SA (2006) Low-frequency fatigue. *Phys Ther* 86: 1146–50.
31 Edwards RH, Hill DK, Jones DA, *et al.* (1977) Fatigue of long duration in human skeletal muscle after exercise. *J Physiol* 272: 769 –78.
32 Trimble MH, Enoka RM (1991) Mechanisms underlying the training effects associated with neuromuscular electrical stimulation. *Phys Ther* 71: 273–80.
33 Gandevia SC (2001) Spinal and supraspinal factors in human muscle fatigue. *Physiol Rev* 81 (4): 1725–89.
34 Warren GL, Lowe DA, Armstrong RB (1999) Measurement tools used in the study of eccentric contraction-induced injury. *Sports Med* 27: 43–59.
35 Martin V, Millet GY, Martin A, *et al.* (2004) Assessment of low-frequency fatigue with two methods of electrical stimulation. *J Appl Physiol* 97: 1923–9.
36 Vøllestad NK, Sejersted OM, Bahr R, *et al.* (1988) Motor drive and metabolic responses during repeated submaximal contractions in man. *J Appl Physiol* 64 (4): 1421–7.
37 Schabort EJ, Hawley JA, Hopkins WG, *et al.* (1998) A new reliable laboratory test of endurance performance for road cyclists. *Med Sci Sports Exerc* 30 (12): 1744–50.
38 McLellan TM, Cheung SS, Jacobs I (1995) Variability of time to exhaustion during submaximal exercise. *Can J Appl Physiol* 20 (1): 39–51.
39 Hinckson EA, Hopkins WG (2005) Reliability of time to exhaustion analyzed with critical-power and log-log modelling. *Med Sci Sports Exerc* 37 (4): 696–701.
40 Bigland-Ritchie B, Jones DA, Woods JJ (1979) Excitation frequency and muscle fatigue: electrical responses during human voluntary and stimulated contractions. *Exp Neurol* 64: 414–27.
41 Mengshoel AM, Saugen E, Førre E, *et al.* (1995) Muscle fatigue in early fibromyalgia. *J Rheumatol* 22: 143–50.
42 Karelis AD, Smith JEW, Passe DH, *et al.* (2010) Carbohydrate administration and exercise performance: what are the potential mechanisms involved? *Sports Med* 40 (9): 747–63.
43 Bangsbo J, Nørregaard L, Thorsø F (1991) Activity profile of competition soccer. *Can J Sport Sci* 16 (2): 110–16.
44 Krustrup P, Mohr M, Steensberg A, *et al.* (2006) Muscle and blood metabolites during a soccer game: implications for sprint performance. *Med Sci Sports Exerc* 38: 1165–74.
45 Borg G (1970) Perceived exertion as an indicator of somatic stress. *Scand J Rehab Med* 2: 92–108.
46 Robertson RJ (2001) Development of the perceived exertion knowledge base: an interdisciplinary process. *Int J Sport Psychol* 32: 189–96.
47 Dunbar CC, Robertson RJ, Baun R, *et al.* (1992) The validity of regulating exercise intensity by rating of perceived exertion. *Med Sci Sports Exerc* 24: 94–9.

48 Eston RG, Williams JG (1988) Reliability of ratings of perceived effort regulation of exercise intensity. *Br J Sports Med* 22: 153–5.
49 Marriott HE, Lamb KL (1996) The use of ratings of perceived exertion for regulating exercise levels in rowing ergometry. *Eur J Appl Physiol* 72 (3): 267–71.
50 Groslambert A, Mahon AD (2006) Perceived exertion: influence of age and cognitive function. *Sports Med* 36 (11): 911–28.
51 Marcora S (2009) Perception of effort during exercise is independent of afferent feedback from skeletal muscles, heart and lungs. *J Appl Physiol* 106 (6): 2060–2.
52 Smirmaul BPC (2012) Sense of effort and other unpleasant sensations during exercise: clarifying concepts and mechanisms. *Br J Sports Med* 46: 308–11.
53 Potteiger JA, Schroeder JM, Goff KL (2000) Influence of music on ratings of perceived exertion during 20 minutes of moderate intensity exercise. *Percept Mot Skills* 91: 848–54.
54 White VB, Potteiger JA (1996) Comparison of passive sensory stimulations on RPE during moderate intensity exercise. *Percept Mot Skills* 82: 819–25.
55 Eston R, Stansfield R, Westoby P, *et al.* (2012) Effect of deception and expected exercise duration on psychological and physiological variables during treadmill running and cycling. *Psychophysiol* 49: 462–9.
56 Swart J, Lindsay TR, Lambert MI, *et al.* (2012) Perceptual cues in the regulation of exercise performance – physical sensations of exercise and awareness of effort interact as separate cues. *Br J Sports Med* 46: 42–8.
57 Eston R (2012) Use of ratings of perceived exertion in sports. *Int J Sports Physiol Perf* 7: 175–82.
58 Krssak M, Petersen KF, Bergeron R, *et al.* (2000) Intramuscular glycogen and intramyocellular lipid utilization during prolonged exercise and recovery in man: A ^{13}C and ^{1}H nuclear magnetic resonance spectroscopy study. *J Clin Endocrin Metab* 85 (2): 748–54.
59 Larson-Meyer DE, Smith SR, Heilbronn LK, *et al.* (2006) Muscle-associated triglyceride measured by computed tomography and magnetic resonance spectroscopy. *Obesity* 14: 73–87.
60 Vanhatalo A, Fulford J, DiMenna FJ, *et al.* (2010) Influence of hyperoxia on muscle metabolic responses and the power–duration relationship during severe-intensity exercise in humans: a ^{31}P magnetic resonance spectroscopy study. *Exp Physiol* 95: 528–40.
61 Sinha U, Sinha S, Hodgson JA, *et al.* (2011) Human soleus muscle architecture at different ankle joint angles from magnetic resonance diffusion tensor imaging. *J Appl Physiol* 110 (3): 807–19.
62 Wilson M, O'Hanlon R, Prasad S, *et al.* (2011) Biological markers of cardiac damage are not related to measures of cardiac systolic and diastolic function using cardiovascular magnetic resonance and echocardiography after an acute bout of prolonged endurance exercise. *Br J Sports Med* 45: 780–4.
63 Chambers ES, Bridge MW, Jones DA (2009) Carbohydrate sensing in the human mouth: effects on exercise performance and brain activity. *J Physiol* 587 (8): 1779–94.
64 Gant N, Stinear CM, Byblow WD (2010) Carbohydrate in the mouth immediately facilitates motor output. *Brain Res* 1350: 151–8.

Part II

What causes (and what does not cause) fatigue in sport and exercise?

Chapter 2

Energy depletion

2.1 Energy metabolism during exercise

It is beyond the scope of this book to provide a detailed overview of energy metabolism. Many excellent undergraduate physiology textbooks discuss this topic in detail, and the reader is recommended to consult such a text as required to support this chapter. However, a brief summary of the importance of adenosine triphosphate (ATP) in human energy metabolism is worthwhile.

Adenosine triphosphate is the most important source of chemical energy in the body (Figure 2.1) Adenosine triphosphate has three components: adenine, ribose, and three phosphates. High-energy bonds attach the three phosphate molecules to each other. The energy in these bonds is released when ATP is broken down in a hydrolysis reaction, and this energy is used by the cell for various functions such as muscle contraction:

$$ATP + H_2O \underset{}{\overset{ATPase}{\longleftrightarrow}} ADP + P_i + H^+ + energy \quad (2.1)$$

where H_2O is water, ADP is adenosine diphosphate, P_i is inorganic phosphate, H^+ is hydrogen, and ATPase is the enzyme adenosine triphosphatease. Only a small amount of ATP is stored in the body at any time (enough to fuel approximately 2 seconds of maximal intensity muscle contraction). Muscle energy turnover can increase 300-fold during explosive muscle contractions, so mechanisms of ATP replenishment are critical to maintenance of muscle performance. This is where food energy comes in. While food energy cannot be used to replenish ATP *directly*, it can do so through three primary metabolic pathways: the phosphocreatine (PCr) pathway, the anaerobic pathway, and the aerobic pathway. In the anaerobic pathway, glucose (from the blood or from glycogen stored in muscle) is metabolised to resynthesise ATP in a series of chemical reactions termed glycolysis. In the aerobic pathway, glucose and fatty acids are metabolised to replenish ATP in two enzymatic systems called the Krebs cycle and the electron transport chain. The PCr pathway does not used stored glucose or fat; instead, it metabolises a compound called PCr (Section 2.2.2). This

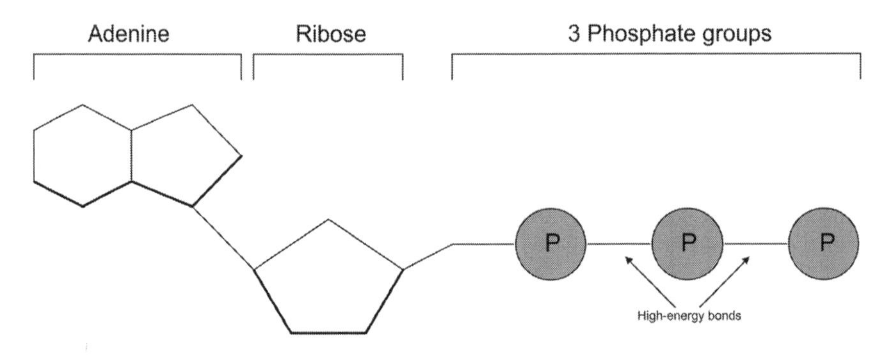

Figure 2.1 Adenosine triphosphate, the most important source of chemical energy in the body. Highlighted are the high-energy bonds between the three phosphate groups. These bonds are broken in a hydrolysis reaction, and the energy released is used for a multitude of processes, including muscle contraction.

compound is present in skeletal muscle and is not significantly influenced by normal dietary intake. The breakdown and resynthesis of ATP is a perpetual cycle, even at rest. Of course, during exercise when energy requirements are greater, ATP turnover is also greater. Therefore, logic dictates that the availability of food energy is critical to ensuring a sufficient supply of ATP for continued exercise performance.

Key point

ATP is the primary source of useable energy. Food energy cannot be used directly to fuel exercise; however, it is required to continually replenish ATP stores.

2.2 Energy metabolism and fatigue during exercise

2.2.1 ATP depletion

As mentioned above, the small endogenous ATP stores must be replenished continuously to avoid ATP depletion (termed the 'energy crisis' hypothesis of exercise fatigue). If ATP stores were to be depleted then the skeletal muscle would enter a state of rigor, a permanently contracted state where the muscles are unable to relax.[1] This is a crucial statement. If exercise fatigue is caused by critical depletion of ATP, then exercise should be terminated due to the muscles entering rigor. However, exercise-induced muscle rigor has never been documented in a human.[1] So the question becomes: is ATP depletion a cause of fatigue during exercise?

Due to the greater rate of ATP turnover at higher exercise intensities, it is logical to think that ATP depletion would be greater during high-intensity exercise. However, repeated 6-second maximal cycle sprints can be achieved without substantial ATP depletion.[2] In fact, significant ATP depletion is not observed at the point of fatigue during progressive exercise to exhaustion (such as would be completed in a VO_{2max} test), high-intensity short duration exercise,[2] or prolonged moderate-intensity exercise.[3–4] Studies conducted on whole muscles or muscle homogenates (muscle tissues that have been mechanically 'broken up' to release their internal structures and substances) show that intramuscular ATP concentrations do not fall below about 60% of resting levels even during intense exercise.[5] It therefore appears that critical ATP depletion is not a viable direct cause of exercise fatigue.

So skeletal muscles appear able to preserve their ATP status.[6] How can they do this? An alternative school of thought is that reduced muscle contraction force (i.e. fatigue) occurs *prior* to a significant fall in muscle ATP levels in order to prevent that very thing from happening: a reduction in ATP to the point where muscle rigor develops and the integrity of the skeletal muscle becomes compromised. Therefore, the suggestion is that the onset of fatigue is an anticipatory, preventative strategy to maintain homeostasis. This is an important concept in fatigue research, and is discussed in detail in Chapter 6.

Key point

In exercising humans, intramuscular ATP concentrations do not fall below about 60% of resting levels, regardless of the intensity or duration of exercise. However, the ATP concentration of single fibres can drop to very low levels.

Key point

The occurrence of ATP depletion and its role in exercise-induced fatigue is open to debate, and more research is required.

Despite the absence of significant ATP depletion at the whole-muscle level, ATP levels in individual muscle fibres can fall to as low as 20% of resting values following maximal exercise,[7] particularly in type II muscle fibres.

Localised ATP depletion may also occur at crucial stages of the excitation-contraction coupling process (the process that enables muscle fibres to contract).[8] It has been suggested that ATP depletion in just a small percentage of muscle fibres may prevent those fibres from contributing to muscle contraction and, thereby, result in fatigue of the whole muscle.[7] Given the conflicting observations regarding ATP depletion at the whole muscle and individual fibre levels, the exact occurrence and influence of ATP depletion on exercise fatigue is still open to debate. However, an important message to take from this discussion is that ATP depletion is far from an accepted cause of exercise-induced fatigue, and in fact is strongly argued against in some of the literature.

2.2.2 Phosphocreatine depletion

Phosphocreatine is a phosphorylated creatine molecule that is particularly important in resynthesising ATP during explosive, high-intensity exercise. ATP resynthesis from PCr is driven by the reaction between PCr and ADP, catalysed by the enzyme creatine kinase:

$$\mathrm{PCr} + \mathrm{ADP} + \mathrm{H}^{+} \xleftrightarrow{\textit{creatine kinase}} \mathrm{ATP} + \mathrm{Cr} \qquad (2.2)$$

where H^+ is hydrogen and Cr is free creatine. Intramuscular PCr stores equate to approximately 80 mmol/kg dry mass. In theory, this is sufficient for approximately 10-seconds of maximal work before PCr stores become depleted (under ideal conditions, PCr stores will be replenished in about 2–4 minutes). To discuss the potential role of PCr depletion in exercise fatigue, it is useful to look at different types of exercise (Chapter 7 discusses in detail the influence of different exercise demands on fatigue processes).

2.2.2.1 *Maximal exercise*

A common protocol for assessing maximal sprint performance is a single cycle or running sprint lasting between 5 – 30 seconds. Studies of this nature have determined that PCr content drops to about 35–55% of resting levels and contributes approximately 50% of the ATP produced during a 6-second sprint,[2] with the remainder supplied by glycolysis, aerobic metabolism, and ATP hydrolysis (Figure 2.2). As the sprint duration increases to 20 seconds PCr content drops to about 27% of resting levels,[9] and to about 20% at the end of a 30 second sprint.[10] The significant reduction in muscle PCr content with increasing sprint duration, and the documented positive relationship between recovery of muscle PCr and muscle power output,[11] suggests that single sprint performance is influenced by PCr availability.[12] However, PCr is not depleted fully in a single sprint. Of course, the majority of people are able to complete a single bout of maximal exercise lasting 5–30 seconds

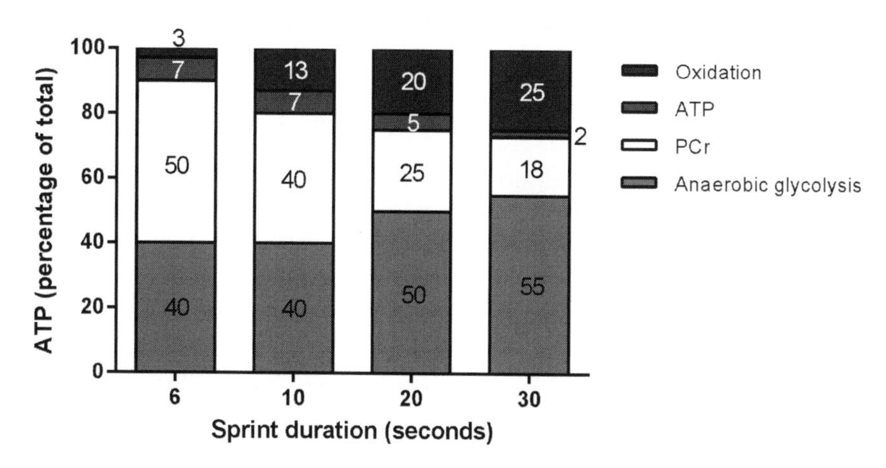

Figure 2.2 Relative energy system contribution to ATP resynthesis, as a percentage of total energy, during sprints of different durations. It is important to remember that this is the contribution of energy systems to *single* sprints at each duration. The energy system contribution to repeated sprints at each duration would change progressively. Adapted from Billaut and Bishop.[12]

without stopping. Despite this, some form of fatigue is still occurring, as the power output / movement speed at the end of the exercise bout will be less than it was earlier on in the bout. The reduction in power output may be partially due to PCr depletion, which would reduce the rate of ATP resynthesis and necessitate a reduction in power output to prevent critical reductions in ATP concentration. However, PCr depletion is probably not the sole cause, as PCr is not fully depleted in a single sprint of this length. Other possible explanations will be discussed in Chapter 6.

Key point

Phosphocreatine levels are not fully depleted during single sprints lasting 5–30 seconds. Therefore, it does not appear that PCr depletion is the sole cause of fatigue during short duration maximal exercise.

2.2.2.2 *Intermittent exercise*

Intermittent exercise refers to short periods of maximal exercise (usually 5–30 seconds long) interspersed with recovery periods, or the variable intensity exercise typical of many team games such as soccer. There is limited data on the metabolic responses to intermittent exercise, however it is known that

ATP provision during intermittent exercise is maintained through the coordinated contribution of the different metabolic energy systems.[12] As intermittent exercise progresses the relative contribution of the energy systems will change based on the previous exercise bouts, and the duration and intensity of the recovery periods.[12] While aerobic and anaerobic energy provision is active during intermittent exercise, the exact contribution of each is still under debate and is likely dependent on the type and intensity of exercise performed (discussed further in Chapter 7), and the individual athlete.

Significant positive relationships have been reported between the ability to resynthesise PCr and the recovery of power output during repeated cycle sprinting.[13–14] Similarly, occlusion of limb blood flow in recovery from intense exercise, which prevents the resynthesis of PCr, prevents the recovery of power output in a subsequent exercise bout.[15–16] These studies provide good evidence that performance during laboratory intermittent exercise is at least partly dependent on PCr contribution. However, it is important to reinforce the phrase *partly dependent*. Studies that have correlated PCr recovery and repeated sprint performance have shown that PCr recovery is associated with 45–71% of the recovery of power output.[13–14] Therefore, alternative factors must explain the other 29–55% variance in power output recovery.

Studies investigating the effect of creatine supplementation on intermittent exercise performance provide further evidence that the influence of PCr on fatigue during this form of exercise is not absolute. Creatine supplementation is thought to improve performance by increasing resting PCr concentration, increasing the rate of PCr resynthesis, or buffering of intramuscular H^+. Some research indicates that creatine supplementation increases PCr stores and improves performance during laboratory repeated sprint protocols of 6 and 30 seconds duration.[17–18] Conversely, other studies have found no effect, or variable effects, of creatine supplementation on laboratory and field-based repeated sprint exercise,[19–22] despite some instances of increased muscle creatine and/or PCr content. These differences in findings, which may be due to differences in sprint protocol and potential placebo effects in some studies, cloud understanding of the role of PCr on intermittent exercise fatigue.

The potential role of PCr in fatigue diminishes as exercise duration increases. This is expected, given the shift towards a predominantly aerobic ATP resynthesis with longer duration exercise. However, PCr may still play a role in fatigue during long duration exercise that includes bouts of short duration high-intensity work, such as team games. As discussed above, PCr contributes approximately half the ATP in a 6-second sprint and is predominantly resynthesised via aerobic metabolism. During team games sprint durations of 2–3 seconds with recovery durations of 2 minutes have been reported.[23–4] Gaitanos *et al.*[2] stated that 30 seconds was sufficient recovery time for continued contribution of PCr to sprinting. Based on the finding that up to 85% of team game time is spent in low-intensity activity[24–5] it would seem that, despite the inherently random pattern of work and recovery, there is ample opportunity for resynthesis of PCr during team games (Section 7.2.2.1.1.2). However, single or multiple sprints with short recovery durations are evident during team games.[24,26] Therefore, while PCr depletion may not cause exercise termination, it cannot be discounted that it may cause a transient loss of muscle force production during this type of exercise (Section 7.2.2.1.1.2).

Key point

Phosphocreatine plays a role in muscle fatigue during single and repeated sprints. The influence of PCr on fatigue diminishes as exercise duration increases, but it may still play a role in long duration exercise that involves bouts of short-duration, high-intensity work.

2.2.3 Glycogen depletion

Carbohydrate, in the form of muscle and liver glycogen and blood glucose, is the primary fuel during exercise. The contribution of carbohydrate to exercising energy metabolism becomes greater with increasing exercise intensity. Carbohydrate is metabolised in glycolysis (anaerobic) and the Krebs cycle (aerobic). Therefore, it is a fuel that can be metabolised to generate ATP across a wide range of exercise demands.

A large amount of research has investigated various aspects of carbohydrate metabolism, far more than can be included in this text. Therefore, discussion will focus on the historical research that first demonstrated the potential link between carbohydrate and exercise performance, subsequent work that reinforced the perception that glycogen depletion causes fatigue, and more recent perceptions of the role of carbohydrate in exercise fatigue.

2.2.3.1 Brief historical perspective

Study into the links between carbohydrate and exercise performance began as far back as the 1920s.[27–8] It was not until the introduction of the muscle biopsy technique in the late 1960s that the study of carbohydrate manipulation became more focused. Two classic studies[29–30] demonstrated that:

1 Prolonged submaximal exercise can deplete muscle glycogen.
2 Following exhaustive exercise, a high-carbohydrate diet can restore muscle glycogen to higher levels than before exercise (supercompensation).

3 The effect of exercise on the muscle glycogen concentration of inactive muscle is negligible, provided blood glucose levels remain fairly stable.
4 Muscle glycogen is the primary fuel source during prolonged moderate- to high-intensity exercise, and muscle glycogen content at the onset of exercise can determine the duration for which exercise can continue (Figure 2.3).

Following this early biopsy work, a wealth of research was published investigating carbohydrate and exercise performance from the perspective of manipulating dietary carbohydrate intake and providing carbohydrate supplements before and during exercise. The overall findings of this research further reinforced the importance of carbohydrate to exercise performance, and the acceptance of key theories behind how carbohydrate exerts its performance-enhancing effects. Some of these theories have over the years, and almost via a word-of-mouth acceptance, become staples for how athletes, coaches, sports science students, and even academics, explain the influence

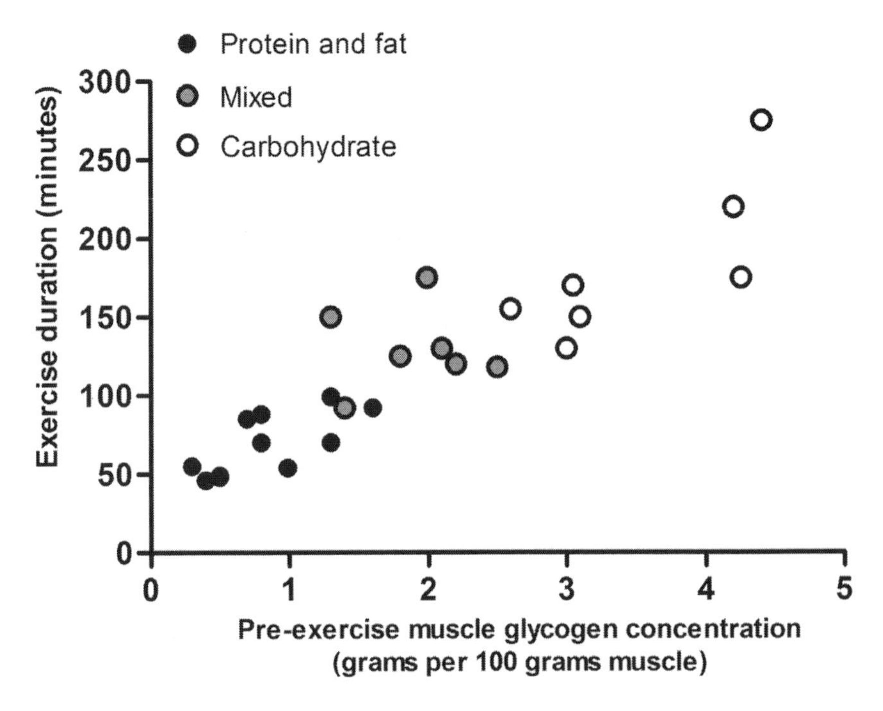

Figure 2.3 Exercise duration at a set work rate on a cycle ergometer following ingestion of one of three different diets (high protein and fat, mixed macronutrient, high carbohydrate). The progressive increase in exercise time with increasing dietary carbohydrate content demonstrates that the ability to continue exercising depends in part on pre-exercise muscle glycogen concentration. Data from Bergström *et al.*[30]

of carbohydrate on exercise performance. To state that carbohydrate does not play a role in fatigue would be indefensible given the wealth of research to the contrary. However, despite the link between muscle glycogen content and exercise performance being made nearly 50 years ago, the fact is that we still do not conclusively know why muscle force is depressed (i.e. fatigue develops) when glycogen levels are low. It is important to look closely at the older research and the more contemporary studies with a critical eye, as doing so may change our opinion of what effect carbohydrate actually has on exercise performance and fatigue, and how it exerts that effect.

Key point

The importance of carbohydrate as a muscle fuel has been known for many decades. However, more recent research is providing knowledge on an expanding number of potential roles for carbohydrate in the regulation of exercise performance.

2.2.3.2 Potential carbohydrate-related causes of fatigue during exercise

One of the most commonly cited reasons for impaired exercise performance, particularly of a long duration, is depletion of muscle glycogen levels leading to an inability to resynthesise ATP at the required rate. This theory has been reported and re-stated so many times that it has taken on the status of fact. Of course, the logic behind it makes sense: glycogen is an important fuel source during exercise – we only have a limited amount of it stored in our body – when it runs out we can no longer exercise at the same intensity – the end result: fatigue. Problem solved?

Unfortunately not. The next sections will take potential carbohydrate-related fatigue mechanisms and provide a contemporary viewpoint of whether the literature supports, refutes, or is equivocal on the veracity of each mechanism.

2.2.3.2.1 GLYCOGEN DEPLETION REDUCES ATP RESYNTHESIS

As shown in Figure 2.3, the link between carbohydrate availability and exercise duration was made several decades ago. We also know that development of fatigue during prolonged exercise often coincides with low muscle glycogen. However, remember the discussion at the beginning of this chapter about ATP resynthesis during exercise (Section 2.2.1). We discussed that if ATP is depleted during exercise (if ATP use far exceeds the rate of

ATP resynthesis), then the muscle will enter a state of rigor: something that has never been documented in an exercising human. In line with this, there is little evidence to support the idea that low muscle glycogen concentrations lead to a reduced ATP supply. In contrast, there is evidence to show that fatigue occurs during prolonged exercise when muscle glycogen levels are low, but ATP levels are not significantly different to levels measured at rest (Figure 2.4).[31–4] This data therefore suggests that reduced ATP resynthesis due to muscle glycogen depletion is not a direct cause of fatigue during prolonged exercise.

However, the observation of high muscle ATP concentrations at fatigue does not rule out the possibility that glycogen depletion reduces ATP concentrations in localised areas of the muscle cell. Contrary to general perceptions, glycogen is not uniformly distributed in a muscle, but rather is localised in clusters. The three primary glycogen clusters are sub-sarcolemmal glycogen (located just under the sarcolemma, or muscle fibre membrane), intermyofibrillar glycogen (located between myofibrils), and intramyofibrillar glycogen (located within the myofibrils, near the muscle z-line).[35] The major glycogen cluster is the intermyofibrillar one (approximately 75% of total glycogen stores), but the exact distributions are dependent on factors such as muscle fibre type, training status, fibre use, and the type of exercise performed.[35] Depletion of specific glycogen clusters may negatively influence ATP levels in such a way that would not be detected by measuring 'whole muscle' ATP concentrations.

Localised ATP depletion has been linked with fatigue via alterations in calcium (Ca^{2+}) release from the sarcoplasmic reticulum. The intramyofibrillar glycogen cluster is preferentially depleted during most forms of exercise.[36] Most intramyofibrillar glycogen is stored close to the triads (a t-tubule surrounded on both sides by an enlarged area of the sarcoplasmic reticulum, termed terminal cisternae; Figure 2.5).[36] This glycogen cluster is thought to generate ATP for the triads so that they are able to perform their important role in the excitation-contraction coupling process,[35–6] namely the release of Ca^{2+} from the sarcoplasmic reticulum (which plays a crucial role in formation of actin-myosin crossbridges and development of muscle force). Depletion of intramyofibrillar glycogen may cause localised ATP depletion at the triads, impairing this important step in the excitation-contraction coupling process. This is supported by research that shows impaired sarcoplasmic reticulum function and Ca^{2+} kinetics following exercise, and an association between muscle glycogen depletion and this impaired function (further discussed in Chapter 5).[36–9] These findings appear to support a metabolic energy deficiency theory of muscle glycogen depletion. However, more research is required to confirm or refute the suggestion, as some studies have not found a link between reduced muscle glycogen concentration and altered Ca^{2+} kinetics. Therefore, a non-metabolic role of muscle glycogen in excitation-contraction coupling cannot be discounted (Section 5.7.1).

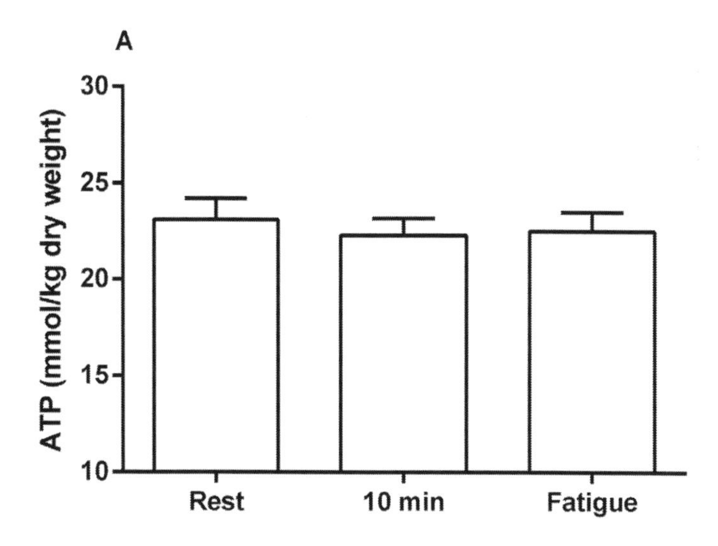

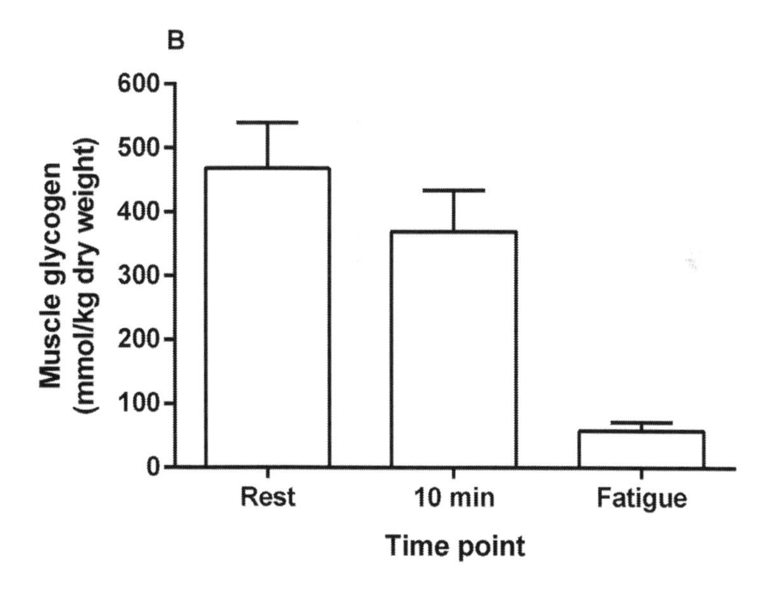

Figure 2.4 Muscle ATP concentration at rest and various stages of prolonged cycling (A) and muscle glycogen concentration at the same points during the same exercise bout (B). It is clear to see that muscle glycogen concentration reaches low levels at fatigue, yet muscle ATP levels do not change significantly from those at rest. Therefore, muscle ATP content is 'defended' even in the presence of low muscle glycogen. This does not support the contention that low muscle glycogen concentrations cause fatigue due to an inability to resynthesise ATP at the required rate. Data in these graphs were created by the author.

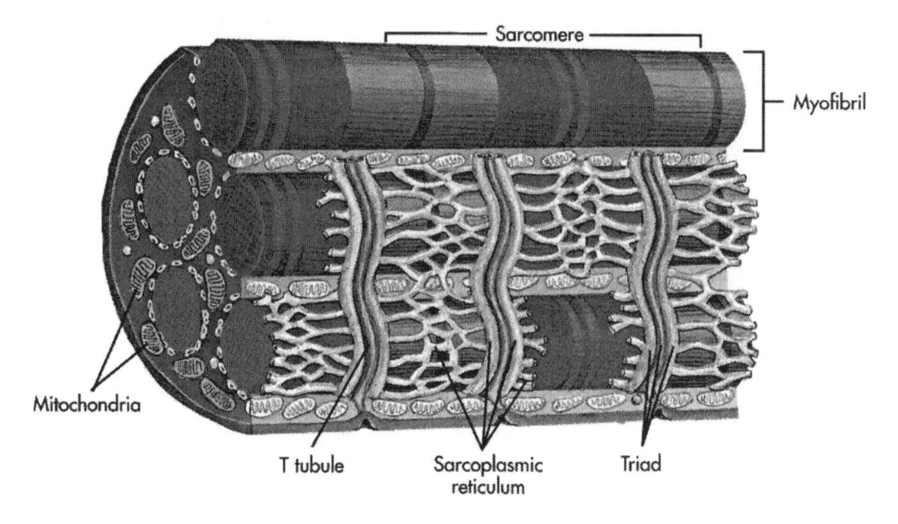

Figure 2.5 Schematic of a muscle sarcomere and surrounding membranes. Identified are the t-tubules, the sarcoplasmic reticulum, and the location of a t-tubule and terminal cisternae of the sarcoplasmic reticulum that forms a triad. From Thibodeau and Patton.[40]

Key point

A popular theory is that muscle glycogen depletion leads to an inability to replenish ATP at the required rate, and hence the development of fatigue. However, there is little evidence to support this hypothesis. In fact, most research shows little change in muscle ATP levels with muscle glycogen depletion.

Key point

Localised muscle glycogen depletion may cause reduced ATP production at specific locations in the excitation-contraction coupling machinery, which could lead to impaired muscle function. This would support an energy deficiency hypothesis of muscle glycogen depletion.

2.2.3.2.2 GLYCOGEN DEPLETION CAUSES HYPOGLYCAEMIA, WHICH LEADS TO FATIGUE

The pattern of use of the four primary fuel sources (muscle glycogen, muscle triglycerides, blood glucose, free fatty acids) during exercise will depend on many factors including the exercise mode, intensity, and duration, the training status, metabolic makeup, and pre-exercise fuel status of the athlete, and environmental conditions, particularly ambient temperature. However, the general pattern of use during moderate-intensity exercise is summarised in Figure 2.6. Intramuscular fuel sources (glycogen and triglycerides) are predominant for approximately the first 90 minutes of exercise. If exercise continues for longer than this, blood-borne fuels (glucose and free fatty acids) become more important, due largely to muscle glycogen depletion. Blood glucose levels during exercise are maintained by the breakdown of liver glycogen (there are other non-carbohydrate sources of glucose, such as amino acids and the glycerol portion of triglycerides, but generally these sources are utilised minimally and will not be discussed here). An increased use of blood glucose as a metabolic fuel will tax the finite liver glycogen stores, potentially

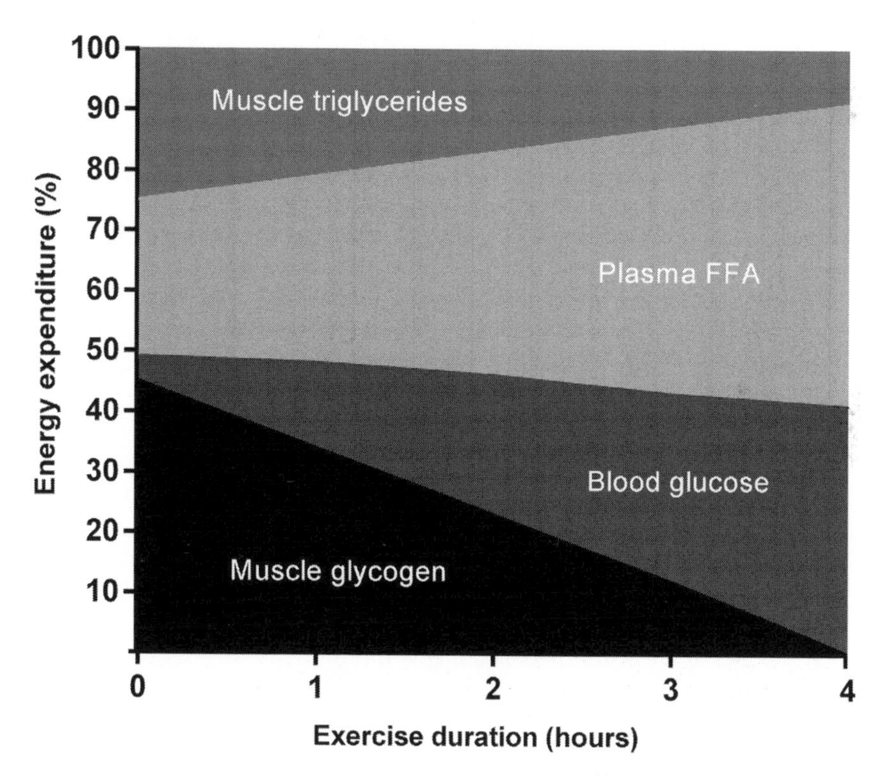

Figure 2.6 Contribution of the four primary energy sources to energy expenditure during moderate-intensity exercise of increasing duration. Note that in the earlier stages of exercise (approximately 0–1.5 hours) intramuscular fuel sources are the primary energy suppliers. If exercise continues for longer, blood-borne fuel sources become predominant. The exact profile of fuel use will depend on factors such as exercise mode and intensity, training status, pre-exercise fuel status, and environmental conditions.

leading to a situation where the liver can no longer maintain blood glucose levels within their optimum range, and hypoglycaemia can develop.

During prolonged exercise, blood glucose is an important fuel for working muscles and the central nervous system (CNS). Brain glucose stores are limited; therefore, the uptake of blood glucose is crucial for the brain. Once blood glucose levels drop below a critical level (approximately 3.6 millimoles/L), brain glucose uptake begins to decline.[41] Therefore, hypoglycaemia may contribute to fatigue in prolonged exercise by limiting fuel supply to the muscles (the periphery; peripheral fatigue) and the brain (CNS; central fatigue).

Several studies appear to support the development of hypoglycaemia as a cause of central fatigue during prolonged exercise. These studies show that hypoglycaemia during prolonged exercise can decrease brain glycogen levels. This may contribute to central fatigue directly or indirectly through other mechanisms that will be discussed in Chapter 6.[42] Muscle force production is also greater after prolonged exercise when blood glucose levels are maintained, with this greater force production related to better neuromuscular drive.[43] Experiments conducted in rats demonstrated that electrically stimulated muscle force production in hypoglycaemia was not different to that in euglycaemia, despite hypoglycaemic rats reaching exhaustion much earlier in the exercise bout.[34] This indicates that low muscle glycogen and hypoglycaemia did not affect the contractile ability of the muscle itself. By electrically stimulating the muscles, therefore bypassing the CNS, the authors concluded that depletion of muscle glycogen and hypoglycaemia contribute to fatigue, but that this fatigue is likely to be central rather than peripheral. However, hypoglycaemia may also contribute to fatigue by impairing fuel availability to the working muscles. As we have already discussed, during prolonged exercise blood glucose becomes a progressively more important fuel source. Improved prolonged submaximal exercise capacity with carbohydrate ingestion in the absence of muscle glycogen sparing has been attributed to a better maintenance of blood glucose and muscle glucose uptake.[44–5]

Interestingly, some studies have found that hypoglycaemia does not negatively affect endurance performance, and that prevention of hypoglycaemia does not consistently delay fatigue during exercise.[46] Exercising in a hypoglycaemic state may not reduce muscle carbohydrate oxidation compared with euglycaemia, and maintenance of euglycaemia can produce a highly variable effect on endurance capacity, with some participants performing similarly whether hypoglycaemic or euglycaemic.[47] It appears that there is an inter-individual response to hypoglycaemia, with some people displaying symptoms such as nausea, confusion, and dizziness, but others showing no outward signs. This makes a consensus on the influence of hypoglycaemia on exercise fatigue difficult, and currently it appears that hypoglycaemia is not a consistent cause of fatigue during exercise.[48]

Key point

While there is evidence that hypoglycaemia may contribute to fatigue via central and peripheral mechanisms during prolonged exercise, this is not consistently observed and the inter-individual response to hypoglycaemia appears to be highly variable.

2.2.3.2.3 WHAT DO CARBOHYDRATE SUPPLEMENTATION STUDIES TELL US ABOUT THE ROLE OF CARBOHYDRATE IN FATIGUE?

It is generally accepted that carbohydrate supplementation can delay the onset of fatigue during exercise. However, much as with glycogen depletion, the exact mechanisms behind this ability are unknown. A classical theory is that carbohydrate supplementation enables sparing of muscle glycogen during exercise, as the body preferentially utilises the carbohydrate entering the systemic circulation from the supplement. Muscle glycogen sparing would then provide a readily available energy store for later in the exercise bout, enabling exercise to continue for longer. Studies have reported a sparing of muscle glycogen with carbohydrate supplementation during various exercise protocols.[49–52] However, a recent review of the literature found that carbohydrate supplementation does not spare muscle glycogen during moderate-intensity exercise.[48] In fact, back in 1986 a study showed that participants could continue cycling for an extra hour when they consumed carbohydrate during exercise, but their muscle glycogen use was almost identical to when they exercised without consuming carbohydrate.[44] The authors attributed this to prevention of hypoglycaemia and associated continued muscle carbohydrate uptake and oxidation. However, as discussed in Section 2.2.3.2.2, there is debate about the exact importance of hypoglycaemia to fatigue. Also, it is interesting to note that in studies demonstrating an association between improved endurance capacity and maintenance of muscle carbohydrate oxidation rates with carbohydrate supplementation, fatigue still occurred despite high oxidation rates. This raises the question of whether maintenance of plasma glucose and/or carbohydrate oxidation rates is actually a mechanism for delaying fatigue.[48] The influence of carbohydrate supplementation on sarcoplasmic reticulum function and Ca^{2+} kinetics during exercise is also equivocal. Clearly, it is difficult to get a straight answer regarding carbohydrate supplementation and exercise performance! This may be further hampered by recent more critical views of the carbohydrate supplement literature. This critique will not be presented in detail, and interested readers are referred to a recent paper for more information.[53] However, in light of the aims of this book, it is relevant to highlight. The fundamental critique of the carbohydrate supplement literature is four-fold:

1 The literature seeks to address an exercise-related concern that has been greatly sensationalised and is in fact not much of a problem at all; namely, dehydration during exercise (Chapter 4 discusses this).
2 A number of prominent authors have close financial and professional ties to large sports drinks manufacturers, suggesting a conflict of interest between research findings and an industry worth hundreds of millions of pounds.
3 The aforementioned links between research and industry is a factor in why there are hardly any published studies showing negative data on carbohydrate supplements and exercise.
4 The quality of the research designs used.

Issues two and three are outside the remit of this book, and the reader is invited to draw their own conclusions after reviewing the evidence. However, the issue of research design quality is worth discussing.

Key point

The common perception is that carbohydrate supplementation delays fatigue by sparing muscle glycogen stores. However, the consensus from the literature is that carbohydrate supplementation does not in fact spare muscle glycogen during moderate-intensity exercise.

The proposed issues with carbohydrate supplementation research designs are in Table 2.1. Small sample sizes are a general feature of sports science research, particularly when compared to clinical or medical research studies. There are many probable reasons for this. For example, a specific subset of people are often required for a study (i.e. males aged 18–25 who have been active soccer players for at least 2 years). This is usually done not to be picky (the researchers life would be much easier if they could recruit anyone onto their study!) but because it will make the data more valid and/or reliable (a single gender removes possible gender differences in responses/outcome measures; a narrow age range reduces performance variability; a specific subject demographic makes the data more applicable to the target population). Recruitment practices are also somewhat different in sports science research, where people are often asked to take part in a tough, time-consuming study with no financial or personal gain, compared with clinical or medical research where there is often access to a much larger population and the research may be carried out across multiple locations/organisations to maximise recruitment.

A small sample size is a critique that can be aimed at most sports science research, but is defensible.

The use of non-specific or unreliable exercise tests, and measurements that have questionable links to fatigue, is a limitation of specific research studies, and it would not be appropriate to speculate on why the researchers chose to use the tests and measures that they did. The use of appropriate blinding techniques is very important to counter the placebo effect, and lack of blinding must be seen as a fundamental limitation. Differences in study approach (exercise protocol, environmental conditions, carbohydrate supplement, etc.), while obviously rationalised as part of the research, is unfortunate as it makes reaching a consensus about the effects of carbohydrate supplementation difficult.

One of the biggest issues associated with carbohydrate supplementation research is the use of a fasting period prior to exercise. Generally, this is done to standardise participants' glycogen levels across trials, thereby removing differences in energy levels between participants as a possible confounding factor in the data. However, fasting will reduce muscle and liver glycogen stores. Therefore, participants will begin exercise with suboptimal glycogen stores, which is likely to enhance the effect of supplementing carbohydrate during exercise. Conducting a fast is not common practice for athletes prior to training or competition, and asking research participants to fast reduces the external validity of the data. It could also be argued that fasting research participants biases the study towards finding a positive effect of the carbohydrate supplement. This goes against the aim of objective research.

The above discussion is included because it is a contemporary viewpoint of an existing body of research. It is also an example that even the most accepted viewpoints should be continually challenged by critically evaluating the research. In doing so, we will gain a better insight and understanding of exactly what we do know, what grey areas exist, how well we can trust the existing viewpoint, and what more we need to learn.

Key point

Specific criticism about research into carbohydrate supplementation during exercise highlights the importance of critically and objectively reviewing research to fully evaluate its veracity.

Hopefully, the discussions above are making you aware that it is far too simple to sum up the influence of carbohydrate on exercise fatigue in a single statement or mechanism. Disagreement between studies could be due to things like the mode and intensity of exercise, training status and muscle fibre type distribution of the participants, and the pre-exercise muscle glycogen

Table 2.1 Some of the methodological and design criticisms of research into carbohydrate supplementation and exercise performance

	Criticism	Explanation
1	Small sample sizes limit generalisability of findings	Low sample size in research means that the study findings cannot be applied beyond people with the characteristics of the study sample. This is a fair criticism of research in general, but it should be noted that most sports science research, particularly physiology research using interventions, is usually done with much smaller sample sizes than, for example, clinical research.
2	Exercise tests used are not externally valid to sports performance	Many studies use time-to-exhaustion tests, which are not valid to real world-sports performance where the goal is usually to complete a set distance in the shortest possible time.
3	Differences in study approach	Much of the research uses different protocols, environmental conditions, work intensities, carbohydrate interventions, and outcome measures. Therefore, comparing studies proves difficult.
4	Lack of solution blinding	A number of studies did not blind participants to the interventions they were receiving, therefore a placebo effect cannot be discounted in these studies.
5	Measurements made not valid to fatigue	Some of the measurements made in the research have questionable validity to fatigue. For example, muscle glycogen sparing has not been clearly correlated with improved performance or delaying of fatigue, and VO_{2max} has been shown to be a poor predictor of sports performance in a homogeneous sample.
6	Pre-testing nutritional manipulation	Many studies put participants on a fast for the night before and on the morning of the study. These fasts usually lasted for 8–16 hours, and would notably reduce liver and muscle glycogen stores which could improve the likelihood of a carbohydrate supplement having a positive effect on performance.

Source: adapted from Cohen.[53]

stores of the participants. For example, we know that during cycling blood glucose levels and total carbohydrate oxidation rates progressively decline prior to fatigue much more than they do during running. This means that carbohydrate supplementation during cycling may improve performance by prevention of hypoglycaemia (Section 2.2.3.2.2) more so than during running. The problem is that few studies which have demonstrated sparing of muscle glycogen have also demonstrated an ability to continue exercise for longer. Therefore, the cause and effect association between muscle glycogen sparing and delayed fatigue is not conclusive, and muscle glycogen sparing may not be a mechanism '*per se* that could explain how the muscle can either sustain or develop more force during exercise and thus increase performance'.[48]

2.2.3.2.4 GLYCOGEN AND EXERCISE FATIGUE: A BRIEF SUMMARY

The above discussions give a lot of information without many clear answers, which while frustrating, is an accurate picture of the current state of knowledge in this field. While it would be tempting to bury our heads in the sand and stick with the comfortable and familiar theory that glycogen depletion leads to an energy crisis in the muscle that causes fatigue, we cannot do this, as we would be ignoring a lot of other research findings. Here is what we do know:

1 Depletion of muscle glycogen is, in some way or ways, associated with the development of fatigue during exercise.
2 Depletion of muscle glycogen probably does not lead to whole-muscle ATP depletion. However, localised glycogen depletion within the muscle may lead to localised ATP depletion, which could disrupt specific steps of the excitation-contraction coupling process and lead to muscle fatigue.
3 Currently, it appears that localised muscle glycogen depletion may interfere with the ATP-dependent process of Ca^{2+} movement into and out of the muscle cell, which would interfere with muscles' ability to produce force.
4 During prolonged exercise, depletion of muscle and liver glycogen may lead to hypoglycaemia. The role of hypoglycaemia on exercise fatigue may be peripheral (less uptake of glucose into the muscle) or central (reduced uptake of glucose by the brain).

In general, focus is beginning to shift from the traditional theories behind carbohydrate-associated fatigue and investigate other potential roles of this important nutrient, such as Ca^{2+} kinetics and central fatigue. In fact, a lot of the contemporary research is pointing more towards central mechanisms of carbohydrate on the fatigue process.

Key point

The importance of glycogen during exercise is well known, and the literature into carbohydrate supplementation during exercise is wide-ranging. Despite this, our knowledge in these areas is far from complete, and the links between glycogen, carbohydrate supplementation, and exercise fatigue still require more study.

2.2.4 Free-fatty acids

Approximately 90% of fat stores are in the form of triglycerides in adipose cells located at various sites around the body. However, there is a smaller but important store of intramuscular triglycerides. Adipose and muscle triglycerides can be used for fuel during exercise. Adipose triglyceride stores are broken down via lipolysis, a process regulated by specific hormone-sensitive lipases that yields one glycerol and three fatty acid molecules from each triglyceride molecule. Glycerol and fatty acids move into the blood, where glycerol can be taken up by the liver and used to form triglyceride, be oxidised and enter glycolysis, or converted to glucose. Free-fatty acids (blood-borne fatty acids that are not bound to the plasma protein albumin) can enter the muscle via a family of fatty acid transporter proteins and the protein fatty acid translocase (FAT/CD36). Once inside the muscle cell, fatty acids are converted to acyl-CoA and enter the mitochondria via the carnitine shuttle. Once inside the mitochondria the fatty acids can undergo β-oxidation, whereby carbon units in the form of acetyl-CoA are removed from the fatty acyl-CoA molecule. Two carbon units are removed for each cycle of β-oxidation. These acetyl-CoAs can then enter the Krebs cycle and contribute to aerobic ATP resynthesis. Fat cannot generate ATP anaerobically.

Fat stores are abundant, even in lean individuals (approximately 60,000–100,000 Kcal in an average young adult male, or enough energy to run at 9-minutes per mile for over 800 miles – theoretically of course!), therefore fatty acid depletion is not a cause of fatigue even during very long duration exercise. However, fat metabolism can still influence fatigue during exercise. The contribution of lipids to energy expenditure increases with the duration of exercise. One of the goals of aerobic training is to improve the body's ability to metabolise fat as a fuel source, due to limited available glycogen stores. Endurance training can increase the rate of appearance of free fatty acids in the blood, suggesting greater lipolysis, and their rate of disappearance from the blood, suggesting greater uptake by the liver/skeletal muscles.[54] Interestingly, though, neither whole-body lipolytic rate nor total fat oxidation were increased by training in this study. The authors attributed this to the dietary interventions employed. Other studies confirm increased oxidation of free-fatty acids during exercise following endurance training,[55–7] increased intensity at which maximal fat oxidation occurs,[58] and that sparing of muscle glycogen can occur when the ability to oxidise fatty acids is enhanced.[59] These metabolic improvements likely relate to training-induced increases in fatty acid transport protein content and localisation at the sarcolemma and mitochondria.[60] Development of a metabolic profile where fatty acid oxidation could delay muscle glycogen depletion may delay fatigue, particularly during prolonged exercise. However, muscle glycogen sparing is not consistently observed with increased fatty acid oxidation.

Key point

Fat is stored as triglyceride, and can be broken down into fatty acids, taken up by the muscles and undergo β-oxidation before being used to generate energy aerobically in the Krebs cycle.

In recent years, some interesting research has been published that suggests training in a fasted state (i.e. with purposely low muscle and/or liver glycogen stores) may be more beneficial for improving fat oxidation during exercise compared with exercising with an abundance of available glycogen. Training in the fasted state may cause a greater disturbance in energy homeostasis within the muscle, triggering adaptations such as increased activity of key enzymes involved in β-oxidation that enable the muscle to use more of the available energy source (i.e. free-fatty acids).[58] Interestingly, training in a fasted state may also stimulate better oxidative metabolism of carbohydrate, suggesting an overall stimulus to oxidative metabolism. Training while fasted also results in lower blood insulin and greater blood epinephrine concentrations, which facilitates greater lipolysis and opportunity for fatty-acid oxidation. Therefore, training in a fasted state may enable athletes to alter their metabolic responses to exercise and, perhaps, delay fatigue. However, whether or not training in a fasted state enables muscle glycogen sparing during exercise is equivocal. Also, training in a fasted state and then undertaking an exercise session with sufficient carbohydrate stores causes the body to shift back to preferentially utilising carbohydrate, even with an improved potential for fat oxidation.[59] As a clear link between training in a fasted state and improved exercise performance has not been made, more research is required before its efficacy as a tool for counteracting fatigue during exercise can be properly examined.

Key point

Training in a fasted state may enable metabolic adaptations that allow the muscle to better oxidise fat for energy, potentially sparing muscle glycogen and delaying fatigue. However, to date this has not been conclusively shown.

2.3 Summary

- Adenosine triphosphate is the most important source of chemical energy in the body and must constantly be replenished from food energy sources, predominantly carbohydrates and fats.
- Significant whole-muscle ATP depletion is not commonly observed during most forms of exercise, regardless of the intensity or duration.
- Significant ATP depletion can occur in individual muscle fibres, particularly fast twitch fibres, which may contribute to fatigue.
- Depletion of PCr stores is associated with fatigue during single short duration maximal exercise efforts, and repeated efforts with short recovery durations. However, PCr depletion does not fully explain the fatigue observed during these forms of exercise.
- While muscle glycogen depletion is associated with fatigue during exercise, the exact mechanisms are still under debate.
- It is unlikely that muscle glycogen depletion causes whole muscle ATP depletion. However, depletion of specific intramuscular glycogen stores may cause localised ATP depletion that could affect specific excitation-contraction coupling processes such as Ca^{2+} release from the sarcoplasmic reticulum.
- Blood glucose is a primary CNS fuel. During prolonged exercise, development of hypoglycaemia due to liver glycogen depletion may contribute to the development of central fatigue and reduced neuromuscular output.
- Hypoglycaemia may also impair muscle glucose uptake and reduce carbohydrate oxidation, thereby impairing muscle function.
- Carbohydrate supplementation studies have reinforced the importance of carbohydrate availability to exercise performance, but have not yet clarified the mechanisms behind carbohydrate efficacy. Many of the commonly cited mechanisms for performance improvement with carbohydrate supplementation, such as muscle glycogen sparing, are open to significant debate.
- Carbohydrate supplement research has recently come under critical scrutiny, and this should be considered prior to evaluating the role of supplementation research in developing our knowledge of carbohydrate and its links to exercise performance and fatigue.
- Fatty acid availability is not a direct factor in the development of fatigue. However, practices such as endurance training and training in a fasted state may promote metabolic adaptations that allow the muscle to oxidise more fat during exercise, thereby sparing muscle glycogen and delaying fatigue, particularly during prolonged exercise. However, the research findings have not been consistent and more work is required in this area.

To think about . . .

You are the coach of a national-level Olympic-distance triathlete (1,500 metre swim, 40 km cycle, 10 km run; approximate duration 2 hours). You would like to develop your athlete's metabolic response to exercise so that you can be sure they are as 'fuel efficient' as possible, thereby minimising their risk of developing fatigue.

Based on the content of this chapter, what strategies would you put in place during training and competition to ensure that your athlete's fuel use was optimal for performance in his event? As you think about this, also think about the justification for your decisions. What prompted you to make each decision? Are your decisions supported by the research? Remember, the onus is on avoidance of fatigue . . .

Test yourself

Answer the following questions to the best of your ability. Try to understand the information gained from answering these questions before you progress with the book.

1 Describe the importance of ATP to energy provision during exercise.
2 Summarise the potential differences between whole-muscle ATP depletion and individual fibre ATP depletion during exercise.
3 What is the role of PCr in fatigue during the following types of exercise: a single maximal-intensity effort; repeated maximal efforts with short recoveries; prolonged exercise that includes bursts of maximal effort with short recoveries?
4 What does our current knowledge indicate about the link between muscle glycogen depletion and ATP resynthesis during exercise?
5 What are the two ways in which hypoglycaemia may influence exercise fatigue?
6 Briefly outline the important considerations we must make when interpreting results of carbohydrate supplementation research and how these results influence our understanding of carbohydrate and exercise fatigue.
7 Explain how altering the metabolism of free fatty acids during exercise many contribute to improved exercise performance and, potentially, delay fatigue.

References

1 Noakes TD, Gibson A (2004) Logical limitations to the 'catastrophe' models of fatigue during exercise in humans. *Br J Sports Med* 38: 648–9.
2 Gaitanos GC, Williams C, Boobis LH, *et al.* (1993) Human muscle metabolism during intermittent maximal exercise. *J Appl Physiol* 75 (2): 712–19.
3 Baldwin J, Snow RJ, Gibala MJ, *et al.* (2003) Glycogen availability does not affect the TCA cycle or TAN pools during prolonged, fatiguing exercise. *J Appl Physiol* 94: 2181–7.
4 Gibala MJ, Gonzalez-Alonson J, Saltin B (2002) Dissociation between muscle tricarboxylic acid cycle pool size and aerobic energy provision during prolonged exercise in humans. *J Physiol* 545: 705–13.
5 Westerblad H, Bruton JD, Katz A (2010) Skeletal muscle: energy metabolism, fiber types, fatigue and adaptability. *Exp Cell Res* 316: 3093–9.
6 MacIntosh BR, Holash RJ, Renaud J (2012) Skeletal muscle fatigue – regulation of excitation-contraction coupling to avoid metabolic catastrophe. *J Cell Sci* 125: 2105–14.
7 Karatzaferi C, de Haan A, Ferguson RA, *et al.* (2001) Phosphocreatine and ATP content in human single muscle fibres before and after maximum dynamic exercise. *Pflugers Arch* 442: 627–41.
8 Jeneson JA, Schmitz JP, van Dijk JH, *et al.* (2010) Exercise ability is determined by muscle ATP buffer content, not Pi or pH. *Proc Intl Soc Mag Reson Med* 18: 864.
9 Bogdanis GC, Nevill ME, Lakomy HKA, *et al.* (1994) Muscle metabolism during repeated sprint exercise in man. *J Physiol* 475: 25–6.
10 Casey A, Constantin-Teodosiu D, Howell S, *et al.* (1996) Metabolic response of type I and II muscle fibres during repeated bouts of maximal exercise in humans. *Am J Physiol* 271 (1 Pt 1): E38–43.
11 Bogdanis GC, Nevill ME, Boobis LH, *et al.* (1995) Recovery of power output and muscle metabolites following 30 s of maximal sprint cycling in man. *J Physiol* 482 (Pt 2): 467–80.
12 Billaut F, Bishop D (2009) Muscle fatigue in males and females during multiple-sprint exercise. *Sports Med* 39 (4): 257–78.
13 Bogdanis GC, Nevill ME, Boobis LH, *et al.* (1996) Contribution of phosphocreatine and aerobic metabolism to energy supply during repeated sprint exercise. *J Appl Physiol* 80 (3): 876–84.
14 Mendez-Villanueva A, Edge J, Suriano R, *et al.* (2013) The recovery of repeated-sprint exercise is associated with PCr resynthesis, while muscle pH and EMG amplitude remain depressed. *PLOS One* 7 (12): 1–10.
15 Harris R, Hultman E, Kaijser L, *et al.* (1975) The effect of circulatory occlusion on isometric exercise capacity and energy metabolism of the quadriceps muscle in man. *Scand J Clin Lab Invest* 35: 87–95.
16 Trump ME, Heigenhauser GJ, Putman CT, *et al.* (1996) Importance of muscle phosphocreatine during intermittent maximal cycling. *J Appl Physiol* 80 (5): 1574–80.
17 Balsom PD, Ekblom B, Söerlund K, *et al.* (1993) Creatine supplementation and dynamic high-intensity intermittent exercise. *Scand J Med Sci Sports* 3 (3): 143–9.
18 Birch R, Noble D, Greenhaff PL (1994) The influence of dietary creatine supplementation on performance during repeated bouts of maximal isokinetic cycling in man. *Eur J Appl Physiol* 69 (3): 268–70.
19 Barnett C, Hinds M, Jenkins DG (1996) Effects of creatine supplementation on multiple sprint cycling performance. *Aust J Sci Med Sport* 28: 35–9.

20 Cox G, Mujika I, Tumilty D, *et al.* (2002) Acute creatine supplementation and performance during a field test simulating match play in elite female soccer players. *Int J Sport Nutr Exerc Metab* 12 (1): 33–46.
21 Dawson B, Cutler M, Moody A, *et al.* (1995) Effects of oral creatine loading on single and repeated maximal short sprints. *Aust J Sci Med Sport* 27: 56–61.
22 McKenna M, Morton J, Selig SE, *et al.* (1999) Creatine supplementation increases muscle total creatine but not maximal intermittent exercise performance. *J Appl Physiol* 87 (6): 2244–52.
23 Mohr M, Krustrup P, Bangsbo J (2003) Match performance of high-standard soccer players with special reference to development of fatigue. *J Sports Sci* 21: 519–28.
24 Spencer M, Lawrence S, Rechichi C, *et al.* (2004) Time-motion analysis of elite field hockey, with special reference to repeated-sprint activity. *J Sports Sci* 22: 843–50.
25 Duthie G, Pyne D, Hooper S (2003) Applied physiology and game analysis of rugby union. *Sports Med* 33 (13): 973–91.
26 Sirotic AC, Coutts AJ, Knowles H, *et al.* (2009) A comparison of match demands between elite and semi-elite rugby league competition. *J Sports Sci* 27 (3): 203–11.
27 Krogh A, Lindhard J (2010) The relative value of fat and carbohydrate as sources of muscular energy. *Biochem J* 14: 290.
28 Levine S, Gordon B, Derick C (1924) Some changes in the chemical constituents of blood following a marathon race: with special reference to the development of hypoglycaemia. *J Am Med Assoc* 82: 1778–9.
29 Bergström J, Hultman E (1967) A study of the glycogen metabolism during exercise in man. *Scand J Clin Lab Invest* 19 (3): 218–28.
30 Bergström J, Hermansen L, Hultman E, *et al.* (1967) Diet, muscle glycogen and physical performance. *Acta Physiol Scand* 71 (2): 140–50.
31 Febbraio MA, Dancey J (1999) Skeletal muscle energy metabolism during prolonged, fatiguing exercise. *J Appl Physiol* 87: 2341–7.
32 Parkin JM, Carey MF, Zhao S, *et al.* (1999) Effect of ambient temperature on human skeletal muscle metabolism during fatiguing submaximal exercise. *J Appl Physiol* 86: 902–8.
33 Vissing J, Haller RG (2003) The effect of oral sucrose on exercise tolerance in patients with McArdle's Disease. *New Eng J Med* 349: 2503–9.
34 Williams JH, Batts TW, Lees S (2012) Reduced muscle glycogen differentially affects exercise performance and muscle fatigue. *ISRN Physiol* (2013): 1–9.
35 Ortenblad N, Nielsen J, Saltin B, *et al.* (2011) Role of glycogen availability in sarcoplasmic reticulum Ca^{2+} kinetics in human skeletal muscle. *J Physiol* 589 (3): 711–25.
36 Ortenblad N, Westerblad H, Nielsen J (2013) Muscle glycogen stores and fatigue. *J Physiol* 591: 4405–13.
37 Chin ER, Allen DG (1997) Effects of reduced muscle glycogen concentration on force, Ca^{2+} release and contractile protein function in intact mouse skeletal muscle. *J Physiol* 498: 17–29.
38 Duhamel TA, Green HJ, Perco JG, *et al.* (2006) Comparative effects of a low-carbohydrate diet and exercise plus a lot-carbohydrate diet on muscle sarcoplasmic reticulum responses in males. *Am J Physiol Cell Physiol* 291: C607–17.
39 Nielsen J, Schrøder HD, Rix CG, *et al.* (2009) Distinct effects of subcellular glycogen localization on tetanic relaxation time and endurance in mechanically skinned rat skeletal muscle fibres. *J Physiol* 587: 3679–90.
40 Thibodeau GA, Patton KT (1999) *Anatomy and Physiology*. 4th ed. p. 317. Maryland Heights, MO: Mosby.
41 Nybo L, Møller K, Pedersen BK, *et al.* (2003) Association between fatigue and failure to preserve cerebral energy turnover during prolonged exercise. *Acta Physiol Scand* 179 (1): 67–74.

42 Matsui T, Soya H (2013) Brain glycogen decrease and supercompensation with prolonged exhaustive exercise. *Social Neuroscience and Public Health*: 253–64.
43 Nybo L (2003) CNS fatigue and prolonged exercise: effect of glucose supplementation. *Med Sci Sports Exerc* 35 (4): 589–94.
44 Coyle EF, Coggan AR, Hemmert MK, *et al.* (1986) Muscle glycogen utilization during prolonged strenuous exercise when fed carbohydrate. *J Appl Physiol* 61 (1): 165–72.
45 Coggan AR, Coyle EF (1987) Reversal of fatigue during prolonged exercise by carbohydrate infusion or ingestion. *J Appl Physiol* 63 (6): 2388–95.
46 Felig P, Cherif A, Minagawa A, *et al.* (1982) Hypoglycaemia during prolonged exercise in normal men. *N Engl J Med* 306 (15): 895–900.
47 Claassen A, Lambert EV, Bosch AN, *et al.* (2005) Variability in exercise capacity and metabolic response during endurance exercise after a low carbohydrate diet. *Int J Sport Nutr Exerc Metab* 15 (2): 97–116.
48 Karelis AD, Smith JW, Passe DH, *et al.* (2010) Carbohydrate administration and exercise performance: what are the mechanisms involved? *Sports Med* 40 (9): 747–63.
49 De Bock K, Derave W, Ramaekers M, *et al.* (2006) Fiber type-specific muscle glycogen sparing due to carbohydrate intake before and during exercise. *J Appl Physiol* 102: 183–8.
50 Hargreaves M, Costill DL, Coggan A, *et al.* (1984) Effect of carbohydrate feedings on muscle glycogen utilization and exercise performance. *Med Sci Sports Exerc* 16 (3): 219–22.
51 Tsintzas OK, Williams C, Boobis L, *et al.* (1995) Carbohydrate ingestion and glycogen utilization in different muscle fibre types in man. *J Physiol* 489 (1): 243–50.
52 Tsintzas K, Williams C, Constantin-Teodosiu D, *et al.* (2001) Phosphocreatine degradation in type I and type II muscle fibres during submaximal exercise in man: effect of carbohydrate ingestion. *J Physiol* 537 (1): 305–11.
53 Cohen D (2012) The truth about sports drinks. *B Med J* 345: 1–8.
54 Friedlander AL, Casazza GA, Horning MA, *et al.* (1999) Endurance training increases fatty acid turnover, but not fat oxidation, in young men. *J Appl Physiol* 86: 2097–105.
55 Friedlander AL, Casazza GA, Horning MA, *et al.* (1998) Effects of exercise intensity and training on lipid metabolism in young women. *Am J Physiol* 275: E853–63.
56 Martin WH, Dalsky GP, Hurley BF, *et al.* (1993) Effect of endurance training on plasma free fatty acid turnover and oxidation during exercise. *Am J Physiol* 265: E708–14.
57 Phillips SM, Green HJ, Tarnolpolsky MA, *et al.* (1996) Effects of training duration on substrate turnover and oxidation during exercise. *J Appl Physiol* 81: 2182–91.
58 Van Proeyen K, Szlufcik K, Nielens H, *et al.* (2011) Beneficial metabolic adaptations due to endurance exercise training in the fasted state. *J Appl Physiol* 110: 236–45.
59 De Bock K, Derave W, Eijnde BO, *et al.* (2008) Effect of training in the fasted state on metabolic responses during exercise with carbohydrate intake. *J Appl Physiol* 104: 1045–55.
60 Talanian JL, Holloway GP, Snook LA, *et al.* (2010) Exercise training increases sarcolemmal and mitochondrial fatty acid transport proteins in human skeletal muscle. *Am J Physiol* 299: E180–8.

Chapter 3

Metabolic acidosis

3.1 Introduction

Metabolic acidosis (a reduction in the normal pH of a fluid or tissue caused by endogenous production of acidic substances) represents an area of confusion with regard to exercise fatigue. Many coaches, athletes, students (and academics) hold the view that the development of acidosis, primarily via lactic acid accumulation, is a key cause of exercise fatigue. This chapter will discuss acidosis from the perspective of lactic acid, lactate, and hydrogen production. The links between these factors and fatigue will be evaluated, and recent research that challenges these links will be discussed. While reading this chapter, it is important to remember that most of the knowledge is still being added to, and the topic remains fiercely debated among academics and researchers. Therefore, the information is not the final word on the topic of metabolic acidosis, but is a summary of where our knowledge currently sits.

Key point

Although our knowledge of the processes involved in metabolic acidosis has developed significantly, the exact causes of metabolic acidosis, and its role in fatigue during exercise, are still keenly debated.

3.2 The role of metabolic acidosis in exercise fatigue: a brief history

The belief that lactic acid is produced in skeletal muscles during exercise and that accumulation of lactic acid causes fatigue can be traced back to research carried out in the early 1900s. By electrically stimulating muscle preparations, researchers reported that the muscles produced lactic acid.[1] When these muscle preparations were incubated following stimulation in nitrogen or oxygen rich environments at different temperatures, lactic acid concentrations increased more in the nitrogen incubation compared with the oxygen incubation. In other words, lactic acid concentrations were lowest in muscles that were exposed to oxygen. Based on these findings, it was concluded that increases in lactic acid were greatest under anaerobic conditions, slower in normal air, and completely absent in a pure oxygen environment.[1] It was also concluded that 'lactic acid is spontaneously developed under anaerobic conditions in muscle' and 'fatigue due to contractions is accompanied by an increase in lactic acid'.[1] Therefore, it appears these early authors were stating that increases in lactic acid cause fatigue in skeletal muscles. However, this is incorrect, as the authors did not state that lactic acid *causes* fatigue; they merely documented the production of lactic acid and the occurrence of muscle fatigue. No cause and effect relationship was implied.[2] This distinction is crucial, as these initial findings may have been misinterpreted to mean that lactic acid has a causative role in muscle fatigue;[2] an interpretation that still influences our views of exercise fatigue today (Section 1.1.1).

Following the early documentation of lactic acid production in skeletal muscle, other researchers reported increased blood lactate concentrations when people exercised to fatigue, and described the biochemistry of glycolysis and its production of lactic acid.[3–4] Perhaps inevitably, given earlier findings and understanding of biochemistry at the time, the conclusion was made that during intense work muscles contract in the absence of an adequate oxygen supply (in 'anaerobiosis'), thereby producing lactic acid which causes muscle acidosis that leads to fatigue. All of these connections were assumed to be cause-and-effect,[4] and the belief that lactic acid production causes acidosis and muscle fatigue was born.

Since this early work, many studies have been published that appear to support the link between lactic acid production, acidosis, and fatigue. In the 1970s, a linear relationship was found between lactate accumulation and loss of muscle force in frogs[5] and later, in human thigh muscle.[6] These studies also indicated that the decline in muscle force and the increase in muscle acidity followed a similar time-course, suggesting that they may have an influence over one another.[7] Both acidosis and the decline in muscle force production occur more slowly following a period of physical training, and in slow twitch compared with fast twitch muscles. These studies appear to provide evidence for a role of lactic acid in muscle fatigue. However, all of these studies used correlation analysis to associate acidosis with fatigue. While correlations do show the association between two variables, they cannot prove a cause and effect relationship between them. Simply put, while acidosis and fatigue may correlate, it cannot be said that acidosis *causes* fatigue. Indeed, much of the research that showed a correlation between lactic acid and fatigue also showed relationships between other metabolic measures and fatigue.[7]

3.2.1 How might lactic acid cause fatigue?

Two main hypotheses were posed for how lactic acid production may cause exercise fatigue. First, a reduced muscle pH, caused by lactic acid production, may impair muscle contraction via a decline in isometric muscle force production and muscle shortening velocity (Section 3.3.2.4). Intramuscular acidosis was thought to do this by reducing sarcoplasmic reticulum calcium (Ca^{2+}) release[8] and calcium sensitivity.[9] However, there is mounting research against this hypothesis (Section 3.3.2.1). Second, intramuscular acidosis could cause fatigue by inhibiting glycolysis (Section 3.3.2.3).[10–13] This hypothesis was developed through observation of reduced activity of key enzymes that regulate glycolysis during exercise that causes notable reductions in muscle pH. Both of these theories gain some support from research that shows making the blood more alkaline can enable better maintenance of work and power during intermittent high-intensity exercise.[14–16] However, as with the influence of acidosis on muscle Ca^{2+} release and sensitivity, there is an important counter-argument to the suggestion that acidosis inhibits glycolysis, and this is presented in Section 3.3.2.3.

Key point

Potential causes of lactic acid-induced fatigue include impaired isometric muscle force and contraction velocity, and inhibition of glycolysis due to a reduction in intramuscular pH.

3.3 Metabolic acidosis and exercise fatigue: the counter-view

The large amount of interest and research effort spent examining metabolic acidosis during exercise and its role in exercise fatigue has not brought all the answers, and metabolic acidosis remains a hotly debated topic. However, these efforts have generated knowledge that, while perhaps not allowing us to completely discount the role of metabolic acidosis in fatigue, certainly allows us to question it.

An important question to answer when discussing the biochemistry of lactic acid is 'What does the body produce during exercise – lactic acid or lactate'? Reading lay articles, or even scientific papers on the subject, you will often see that the terms lactic acid and lactate are used interchangeably as though they mean the same thing. Importantly, they do not. Lactic acid is, as the name suggests, an acidic compound that has the potential to release a proton (hydrogen ion, H^+) into a solution, thereby making that solution more acidic (Figure 3.1). Conversely, lactate does not release H^+; therefore, it is termed an acid salt. As lactate does not have a H^+ to donate, it does not directly make its environment more acidic (Figure 3.1).

During exercise, ATP is resynthesised via anaerobic glycolysis (Figure 3.2) and oxidative phosphorylation via β-oxidation of fatty acids and breakdown of pyruvate in the Krebs cycle and electron transport chain. Anaerobic glycolysis is always active, regardless of the intensity of exercise or the extent of the oxidative contribution to ATP resynthesis. This is because carbohydrate needs to be converted to pyruvate, which is then converted to acetyl CoA for entry into the Krebs cycle. The conversion of carbohydrate to pyruvate occurs via glycolysis (Figure 3.2). Specific stages of glycolysis, particularly those involving ATP hydrolysis, produce H^+ (equation 2.1 and Figure 3.2). A greater flux (or activity) of glycolysis will lead to greater H^+ production. During intense exercise, the mitochondria are not able to metabolise all of the pyruvate that is produced in glycolysis (in other words, the activity of the mitochondria lags behind the activity of glycolysis). To prevent pyruvate accumulation, which would inhibit glycolysis and thereby impair both anaerobic and oxidative ATP resynthesis, pyruvate can be converted, via the lactate dehydrogenase reaction, to lactate (Figure 3.2). This is crucial: lactate, not lactic acid, is produced via glycolysis.[17] The lactate dehydrogenase reaction also consumes H^+, and generates the H^+ carrier molecule nicotinamide adenine dinucleotide (NAD^+), which is able to take up H^+ from the cytosol and transport it into the electron transport chain where it plays a critical role in ATP resynthesis. The conversion of pyruvate to lactate, involving use of NADH and H^+ and the production of NAD^+, is summarised in the following equation:

$$\text{Pyruvate} + \text{NADH} + H^+ \xrightarrow{\text{lactate dehydrogenase}} \text{Lactate} + NAD^+ \qquad (3.1)$$

where NADH is the reduced form of NAD^+ (meaning it has H^+ attached to it), and NAD^+ oxidised form of NAD (it does not have H^+ attached to it, and is therefore ready to accept H^+).

Increased glycolytic flux can also cause production of H^+ at a rate faster than it can be removed by NAD^+. In this situation, NAD^+ may become saturated with H^+ ions. This saturation could lead to H^+ accumulation in the cytosol that, if unchecked, could reduce intramuscular acidity to the extent that the integrity and function of the tissue may be compromised. The lactate dehydrogenase reaction acts as a buffer against this cellular H^+ accumulation by consuming H^+ and recycling NAD^+ (Figure 3.2) in the process of converting pyruvate to lactate.[4] Simply put, the production of lactate via the lactate dehydrogenase reaction is alkalinising to the cell, not acidifying. Lactate may also facilitate H^+ removal from the cell via monocarboxylate (MCT) transporters present in cell membranes (Section 3.3.1). These transporters also serve to remove H^+ from the cell, meaning that the removal of lactate also removes H^+ from the muscle.

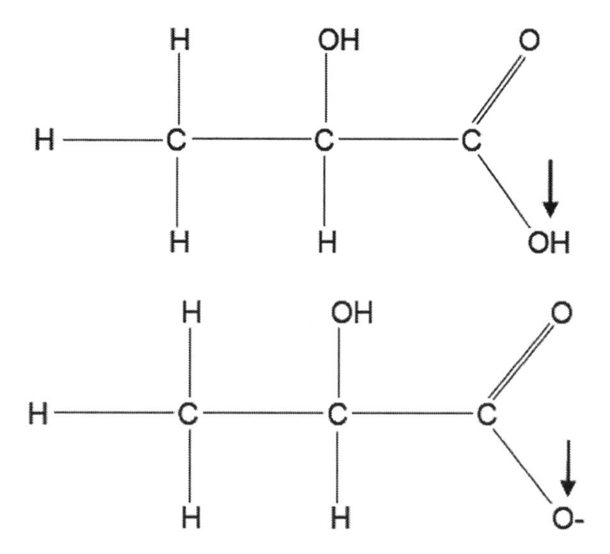

Figure 3.1 The chemical structure of lactic acid (top) and lactate (bottom). Lactic acid contains hydrogen that dissociates and moves into the surrounding solution as a hydrogen ion (H^+), increasing its acidity. However, as we have discussed, it is lactate and not lactic acid that is produced in muscle during exercise. Lactate does not release H^+ and cannot directly increase the acidity of its environment.

As already discussed, lactate does not directly make the internal environment more acidic; therefore, its production cannot directly contribute to intramuscular acidosis. This would appear to clarify the issue, and suggest that the lack of lactic acid production during intense exercise means that lactic acidosis cannot be considered a cause of fatigue. However, it is possible that lactate, as a strong acid anion (negatively charged ion) may cause hydrogen formation from water.[7] Therefore, lactate production may still indirectly cause some intramuscular acidosis. However, it is highly unlikely that this would contribute meaningfully to exercise fatigue.

Key point

Lactate, not lactic acid, is produced in glycolysis. Lactic acid has the potential to make its environment more acidic by releasing a hydrogen ion, whereas lactate does not. This has important implications for the role of lactate/lactic acid in fatigue.

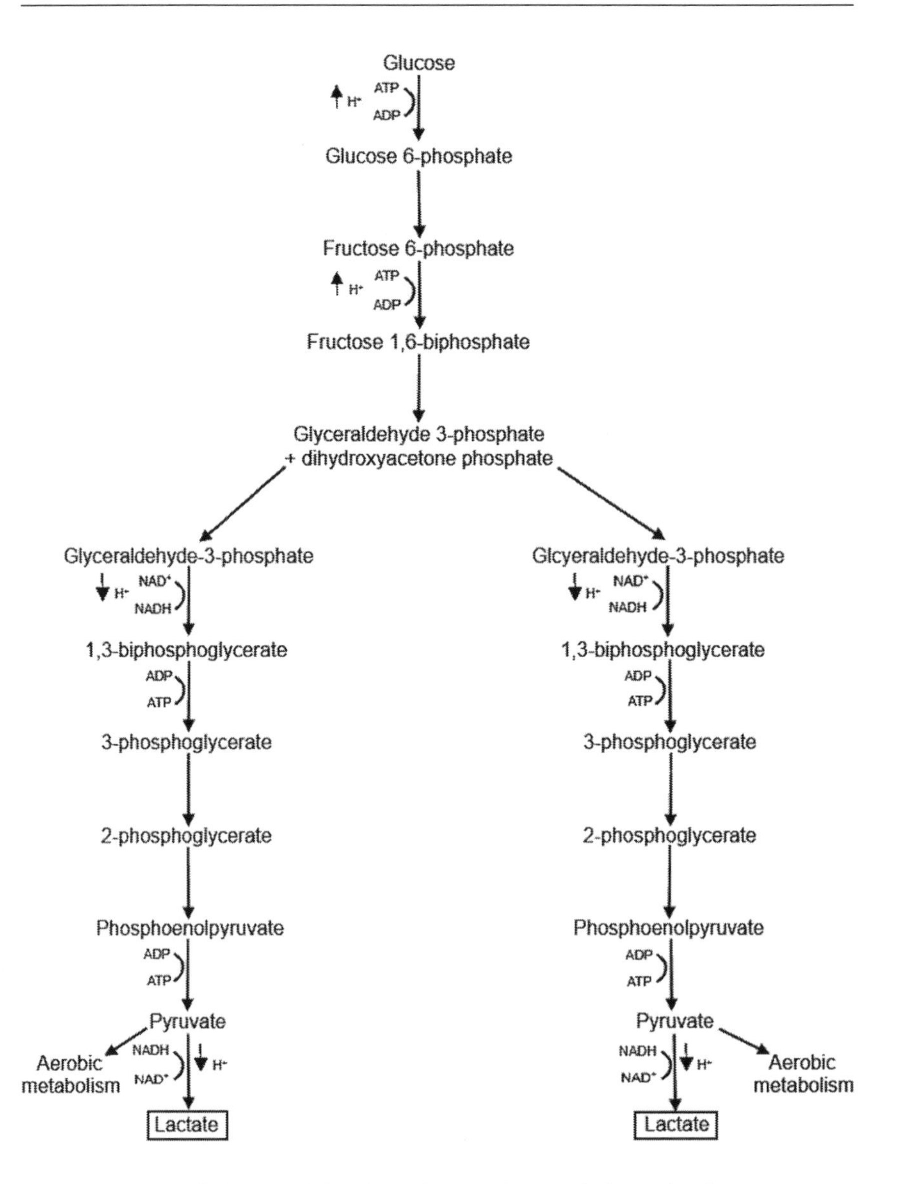

Figure 3.2 A simplified view of glycolysis, showing the metabolism of a glucose molecule to pyruvate for entry into the Krebs cycle (aerobic metabolism). Also highlighted are the reactions of glycolysis that produce hydrogen (↑H^+) and those that consume or remove hydrogen (↓H^+).

As stated above and shown in Figure 3.2, lactate, not lactic acid, is produced in glycolysis. In fact, virtually no lactic acid exists in the body,[7] as the acid dissociation constant of lactic acid is lower than the normal pH of body tissues and fluids. This means that any lactic acid present in the body would dissociate to lactate and H^+. The relationship between these two ions, in terms of how they are produced and what effect they have on their environment and on one-another, are crucial to understanding the counter-argument to the lactic acidosis hypothesis. We have discussed (and will continue to do so) lactate, and we have mentioned H^+, specifically that it can make the environment it is placed in more acidic. Let us discuss this further.

A H^+ ion is essentially a hydrogen atom that has donated its single electron in a chemical reaction (termed an oxidation reaction). The structure of a hydrogen atom is a nucleus containing a single proton, and a single electron 'spinning' around that nucleus (Figure 3.3). If the hydrogen atom loses its electron, all that remains is a single proton. That is why H^+ ions are also referred to as protons. The plus sign in H^+ refers to the fact that the ion is now positively charged as it only contains a proton. Hydrogen ions (protons) are acidic (an acid is any substance that donates protons), and therefore make the solution they are placed in (water, blood, or intracellular fluid) acidic.

A traditional viewpoint is that production of lactate is also associated with production of H^+ ions, which causes a reduction in the pH of the intramuscular environment. Simply put, this view states that production of lactate is a cause of acidosis. However, this view has been challenged by numerous researchers who state that lactate has no involvement in H^+ production (and vice versa), and that in fact H^+ is produced during glycolysis from the hydrolysis of ATP (see Figure 3.2 and equation 2.1).[18–20] This would appear to absolve lactate from any role in the development of acidosis during exercise. However,

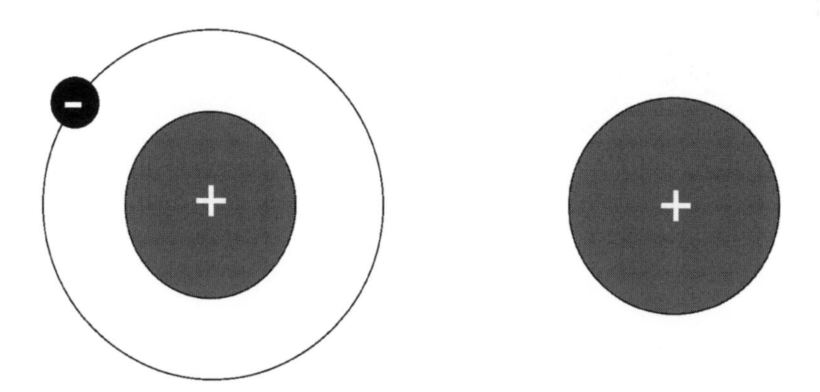

Figure 3.3 A hydrogen atom (left), composed of a single proton (positive charge, +) and a single electron (negative charge, –). The loss of the single electron in an oxidation reaction leaves the single positively charged proton remaining (right). This single proton is referred to by the abbreviation H^+.

as with most topics in this book the picture is not black and white, as other researchers contend that lactate production does cause acidosis by altering the behaviour of water so that it releases H^+ into the intracellular environment, and that the coincidental production of lactate and H^+ during exercise is, essentially, the production of lactic acid.[17,21–3] Some of the confusion may relate to the experimental design used by research studies in this topic. Some studies use small amounts of human tissue in a laboratory environment in an attempt to artificially re-create the internal environment of the body (termed *in vitro* research), whereas other studies actually use an entire, living human or animal (*in vivo* research). It is extremely difficult to replicate the complex functioning of animal tissue *in vitro*; therefore, this type of research may not produce a full picture of biochemical processes. A good example is that some *in vitro* research examining the role of pH reduction on muscle function carried out experiments at tissue temperatures notably lower than that of an intact, *in vivo* muscle. Acid–base regulation is influenced by temperature, and studies conducted at temperatures much nearer to normal physiological temperatures have reported very little effect of reduced pH on muscle function (see Section 3.3.2). Also, looking at the complex biochemical reactions underpinning metabolic processes in isolation may limit our understanding of exactly what is going on, as these reactions are interdependent and influence one another.[17] It is therefore more appropriate to study them as a group event – something that is very difficult to do. The key message here is that the methods used by researchers should be considered when reading research into the biochemistry of metabolic acidosis. Regardless of the exact cause of its production, what is important is that accumulation of H^+ can reduce the pH of the muscle and blood. This pH reduction (acidosis) has long been considered a cause of muscle fatigue during intense exercise.

Key point

A H^+ ion is a hydrogen atom that has donated its single electron, leaving behind a single proton. Hydrogen ions are acidic, and will make the solution they are placed in more acidic.

Key point

The production of lactate does not produce H^+, and therefore does not directly make its environment more acidic. However, lactate production may alter the behaviour of intracellular water, thereby indirectly causing H^+ production.

3.3.1 Lactate: misconceptions and benefits

Lactate remains a misunderstood substance for many. The most important misconception is that lactate is directly responsible for fatigue during exercise. However, there are other common misconceptions, as well as some important benefits, of lactate production that should be addressed:

1 *Lactate is a waste product that serves no useful purpose.*

This is an often repeated, and probably not much thought about, statement. As a general rule, the body does not 'waste' much of its energy or resources. Even things that appear at first to be wasteful (example: the large amount of metabolic energy that is released as heat) actually serve an important role (this heat keeps us warm and regulates our body temperature, enabling our body systems to function optimally). Therefore, it does not make sense to view lactate as an unwanted fatigue-inducing agent; a by-product that through some flawed metabolic evolution has to be tolerated and its damaging effects minimised. Indeed, this view is no longer relevant, for at least two reasons. The first is that lactate production actually serves to reduce acidosis within skeletal muscle, potentially enhancing or at least maintaining function and improving exercise performance. Lactate production is observed during hard exercise due to the production and transport of lactate as described in Section 3.3. However, the traditional interpretation that lactate accumulation is the cause of fatigue is erroneous, and a classic example of the misapplication of the cause and effect phenomenon. As we know, the existence of a correlation between two variables does not imply that one variable causes the change in the other variable. In other words, just because increased muscle/blood lactate and impaired performance are correlated, does not mean that increased muscle/blood lactate *causes* impaired performance. This is further clarified if we consider that production of lactate consumes H^+, meaning that lactate production acts to reduce the acidity of the muscle. Larger amounts of lactate are detected during periods of high-intensity work when some performance decrement may also be seen; however, lactate production is high due to its role in buffering excess pyruvate and H^+, and is not impairing performance. Therefore, increased lactate production is the result of the body attempting to prevent increases in intramuscular acidity, and its occurrence at fatigue is coincidental.

The benefit of glycolysis and lactate production is further evidenced by observations made in patients with McArdle's disease, which is a genetic condition characterised by an inability to break down glycogen via glycolysis, and therefore an inability to produce lactate. People with this condition actually fatigue more quickly during exercise than people who do produce lactate, providing strong evidence that lactate production is actually beneficial to performance. Therefore, the substance that has been demonised for so long as the cause of fatigue during exercise actually does the opposite: it helps us to keep exercising for longer.

The second reason why lactate is not simply a waste product is that it is a fuel source during and after exercise. Approximately 75% of all lactate produced during exercise is used as muscle fuel, and up to 25% of the energy needed during a 1,500-metre run is supplied by lactate.[24] The use of lactate as a fuel is facilitated by the presence of the specialised MCT proteins present in the sarcolemma and the mitochondria of muscle fibres which facilitate the transport of lactate from fibre to fibre, and into the mitochondria for conversion back to pyruvate and subsequent oxidation for energy. Lactate is also converted to glucose post-exercise in the liver in a process called gluconeogenesis, which helps to replenish the finite carbohydrate stores that have been depleted during exercise.[25] It also appears that the brain, previously thought to exclusively use glucose as a fuel source, may also use lactate to generate energy both before and after exercise.[26–7]

The functional importance of lactate is being further understood by studies investigating its ergogenic effects as a supplement during exercise. In particular, supplementation with lactate during high-intensity, short duration exercise has been shown to significantly improve performance.[28] The primary mechanism behind this performance improvement appears to be an alkalinising effect of lactate on the blood, as lactate is buffered to bicarbonate, and bicarbonate is a primary blood-based acid buffering system. Therefore, lactate consumption may increase the pH gradient between the muscle and blood, which would facilitate the movement of H^+ out of the muscle and into the blood, where it could then be buffered by bicarbonate.

2 *Lactate causes muscle soreness, pain, and other uncomfortable symptoms during and after exercise.*

There is no scientific theory or rationale suggesting that lactate contributes to the uncomfortable muscular sensations typically felt during and in the hours and days after hard and/or unaccustomed exercise. In fact, as lactate produced during exercise is removed from muscle within approximately 1 hour after exercise,[29] it cannot be the cause of delayed muscle soreness. The unpleasant muscle symptoms sometimes felt during exercise, such as soreness and burning, do not have a clearly accepted cause. However, these sensations may be due to stimulation of pain-generating (nociceptive) free nerve endings in the muscle (termed group III and IV muscle afferents) by biochemical substances such as H^+, and by mechanical stress associated with contraction.[30] The muscle soreness sometimes felt in the hours and days following exercise is likely due to a pathway effect involving micro trauma of the muscle architecture that leads to inflammation, intramuscular oedema (swelling), and the hormone-mediated sensitisation of free nerve endings in the muscle.[31–2]

3.3.2 The impact of hydrogen production on muscle function

3.3.2.1 Sarcoplasmic reticulum Ca^{2+} release and Ca^{2+} binding to troponin C

Originally, it was thought that metabolic acidosis caused a reduction in muscle force by reducing the rate of Ca^{2+} release from the sarcoplasmic reticulum. The release of Ca^{2+} is crucial for muscle contraction, and if insufficient Ca^{2+} is released the muscle may contract with less force. However, it appears that the normal processes of Ca^{2+} release from the sarcoplasmic reticulum are not impaired, even when muscle pH levels are as low as 6.2 (from a normal resting pH of ~7.1).[33] It therefore appears that the influence of acidosis on Ca^{2+} movement from its intramuscular storage site is minimal.

Once Ca^{2+} has been released from the sarcoplasmic reticulum, it must bind with troponin C, part of a complex of three proteins that play a crucial role in initiating the process of cross-bridging of the two primary contractile filaments in skeletal muscle, actin and myosin (Figure 3.4). This cross-bridging is necessary for muscle contraction. If Ca^{2+} cannot bind to troponin C, then actin and myosin cannot interact and muscle contraction will not occur. Hydrogen competes with Ca^{2+} to bind to troponin C, and for this reason it was thought that intramuscular H^+ accumulation would reduce muscle force. However, increased intramuscular acidity also causes a reduction in the binding of Ca^{2+} to other locations in the muscle fibre, such as the sarcoplasmic reticulum Ca^{2+} pump. In fact, the reduction in Ca^{2+} binding to the Ca^{2+} pump is much greater than the reduction in Ca^{2+} binding to troponin C. Therefore, the amount of Ca^{2+} in the muscle fibre that is free to bind to troponin C actually increases in acidic conditions. As a result, muscle force production may actually increase in an acidic muscle. In short, acidosis has a much smaller influence on the muscle contractile mechanism than originally thought, and may even favour a greater force development than under normal pH conditions.

Key point

Intramuscular acidosis causes changes to Ca^{2+} kinetics, but these changes have, at most, only a small effect on muscle force production. In fact, some of these changes may actually favour an increase in muscle force development under acidic conditions.

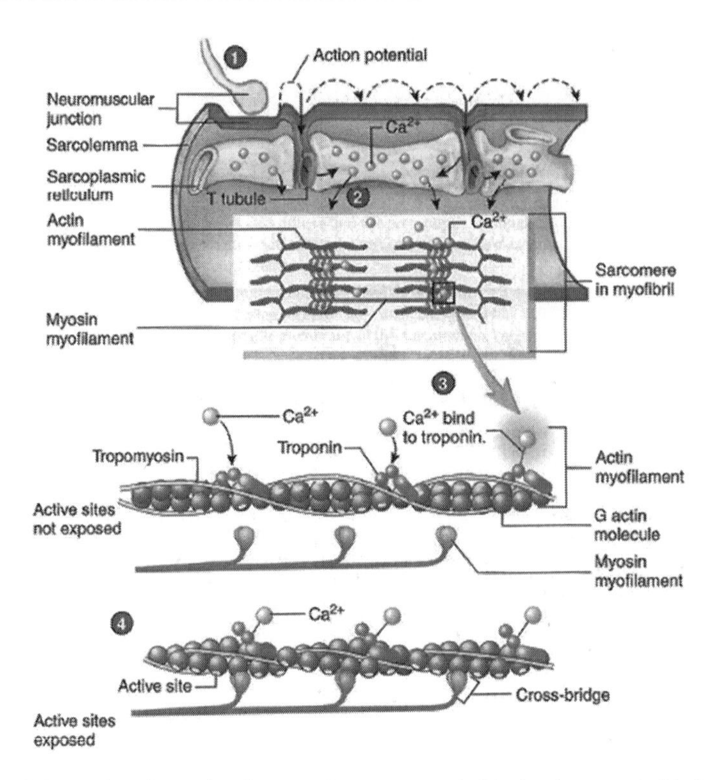

Figure 3.4 In a relaxed muscle, the protein tropomyosin blocks the myosin binding sites on actin, preventing actin and myosin from interacting. When an action potential spreads through the t tubules (1), the t tubules depolarise, causing channels in the sarcoplasmic reticulum to open, releasing Ca^{2+} into the myoplasm (2). Ca^{2+} ions then bind to troponin C, causing a shape change in troponin that pushes tropomyosin away from the myosin binding sites of the actin filaments (3). This allows actin and myosin to interact and muscle contraction to occur (4).

Source: Tate.[58] Permission has been granted to replicate the figure from this book.

3.3.2.2 Muscle membrane excitability

Research into the effect of H^+ on the excitability of skeletal muscle (the ability of the electrical signal to move across the muscle membrane and into the muscle to stimulate Ca^{2+} release) is a good example of how H^+ can exert positive effects on muscle function. During repeated muscle contractions, potassium (K^+) is lost from the intramuscular environment and accumulates in the extracellular environment (this will be discussed in more detail in Chapter 5). Accumulation of K^+ in the extracellular space can impair the excitability of the muscle fibre, reducing contraction force. Intramuscular acidity can help to maintain muscle fibre excitability and force production during repeated contractions, perhaps by counteracting the force-depressing effects of extracellular K^+ accumulation.[34] However, studies investigating the relationship between acidosis and K^+ kinetics *in vitro* often cannot replicate the exact conditions in which muscles contract. Therefore, there may be a discrepancy between research findings and actual *in vivo* responses. This discrepancy may explain why a protective effect of acidosis can be absent during repeated *in vivo* muscle contractions.[35] Other work suggests that acidosis causes a reduction in the activity of muscle membrane chloride channels.[36] Movement of chloride through these channels has an inhibitory effect on muscle excitability. The reduction in chloride channel activity caused by acidosis could thereby reduce this inhibition and increase muscle excitability.

Key point

Acidosis may help to maintain muscle membrane excitability and force production, perhaps by counteracting the force-depressing effects of extracellular K^+ accumulation, or by reducing the activity of muscle membrane chloride channels.

3.3.2.3 The rate of glycolysis

During maximal intermittent exercise, significant relationships have been reported between reduced muscle pH and reduced power output or work performed.[37–9] It has been suggested that intramuscular acidosis may negatively affect the function of key enzymes involved in glycolysis (primarily phosphofructokinase and glycogen phosphorylase). Enzymes function optimally at the normal pH of the tissue they are located in. Reducing this pH may impair enzyme function and, in the case of glycolysis, reduce the ability of the muscle to generate energy.[40] While there is evidence to show that during intense exercise, particularly consisting of short repeated bouts of work, the contribution of glycolysis to energy requirement progressively declines,[40–2] the role of acidosis in this process is questionable. As discussed in Section 3.2.1, making the blood more alkaline appears to enable greater removal of H^+ from the working muscle, leading to improved exercise performance. However, some studies have found no effect of increased blood alkalinity on exercise performance.[39,41,43] Discrepancies in results may be due to the exercise intensity and duration, use of short recovery durations between exercise bouts; and the *in vivo* buffer capacity of research participants. As a result, this research alone should not be used to form a conclusion about the effect of acidosis on the rate of glycolysis.

Some authors have found no influence of acidosis on muscle glycolytic rate,[44–5] and have suggested that muscle pH reductions typically found during exercise have no effect on glycolysis. This view is further supported by the following observations:

1 The time course of muscle force recovery after intense exercise is much faster than the time course of pH recovery.
2 People are able to produce high muscle force/power under conditions of acidosis.
3 No significant correlations have been found between recovery of muscle pH and recovery of sprint performance.[46]

Clearly, there is conflict in the available literature regarding the effects of acidosis on the function of glycolysis. More research needs to be carried out to enable a clearer picture to form, but the important message is again that the perceived negative effects of H^+ accumulation and associated acidosis are in no way universally accepted.

Key point

The suggestion that acidosis inhibits glycolytic enzymes and therefore slows the rate of glycolysis is controversial, with some research demonstrating no associations between muscle pH and muscle force production or high intensity exercise performance.

3.3.2.4 The cross-bridge cycle

Reductions in muscle pH can impair force production at the cross-bridges (where the myofilaments actin and myosin bind together) when in the high-force state (when actin and myosin are strongly bound together and muscle contraction is occurring).[9] During intense exercise, muscle pH can reach sufficiently low levels (approximately pH 6.2) for impairment of cross-bridge force production to occur.[47] Hydrogen may impair cross-bridge force production by reducing the number of cross-bridges that form and/or the force produced per cross-bridge, although the more likely effect is a reduced force production per cross-bridge.[9] The depressive effect of H^+ on cross-bridge force production persists even when sufficient Ca^{2+} is present to saturate troponin C binding sites, suggesting that the influence of H^+ on cross-bridge force is independent of any potential role of H^+ in impaired Ca^{2+}-binding to troponin C.[48–9] It is also likely that the influence of H^+ on cross-bridge force production is affected by exercise intensity and is greatest in type II fibres, as these fibres show the lowest pH values.[50]

Hydrogen production and associated pH reduction may also reduce the maximum velocity of muscle contraction. Currently, the mechanism behind this potential effect is unknown. There is also controversy in the literature as to the importance of reduced pH on fibre velocity.[51] Muscle shortening velocity may not be impaired until pH decreases below 6.7,[9] which can happen during intense exercise. Therefore, the influence of pH on muscle fibre velocity is probably dependent on the extent of H^+ production, muscle temperature, and muscle Ca^{2+} kinetics.[9]

As H^+ production may impair both muscle force and velocity, it is unsurprising that it may also impair muscle power.[9] In type I fibres, H^+ production appears to inhibit power to a greater extent at warmer temperatures (perhaps due to greater reductions in velocity at warmer temperatures), and to a greater extent at colder temperatures in type II fibres.[9] However, much of the data examining fibre type differences was collected *in vitro*, and should be interpreted with this in mind.[9]

Key point

Hydrogen production can impair cross-bridge force production, thereby reducing muscle force. Hydrogen production may also reduce the maximum velocity of muscle contraction, although this is dependent on the extent of acidosis, muscle temperature, and Ca^{2+} kinetics. The potential influence of H^+ on muscle force and velocity indicates that it may also impair muscle power output.

3.3.2.5 Central nervous system drive

High-intensity exercise can lead to large amounts of H^+ moving from the muscle into the blood. If H^+ enters the blood at too high a rate, it can exceed the buffering capacity of the blood and an extracellular (i.e. blood) acidosis can develop. Extracellular acidosis can desaturate arterial haemoglobin (i.e. reduce the amount of oxygen being transported in the blood), termed the Bohr effect. Reduced arterial saturation of haemoglobin can impair oxygen delivery to the brain.[52] This may in turn induce a cerebral hypoxia that could contribute to central fatigue.[7,52–5] Indeed, fatigue of a central origin has been shown to occur within a few seconds of maximal force production.[56] Therefore, the blood alkalinising effect of substances such as sodium bicarbonate may attenuate arterial haemoglobin desaturation and reduce central fatigue.[7] This suggestion has support from studies showing that blood acidosis increases ratings of perceived exertion (RPE) and reduces exercise tolerance, and that ingestion of bicarbonate attenuates increases in RPE.[52,57] The role of sodium bicarbonate in maintaining CNS drive may help to explain why a direct beneficial effect of sodium bicarbonate on muscle contractile performance is not always seen.

Key point

Extracellular acidosis caused by blood H^+ accumulation can lead to arterial haemoglobin desaturation. This desaturation can impair oxygen delivery to the brain, inducing a cerebral hypoxia that could contribute to the development of central fatigue, increasing effort perception and impairing exercise tolerance.

3.3.3 Lactate, hydrogen, acidosis and fatigue: a brief summary

Explaining the potential influence of metabolic acidosis on exercise fatigue is tricky, not least because there is still much ongoing debate on the topic. Regarding lactate, here are some key things to remember (also see Table 3.1):

1. Lactate, not lactic acid, is produced in the muscles during intense exercise.
2. Lactate and lactic acid should not be thought of as the same thing: they are different substances.
3. Lactate is produced *in response to* the muscle becoming more acidic due to production of H^+. Lactate production is *not* the cause of muscle acidity.
4. Lactate production *reduces* muscle acidity by consuming H^+, allowing intense exercise to continue for longer.
5. Lactate is an important source of fuel for exercising muscles and the brain.
6. During intense exercise, fatigue would occur sooner if lactate were not produced.

Based on current research evidence, it appears that metabolic acidosis stemming from H^+ production has a much smaller influence on fatigue during exercise than previously thought. In fact, there is evidence that a reduced pH can actually increase muscle force production and help to maintain muscle excitability. However, the small direct influence of H^+ on muscle performance (thought to be less than a 10% performance reduction) may still be sufficient to contribute to performance impairment during whole body exercise,[7] particularly at the elite performance level. Furthermore, H^+ production may impact performance in ways other than direct muscle impairment, such as by reducing CNS drive and increasing effort perception. Therefore, H^+ should still be considered in discussions on exercise fatigue, but it is not the 'go to' culprit for all things fatigue-related.

Table 3.1 Some common misconceptions about the nature and roles of lactate, and the more contemporary counter-views

Misconception	*Counter-view*
1 Lactic acid and lactate are the same substance.	1 Lactic acid contains a H^+ ion that can dissociate from lactic acid and increase acidity of the surrounding tissue/fluid. Lactate does not contain a H^+ ion that can dissociate; therefore, it does not directly make its environment more acidic.
2 Lactic acid is produced in large amounts during exercise.	2 Hardly any lactic acid is present in the body. During exercise, two separate ions are produced: lactate and H^+.
3 Lactate is the cause of muscle burn and muscle fatigue during exercise.	3 There is no evidence for lactate contributing to the burning sensation sometimes experienced during exercise. Lactate actually extends exercise performance via its roles as a H^+ buffer and as a source of metabolic fuel.
4 Lactate is a waste product that has no benefit during exercise.	4 See point 3. Lactate is a H^+ buffer and a source of fuel during exercise across a range of intensities and durations.
5 Lactate is responsible for the muscle soreness sometimes experienced in the hours or days following exercise.	5 See point 3. Furthermore, the additional lactate produced during exercise is metabolised within the first hour of recovery. Therefore, it cannot contribute to muscle soreness several hours or days following exercise.

3.4 Summary

- Research conducted in the early 1900s on muscle preparations identified the production of lactic acid in anaerobic conditions and elevated lactic acid concentration at the point of muscle fatigue.
- This research may have been misinterpreted to mean that lactic acid production causes muscle fatigue.
- Lactic acid was suggested to contribute to fatigue by impairing isometric muscle force production and muscle shortening velocity, and by inhibiting glycolysis via reduced activity of important glycolytic enzymes.
- An important distinction is that lactate, not lactic acid, is produced via glycolysis at rest and during exercise. Virtually no lactic acid exists in the body.
- Lactate does not release H^+ into the surrounding environment. Therefore, lactate does not directly make its environment more acidic.
- Lactate does not directly produce H^+ ions. The breakdown of ATP during glycolysis is a primary source of H^+ production.

- Hydrogen ions are hydrogen atoms that have lost their single electron, leaving behind a single proton. Hydrogen ions are acidic, and make the solution they are placed in more acidic.
- It was traditionally thought that lactate production increased H^+ production. However, contemporary viewpoints suggest that at no point does lactate production cause an increase in H^+ concentration.
- Lactate is an important source of fuel for skeletal muscles and the brain, and acts as a H^+ buffer. Therefore, lactate production serves to reduce tissue acidity, in opposition to the traditional perspective.
- Hydrogen production was thought to impair exercise performance by reducing Ca^{2+} release from the sarcoplasmic reticulum, impairing muscle excitability, and reducing the activity of glycolysis. However, at normal physiological temperatures the influence of H^+ accumulation on these mechanisms is minimal.
- Hydrogen production may impair cross-bridge force production, muscle contraction velocity, and muscle power. However, the influence of H^+ on these outcomes would depend on the extent of acidosis, muscle temperature, muscle Ca^{2+} kinetics, and muscle fibre type.
- Hydrogen production may contribute to reduced CNS drive and the development of central fatigue by causing a desaturation of arterial haemoglobin.
- While the role of H^+ on muscle fatigue is less than previously thought, it may still be sufficient to contribute to limitations in whole-body exercise performance.

To think about . . .

The production of lactate rather than lactic acid, the beneficial roles of lactate production during exercise (as a fuel source and metabolic buffer) and the minimal role of acidosis in exercise fatigue have been known for quite some time. Despite this wealth of scientific research, it is still common to hear many athletes, coaches, sports commentators (many of whom are former elite athletes) and sport and exercise science students place the blame for sore, tired muscles and impaired exercise performance on 'lactic acid build-up'.

Why is there still such a reliance on outdated explanations for a particular phenomenon? Is it because people feel more comfortable with established explanations that the majority believe to be correct, despite evidence to the contrary? Or is it because the findings and messages produced by scientific research are not getting through to the people that can learn from them and make use of them? If the messages aren't getting through, why not? How do you think scientists and researchers should make themselves heard?

Test yourself

Answer the following questions to the best of your ability. Try to understand the information gained from answering these questions before you progress with the book.

1 How did the perception develop that an increased production of lactic acid contributed to fatigue during exercise?
2 What are the two primary ways in which lactic acid production was thought to contribute to exercise fatigue?
3 What is the difference between a lactic acid molecule and a lactate molecule? What is the importance of this difference for the development of acidosis?
4 What is the difference between a hydrogen atom and a proton? What is the importance of this difference for the development of acidosis?
5 List the main misconceptions about, and benefits of, lactate that were discussed in the chapter.
6 What are the main ways in which acidosis is thought to impair exercise performance?

References

1 Fletcher WM, Hopkins FG (1907) Lactic acid in amphibian muscle. *J Physiol* 35: 247–309.
2 Noakes TD, Gibson A (2004) Logical limitations to the 'catastrophe' models of fatigue during exercise in humans. *Br J Sports Med* 38: 648–9.
3 Hill AV, Lupton H (1923) Muscular exercise, lactic acid, and the supply and utilization of oxygen. *Q J Med* 16: 135–71.
4 Robergs RA, Ghiasvand F, Parker D (2004) Biochemistry of exercise-induced metabolic acidosis. *Am J Physiol Regul Integr Comp Physiol* 287: R502–16.
5 Fitts RH, Holloszy JO (1976) Lactate and contractile force in frog muscle during development of fatigue and recovery. *Am J Physiol* 231: 430–3.
6 Spriet LL, Sodeland K, Bergstrom M, *et al.* (1987) Skeletal muscle glycogenolysis, glycolysis, and pH during electrical stimulation in men. *J Appl Physiol* 62: 616–21.
7 Cairns SP (2006) Lactic acid and exercise performance: culprit or friend? *Sports Med* 36 (4): 279–91.
8 Lamb GD, Recupero E, Stephenson DG (1992) Effect of myoplasmic pH on excitation-contraction coupling in skeletal muscle fibres of the toad. *J Physiol* 448: 211–24.
9 Fitts RH (2008) The cross-bridge cycle and skeletal muscle fatigue. *J Appl Physiol* 104: 551–8.
10 Balsom PD, Seger JY, Sjödin B, *et al.* (1992) Physiological responses to maximal intensity intermittent exercise. *Eur J Appl Physiol* 65: 144–9.
11 Brooks S, Nevill ME, Meleagros L, *et al.* (1990) The hormonal responses to repetitive brief maximal exercise in humans. *Eur J Appl Physiol* 60: 144–8.
12 Christmass MA, Dawson B, Arthur PG (1999) Effect of work and recovery duration on skeletal muscle oxygenation and fuel use during sustained intermittent exercise. *Eur J Appl Physiol* 80: 436–47.
13 Gaitanos GC, Williams C, Boobis LH, *et al.* (1993) Human muscle metabolism during intermittent maximal exercise. *J Appl Physiol* 75: 712–9.

14 Bishop D, Edge J, Davis C, *et al.* (2004) Induced metabolic alkalosis affects muscle metabolism and repeated sprint ability. *Med Sci Sports Exerc* 36: 807–13.
15 Bishop D, Claudius B (2005) Effects of induced metabolic alkalosis on prolonged intermittent-sprint performance. *Med Sci Sports Exerc* 37: 759–67.
16 Lavender G, Bird SR (1989) Effect of sodium bicarbonate ingestion upon repeated sprints. *Br J Sports Med* 23: 41–5.
17 Lindinger MI, Kowalchuk JM, Heigenhauser GJF (2005) Applying physiochemical principles to skeletal muscle acid-base status. *Am J Physiol Regul Integr Comp Physiol* 289: R891–4.
18 Brooks GA (2010) What does glycolysis make and why is it important? *J Appl Physiol* 108: 1450–1.
19 Robergs RA, Ghiasvand F, Parker D (2004) Biochemistry of exercise-induced metabolic acidosis. *Am J Physiol Regul Integr Comp Physiol* 287: R502–16.
20 Robergs RA, Ghiasvand F, Parker D (2005) Lingering construct of lactic acidosis. *Am J Physiol Regul Integr Comp Physiol* 289: R904–10.
21 Böning D, Strobel G, Beneke R, *et al.* (2005) Lactic acid still remains the real cause of exercise-induced metabolic acidosis. *Am J Physiol Regul Integr Comp Physiol* 289: R902–3.
22 Böning D, Maassen N (2008) Point: counterpoint: lactic acid is/is not the only physiochemical contributor to the acidosis of exercise. *J Appl Physiol* 105: 358–9.
23 Lindinger MI (2011) Lactate: metabolic fuel or poison? *Exp Physiol* 96: 1099–100.
24 Brooks GA (2007) Lactate: link between glycolytic and oxidative metabolism. *Sports Med* 37: 341–3.
25 Brooks GA (2009) Cell-cell and intracellular lactate shuttles. *J Physiol* 587: 5591–600.
26 Ide K, Schmalbruch IK, Quistorff B, Horn A, Secher NH (2000) Lactate, glucose and O_2 uptake in human brain during recovery from maximal exercise. *J Physiol* 522: 159–64.
27 Quistorff B, Secher NH, Van Lieshout JJ (2008) Lactate fuels the human brain during exercise. *Journal Fed Am Soc Exp Biol* 22: 3443–9.
28 Morris DM, Schafer RS, Fairbrother KR, Woodall MW (2011) Effects of lactate consumption on blood bicarbonate levels and performance during high-intensity exercise. *Int J Sport Nutr Exerc Metab* 21: 311–7.
29 Monedero J, Donne B (2000) Effect of recovery interventions on lactate removal and subsequent performance. *Int J Sports Med* 21: 593–7.
30 Mense S (2009) Algesic agents exciting muscle nociceptors. *Exp Brain Res* 196: 89–100.
31 Aminian-Far A, Hadian M, Olyaei G, Talebian S, Bakhtiary A (2011) Whole-body vibration and the prevention and treatment of delayed-onset muscle soreness. *J Athl Perf* 46: 43–9.
32 Lewis PB, Ruby D, Bush-Joseph CA (2012) Muscle soreness and delayed onset muscle soreness. *Clin Sports Med* 31: 255–62.
33 Wada M, Kuratani M, Kanzaki K (2013) Calcium kinetics of sarcoplasmic reticulum and muscle fatigue. *J Phys Fitness Sports Med* 2: 169–78.
34 Nielsen OB, de Paoli F, Overgaard K (2001) Protective effects of lactic acid on force production in rat skeletal muscle. *J Physiol* 536: 161–6.
35 Kristensen, M, Albertsen, J, Rentsch, M, Juel, C (2005) Lactate and force production in skeletal muscle, *J Physiol* 562: 521–6.
36 Pedersen TH, de Paoli F, Nielsen OB (2005) Increased excitability of acidified skeletal muscle: role of chloride conductance. *J Gen Physiol* 125: 237–46.
37 Bishop D, Edge J, Goodman C (2004) Muscle buffer capacity and aerobic fitness are associated with repeated-sprint ability in women. *Eur J Appl Physiol* 92: 540–7.

38 Krustrup (2003) Muscle metabolites during a football match in relation to a decreased sprinting ability. Communication to the Fifth World Congress of Soccer and Science, Lisbon, Portugal.
39 Messonnier L, Denis C, Féasson L, *et al.* (2006) An elevated sarcolemmal lactate (and proton) transport capacity is an advantage during muscle activity in healthy humans. *J Appl Physiol.* DOI: 10.1152/japplphysiol.00807.2006.
40 Spriet LL, Lindinger MI, McKelvie RS, *et al.* (1989) Muscle glycogenolysis and H+ concentration during maximal intermittent cycling. *J Appl Physiol* 66: 8–13.
41 Gaitanos GC, Williams C, Boobis LH, Brooks S (1993) Human muscle metabolism during intermittent maximal exercise. *J Appl Physiol* 75: 712–9.
42 McCartney N, Spriet LL, Heigenhauser GJF, Kowalchuk JM, Sutton JR, Jones NL (1986) Muscle power and metabolism in maximal intermittent exercise. *J Appl Physiol* 60: 1164–9.
43 Katz, A, Costill, DL, King, DS, Hargreaves, M, Fink, WJ (1984) Maximal exercise tolerance after induced alkalosis. *Int J Sports Med* 5: 107–10.
44 Bangsbo, J, Madsen, K, Kiens, B, Richter, EA (1996) Effect of muscle acidity on muscle metabolism and fatigue during intense exercise in man. *J Physiol* 492: 587–96.
45 Lamb, GD, Stephenson, DG, Bangsbo, J, Juel, C (2006) Point: Counterpoint: Lactic acid accumulation is an advantage/disadvantage during muscle activity. *J App Physiol* 100: 1410–14.
46 Girard O, Mendez-Villanueva A, Bishop D (2011) Repeated-sprint ability. Part 1: factors contributing to fatigue. *Sports Med* 41: 673–94.
47 Cady EB, Jones DA, Moll A (1989) Changes in force and intracellular metabolites during fatigue of human skeletal muscle. *J Physiol* 418: 327–37.
48 Debold EP, Dave H, Fitts RH (2004) Fiber type and temperature dependence of inorganic phosphate: implications for fatigue. *Am J Physiol* 287: C673–81.
49 Metzger JM, Moss RL (1990) Calcium-sensitive cross-bridge transitions in mammalian fast and slow twitch skeletal muscle fibers. *Science* 247: 1088–90.
50 Fitts RH (1994) Cellular mechanisms of muscle fatigue. *Physiol Rev* 74: 49–94.
51 Knuth ST, Dave H, Peters JR, Fitts RH (2006) Low cell pH depresses peak power in rat skeletal muscle fibres at both 30°C and 15°C: implications for muscle fatigue. *J Physiol* 575: 887–99.
52 Nielsen HB, Bredmose PP, Stromstad M, Volianitis S, Quistorff B, Secher NH (2002) Bicarbonate attenuates arterial desaturation during maximal exercise in humans. *J Appl Physiol* 93: 724–31.
53 Knicker AJ, Renshaw I, Oldham ARH, Cairns SP (2011) Interactive processes link the multiple symptoms of fatigue in sport competition. *Sports Med* 41: 307–28.
54 Nybo L, Secher NH (2004) Cerebral perturbations provoked by prolonged exercise. *Prog Neurobiol* 72: 223–61.
55 Amann M, Calbert JAL (2008) Convective oxygen transport and fatigue. *J Appl Physiol* 104: 861–70.
56 Gandevia SC, Allen GM, Butler JE, Taylor JL (1996) Supraspinal factors in human muscle fatigue: evidence for suboptimal output from the motor cortex. *J Physiol* 490: 529–36.
57 Swank A, Robertson RJ (1989) Effect of induced alkalosis on perception of exertion during intermittent exercise. *J Appl Physiol* 67: 1862–7.
58 Tate P (2009) *Seeley's Principles of Anatomy and Physiology*. McGraw Hill, New York.

Chapter 4

Dehydration and hyperthermia

4.1 Introduction

This chapter will follow a similar approach to Chapter 3, as dehydration and hyperthermia are as much a cause of fatigue during exercise as acidosis in the minds of many. The concepts of dehydration and hyperthermia are often linked as though one cannot exist without the other. This is not the case. Therefore, the chapter will address them as separate issues but will combine them as necessary. The chapter will first discuss dehydration. The classical mechanisms of dehydration-induced fatigue will be highlighted, along with other less well known potential mechanisms of dehydration-induced fatigue. The evolution of knowledge regarding dehydration and exercise fatigue will then be discussed, culminating in an overview of current thinking on this topic.

The section on hyperthermia will follow a similar approach. Classical theories will be discussed. This will include the concept of a 'critical' core temperature that, once attained, impairs exercise performance. The link between dehydration and hyperthermia will also be highlighted, as will the potential roles of dehydration and hyperthermia, alone and in combination, on exercise fatigue. By the end of the chapter, the reader should have a greater *critical* understanding of the potential influence that these two commonly cited factors have on exercise fatigue.

4.2 Dehydration and exercise fatigue

4.2.1 Defining terms

Before progressing, it would be useful to define some of the key terms that will be used throughout this chapter. *Hydration* or *euhydration* refers to a normal (or, more accurately, appropriate) body water content for an individual. It is the absence of hyper or hypohydration. *Hyperhydration* refers to a state of excess body water content. Hyperhydration can be a potentially serious condition, and will be discussed in this chapter. The dynamic process of losing body water is termed *dehydration*. Finally, the level of hydration of the body following a given fluid loss is termed *hypohydration*. Dehydration and hypohydration are closely related, but do not mean the same thing. For example, during exercise a person loses fluid, primarily through sweat. At the end of exercise, they may have lost a volume of fluid that is equivalent to 1.5% of their body mass (BM). Therefore, through the process of dehydration, the person has become hypohydrated by 1.5%. Dehydration is the process of body water loss; hypohydration is the end result of this loss.

Key point

The terms dehydration and hypohydration do not mean the same thing. Dehydration is the process of losing water from the body; hypohydration is the end result of this water loss.

4.2.2 The importance of water in the body

Despite having no caloric value, water is one of the most important nutrients for life, second only to oxygen. A person can survive for several weeks without consuming food, and can survive losses of up to 40% of their BM in fat, carbohydrate, and protein. However, a matter of days without water, or a water loss of only 9–12% of BM, can be fatal. Our reliance on water is due to its prevalence in the body and the number of important roles that it carries out to enable optimal bodily function. When euhydrated, water comprises approximately 60% of the BM of an adult male, and 50% of an adult female (this figure is partly dependent on body composition; lean tissue contains much more water than fat (approx. 73% versus 10%), therefore a person with a greater amount of lean tissue will have greater body water content). Approximately two thirds of body water content is contained inside our cells (intracellular fluid), with the other third outside the cells (extracellular fluid).

Water is the medium in which most of the life preserving processes in cells, tissues, and organ systems occur (Table 4.1). The importance of water means it is critical to ensure an appropriate water balance, defined as the balance between water intake and water loss (Figure 4.1). Most of the factors highlighted in Table 4.1 are important during exercise as well as at rest. Therefore, it is easy to see why body water content and its loss during exercise have been considered for so long a critical determinant of exercise performance.

A complication when trying to understand concepts associated with water balance is that most of the factors that influence water balance (levels of exercise/physical activity, sweat rate, body composition, diet, fluid intake) are individual. As a result, water losses and requirements differ significantly between people. One of the most important factors influencing water balance is sweat loss during physical activity/exercise. The influence of physical

Table 4.1 Important functions of water within the human body

1	Forms the fluid portion of blood, allowing the transport of nutrients, waste products, oxygen, and immune cells to all parts of the body.
2	Maintains appropriate blood volume; crucial for function of the cardiovascular system.
3	Plays a role in metabolic reactions.
4	Acts as a solvent for proteins, glucose, vitamins and minerals.
5	Plays an important role in maintenance of electrolyte balance.
6	Forms the fluid portion of sweat, allowing thermoregulation to occur.
7	Transports heat from deeper regions of the body to the skin surface, further assisting thermoregulation.
8	Helps to lubricate joints.
9	Major constituent of spinal and eye fluid.

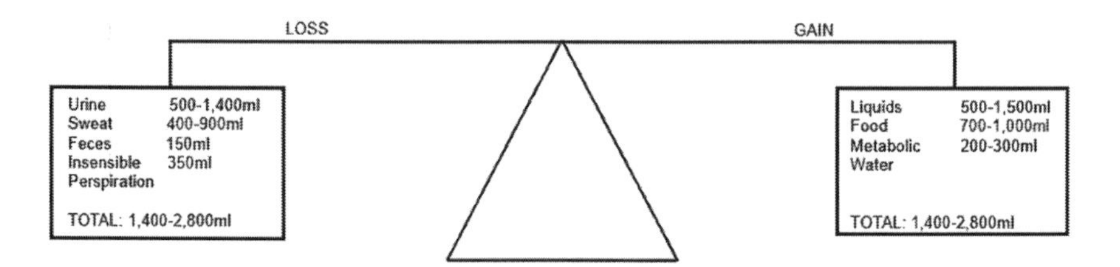

Figure 4.1 Typical daily water loss and gain for an average adult. The figures for water loss and gain will be influenced by diet, fluid ingestion, body mass, body composition, environmental conditions, and level of physical activity/exercise. The scale can tip to the left (negative water balance; greater water loss than gain: dehydration/hypohydration) or to the right (positive water balance, greater water gain than loss: hyperhydration).

activity on body water loss has led to the recommendation that water requirements should be calculated with reference to the amount of daily physical activity someone is engaged in. It is recommended that normal adults should consume 1–1.5 ml of water for every Kcal expended, and athletes should consume 1.5 ml of water for every Kcal expended. Therefore, an athlete who expends 4000 Kcal per day would require 6000 ml, or 6 L, of water (from food and fluid sources combined) per day (4000 × 1.5 = 6000). However, as you will see as you read this chapter, current fluid intake recommendations for athletes and the general population are being challenged.

Key point

Body water balance is influenced by factors that vary greatly between people. As a result, water requirements can vary significantly from person to person.

4.2.3 Classical mechanism of dehydration-induced performance decrement

During exercise, sweat rate greatly increases. Sweating is the main way that the body dissipates heat produced from the increase in energy metabolism during exercise. The fluid portion of sweat comes from blood plasma, muscle tissue, skin and other internal organs. The loss of fluid from blood plasma causes a decrease in plasma volume. Reduced plasma volume means that less blood enters the heart in each cardiac cycle (termed reduced cardiac filling pressure). Reduced cardiac filling pressure contributes to a reduction in stroke volume (the volume of blood pumped from the heart in each beat) and cardiac output (the volume of blood pumped from the heart per minute), meaning that heart rate has to increase to maintain appropriate blood and oxygen delivery to working tissue. This reduction in cardiac efficiency may in itself lead to impaired exercise performance, with an approximate increase in exercising heart rate of 3–5 beats per minute for every 1% loss of BM due to dehydration.[1] However, if water loss and exercise continue, the reduced plasma volume may lead to competition for blood flow between core organs and tissues and the skin (termed circulatory stress). This competition could lead to reduced skin blood flow, impairing evaporative heat loss and leading to an increase in core body temperature (hyperthermia). Therefore, according to the classical theory, dehydration may impair performance directly through alterations in cardiac efficiency, and indirectly by contributing to the development of hyperthermia. An overview of the classical theory of dehydration-induced performance decrement is in Figure 4.2.

Key point

Dehydration may contribute to performance decrement directly by reducing cardiac efficiency and indirectly by contributing to the development of hyperthermia.

4.2.4 Other potential mechanisms of dehydration-induced performance decrement

Dehydration can alter metabolic function by increasing liver glucose output and the reliance on carbohydrate metabolism via increased oxidation of muscle glycogen, which leads to greater blood lactate levels at a given exercise intensity.[2] The greater reliance on carbohydrate oxidation when hypohydrated may be due to increased core temperature, which can alter metabolic enzyme activity and mitochondrial function,[3–4] suggesting that dehydration without hyperthermia may not influence exercise metabolism. Greater reliance on carbohydrate oxidation could contribute to fatigue via glycogen depletion (see Chapter 2 for a detailed discussion of the role of glycogen depletion as a cause of fatigue during exercise).

Perceived exertion during exercise may increase when hypohydrated compared to the same exercise workload in a euhydrated state.[1] Similarly, cognitive function (vision, attention, memory etc) may be impaired when hypohydrated.[5] If hypohydration does alter the perception of effort and mental processes during exercise, this could contribute to decreased performance by altering factors such as motivation, decision making, and pacing strategies. The impact of various factors including hypohydration

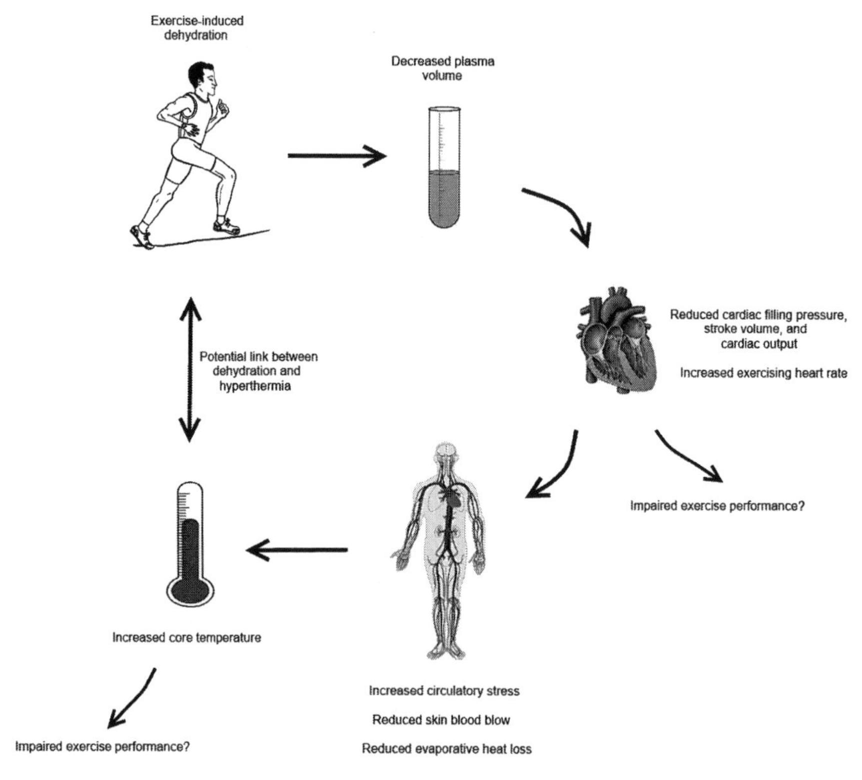

Figure 4.2 The classical proposed mechanism of impaired exercise performance with dehydration. Body water loss during exercise decreases plasma volume, leading to reduced cardiac filling pressure, stroke volume and cardiac output. This impaired cardiac efficiency means that heart rate has to increase to maintain appropriate blood and oxygen delivery to working tissue. Elevated heart rate could in itself lead to impaired exercise performance. However, if water loss and exercise continue, reduced plasma volume may lead to competition for blood flow between the core organs and tissues and the skin (circulatory stress). This competition could lead to reduced skin blood flow, impairing evaporative heat loss and leading to an increase in core body temperature.

on perceptual responses to exercise will be discussed in this chapter and Chapter 6. Causes of fatigue attributable to dehydration can be central or peripheral in origin, and are further discussed in Section 4.6 and summarised in Figure 4.3.

> **Key point**
>
> Dehydration may contribute to performance decrement, directly or indirectly, by altering the perception of effort, cognitive function, and energy metabolism.

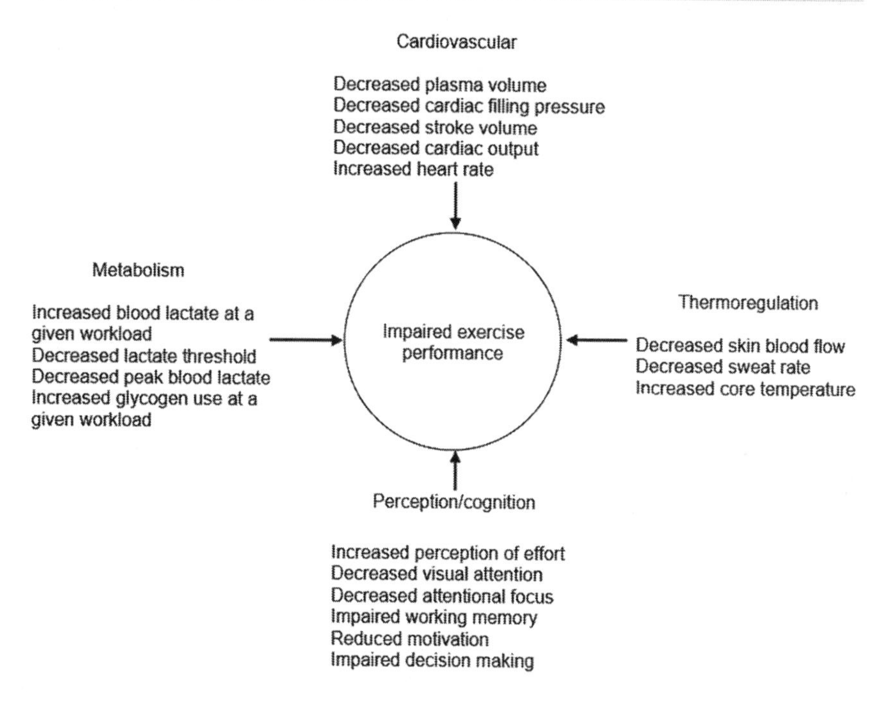

Figure 4.3 A summary of the factors associated with dehydration that could contribute to impaired exercise performance.

4.3 Dehydration and exercise fatigue: research issues

There is an abundance of research showing that dehydration during exercise can lead to performance decrements.[6–7] The potential negative consequences of dehydration discussed in Sections 4.2.3 and 4.2.4 have informed published guidelines for fluid intake during exercise. The most up to date guidelines are fundamentally quite simple. The guidelines recommend that people should develop customised fluid replacement programmes that enable them to begin exercise euhydrated, and that prevent excessive fluid losses during exercise.[8] An obvious question is: what is classed as 'excessive' fluid losses? Early literature that provided the foundation for study into hydration and exercise identified an apparent 'threshold' fluid decrement of 2% of a person's BM, above which aerobic exercise performance appeared to be impaired.[7–9] Over the years, this 2% dehydration threshold has become firmly established as a principle on which fluid intake recommendations are based.

Key point

Early research established an apparent 'threshold' hypohydration level of 2% body mass, above which aerobic exercise performance is impaired. This threshold has become established as a cornerstone of fluid intake recommendations and guidelines.

However, as has been mentioned in previous chapters, it is important to consider how research was carried out so that we can better interpret its results. Research into fluid balance and exercise performance began to be published about 25–30 years ago, and some of the earlier studies are regularly cited as classic papers in the field. More specifically, some of these studies are cited to support the notion that dehydration impairs exercise performance. A limitation of some of these studies is the manner in which dehydration was 'achieved'. Some studies required people to sit for extended periods of time in a hot environment without drinking anything.[10] Some studies required participants to complete 2 hours of exercise in a hot environment with limited fluid intake, followed by 1 hour of rest in a normal temperature environment with restricted fluid intake, *then* undertake another exercise session.[11] Some studies also used diuretics to stimulate fluid loss by increasing urine output.[12] These approaches essentially ensure that a person *begins* exercise in a hypohydrated state, rather than losing fluid and potentially becoming hypohydrated *during* exercise. Clearly, none of these pre-exercise approaches would be carried out by a person preparing to exercise in the real world. Using these study designs, it also may not be possible to separate the effects of hypohydration on exercise performance from possible effects of the procedures used to achieve hypohydration.[8] Due to this concern, it has been suggested that only studies in which hypohydration develops during exercise provide a valid measure of the effects of hypohydration.[8]

If research is carried out with the aim of studying the effect of fluid restriction on exercise performance, then it is probable that the people taking part in that research will know that they are going to have to exercise with no fluid intake, or a greatly reduced fluid intake compared to that they would normally choose to consume. This foreknowledge may give the participants a different mind-set about the exercise they were about to do, perhaps making them anticipate a poorer performance.[8] In fact, it has been shown that when people are aware at the beginning of exercise that their fluid intake is going to be restricted, they begin exercise at a lower intensity than when they are able to drink *ad libitum*.[13] This shows that the negative influence of performance attributed to hypohydration can, depending on the research approach taken, be due to other factors.

Many research participants come from what is termed a 'convenience' sample, meaning a group of people to which the researchers have easy access. As a result, participants are often not of a high athletic ability. Athletes may differ in many ways, physiologically and psychologically, from convenience participants. Therefore, results produced from research using convenience samples may not be relevant to different groups of people such as competitive athletes.

Perhaps the most important consideration to make when interpreting dehydration research is the type of exercise undertaken. Much of the research used fixed intensity exercise, and/or protocols requiring participants to exercise to exhaustion. These are understandable choices, as this form of exercise allows researchers to control for many factors that can influence study results. However, protocols requiring exercise to exhaustion are notoriously unreliable (Section 1.3.1).[14–15] If participants' performance in these tests varied to a great extent, it may over-state the influence of factors such as dehydration on performance, or it could have the opposite effect and mask the effects of such interventions. Also, fixed-intensity exercise (whether to exhaustion or not) is not representative of the majority of real-world exercise scenarios. In most competitive sports, the aim is to complete a set distance in the fastest possible time, rather than perform for as long as possible. Real-world exercise is also usually self-paced, meaning the athlete has the choice of whether to increase or decrease their workload at any time. Therefore, while fixed-intensity exercise allows only one of two choices (keep going vs stop), self-paced exercise allows continual changes in effort that could affect exercise performance.[15]

Key point

The way in which research into dehydration and exercise performance is carried out should be considered when interpreting the results of such research.

The issues with some previous research into the effects of dehydration on exercise performance are further highlighted when we consider more recent investigations. A number of recent studies have shown that dehydration does not impair exercise performance lasting from 60 minutes to more than 4 hours, in both normal and warm environments, despite participants losing 1.7–3.1% of their pre-exercise BM.[16–19] These losses exceed that stated by earlier research to impair exercise performance (i.e. the 2% 'threshold'), so why was exercise performance not impaired? To explain the likely reasons, it would be useful to summarise each of the studies in turn, and then bring this information together into a final summary:

Marino et al.[17] These authors found that ingesting no fluid during 60 minutes of self-paced high-intensity cycling in moderate (hypohydration 1.7% BM) or warm (hypohydration 2.1% BM) conditions did not impair performance compared with consuming enough fluid to maintain BM. Interestingly, the authors provided evidence to suggest that the neuromuscular system altered muscle recruitment in response to different hydration levels, thereby enabling a similar performance level despite differences in hydration status.

Nolte et al.[18] This study was a little different to some of the other hydration research, as it investigated the relationship between fluid intake and time to complete a 14.5 km march in soldiers. Interestingly, no relationship between fluid intake and exercise time, or BM loss and exercise time, was found. Furthermore, the soldiers' hydration status was maintained despite BM losses of around 2%.

Zouhal et al.[19] This study investigated the relationship between BM change (as an indicator of hydration) and marathon finishing time. The authors found that the greater the BM loss, the faster the marathon finishing time. Put another way, the people who lost more weight, and therefore were, perhaps, more hypohydrated, tended to perform better than those who maintained a stable hydration status or who drank more fluid than they lost during the run.

Dion et al.[16] These authors reported that the time to complete a half-marathon was not different when people either drank enough water to maintain BM or drank according to the dictate of their thirst (in other words, they drank as much water as they wanted to when they felt thirsty). People drank much less water, and lost an average of 3.1% BM, when drinking to thirst. However, there was no difference in performance, sweat loss, sweat rate, body temperature, or heart rate between the trials.

Overall summary The research studies discussed above, and others that have found either no effect or a minimal effect of dehydration on exercise performance,[20–2] have one thing in common: they all used self-paced, real world exercise (meaning the studies were either conducted in natural exercise situations, or natural exercise was well replicated in a laboratory setting). As discussed above, self-paced exercise gives the participant more options about how they regulate their performance, making this a more appropriate type of exercise with which to test the influence of factors such as dehydration on performance. In fact, an analysis of dehydration research shows that dehydration only impairs exercise performance when fixed-workload exercise (which does not mimic real-world exercise) is used.[23]

Key point

Studies using self-paced exercise demonstrate that fluid loss does not impair exercise performance. A review of the literature further states that dehydration only impairs exercise performance during fixed-workload exercise.

Another interesting point from the above studies is that a BM loss of, say, 2% during exercise does not necessarily mean that a person has become notably hypohydrated. For example, participants in the study by Nolte *et al.*[18] lost on average 1.98% of their BM. Yet, according to urinary measures, the hydration status of those participants was not affected. This suggests that BM changes may not accurately reflect body water loss. During exercise, additions can be made to total body water content by production of water from aerobic energy metabolism, and the release of water from the breakdown of stored muscle and liver glycogen.[24] Similarly, BM losses can occur through substrate oxidation, independent of fluid loss. Therefore, processes are at work during exercise that can reduce BM, but at the same time increase total body water content. As a result, BM loss can decrease by as much as 1–3% without notable dehydration occurring.[24]

Key point

Reduced body mass during exercise does not necessarily mean that a person's hydration status has been negatively affected. Body mass loss does not necessarily equate with fluid loss.

The fact that BM loss can occur during exercise without the onset of hypohydration suggests that it may not be necessary to drink sufficient fluid during exercise to prevent BM loss. In fact, some researchers suggest that the athletes who finish races fastest tend to be the athletes who drink more to the dictates of their own thirst rather than in an attempt to prevent BM loss,[19] and that drinking to thirst is the most effective hydration strategy during exercise.[16] Body mass loss without hypohydration would actually be beneficial from a performance perspective, as the athlete would have less mass to transport during their event, enabling them to compete at a given intensity while expending less effort and energy. In support of this suggestion, it is frequently observed (but not well advertised) that the fastest finishers in endurance activities are often those who lose the most BM during the event.[7,19,25]

Therefore, should we recommend that people taking part in endurance exercise actually aim to lose BM, thereby making the exercise 'easier'? Certainly not. As one study puts it: 'the possibility remains that high levels of body weight loss in *certain unique individuals* might enhance exercise performance simply as the result of a lesser body weight that needs to be transported' (emphasis by the author of this book).[19] This statement draws attention to the fact that a lot of the research that has found a relationship between BM loss and improved performance during endurance exercise has used participants that are either well trained, experienced endurance athletes, well acclimated to the environmental conditions in which the study took place, or all of these things. These factors may allow them to respond to BM loss differently than individuals who do not have these characteristics. It is also important to note that some of the relationships between BM loss and endurance performance, while statistically significant, are actually quite small. For example, in their study of 643 marathon runners Zouhal *et al.*[19] reported a correlation coefficient of $r = 0.21$ between BM change and marathon finishing time. Statistically, this correlation was significant and suggested that greater BM loss led to a faster finishing time. However, this correlation indicates that only 4% of the change in marathon finishing time could be explained by changes in BM during the event (0.21^2 to calculate the coefficient of determination, $r^2 = 0.04$). Indeed, restricting fluid during exercise probably does not provide a performance benefit, but neither does consuming more fluid than would be ingested under normal conditions.[16] Therefore, drinking according to thirst may be the most effective strategy.

Key point

Only people with specific characteristics may show improved exercise performance with high levels of body mass loss. Therefore, intentional body mass loss should not be recommended as a general strategy for improving performance.

Clearly, there is evidence that dehydration induced BM loss during exercise does not impair exercise performance. There is also evidence against the long-held belief that dehydration increases cardiovascular and thermoregulatory strain during exercise, and that this leads to impaired performance (Figure 4.2). During self-paced exercise, increases in core temperature and heart rate associated with dehydration do not appear to influence performance,[16,26–7] ratings of perceived exertion, or heat stress during exercise.[16]

It is often difficult to see the 'big picture' regarding research findings in a given area, particularly one as large as hydration and exercise performance. Luckily, a recent meta-analysis (combining results from many research studies to identify patterns) has made the job easier.[28] This analysis reviewed 13 studies that used 60-minute cycle time trials under real-world exercise conditions. None of the studies reported a statistically significant negative effect of dehydration on exercise performance. In fact, one study actually found that a BM loss of 2.3% significantly improved performance during a 1-hour cycle time trial compared to maintaining euhydration. Other important findings from this meta-analysis were:

- Hypohydration during exercise by an average of about 2.2% BM does not impair exercise performance, and in fact may cause a performance improvement (albeit trivial). Therefore, the overriding view is that dehydration during exercise will not cause a notable improvement or decrement in performance.
- Drinking to thirst increases power output during cycle time trials by an average of about 5% compared to drinking below thirst, and by an average of about 2.5% compared to drinking more than dictated by thirst alone.
- The probability that drinking to thirst alone confers a general advantage during cycle time trials is 98% compared to drinking below thirst, and 62% compared to drinking above thirst.
- There is no relationship between percentage change in BM and percentage change in power output during exercise.
- Both exercise duration and intensity are more important determinants of performance than dehydration.
- There is no significant difference in performance between exercise that results in a BM loss of less than 2% or a BM loss of more than 2%. This appears to do away with the often cited dehydration 'threshold' of 2% BM.
- It is not dehydration itself that is responsible for performance decrements during exercise, but rather drinking insufficiently to satisfy thirst. Therefore, drinking 'ahead' of thirst in order to prevent BM loss and performance decrement, as has become a much believed dogma, is not necessary.
- Following thirst sensation during real-word exercise is the most effective way to maximise performance.

The study of Goulet[28] is an excellent summary of research findings about the *real world* effect of dehydration on endurance exercise performance. However, it is important to note that Goulet[28] only reviewed studies that involved one hour of cycle exercise in trained cyclists or endurance trained people. As was mentioned earlier, a particular set of characteristics may be required for notable BM loss not to impair exercise performance. This should be considered when applying the findings of this study to other populations.

Key point

Performance is not different with body mass losses less than or greater than 2% BM. Therefore, the often cited dehydration 'threshold' of 2% BM appears irrelevant.

Key point

Research suggests that neither under- nor over-drinking during exercise will significantly improve performance. Therefore, drinking to thirst may be the most effective strategy.

4.4 Hyperhydration during exercise

Section 4.3 discussed how drinking to thirst, rather than to prevent BM loss, may be the most effective way to maximise exercise performance. There is also another issue that suggests drinking to thirst may be more appropriate and, perhaps, safer than consuming large volumes of fluid; the issue of hyperhydration (defined in Section 4.2.1).

There are several potential issues with hyperhydration. First, hyperhydration will increase BM, which may be detrimental to performance particularly during weight bearing exercise. Second, there have been many instances of people reporting a variety of gastrointestinal symptoms of differing severities when trying to drink more than they would through choice during exercise, usually in an attempt to prevent BM loss. Clearly, gastrointestinal problems will hamper exercise performance. However, a potentially more serious consequence of hyperhydration is the development of *hypervolemia* (abnormal increases in blood plasma volume) or *hyponatraemia* (an abnormally low blood sodium level).

First, it is important to note that modest hypervolaemia is a normal, desirable chronic adaptation to endurance exercise training. Increases in plasma volume, and hence blood volume, contribute to the improved cardiac (greater stroke volume, maximal cardiac output, and lower heart rate) and thermoregulatory (increased sweating sensitivity and sweat rate) function characteristic of improved fitness.[29] However, excessive hypervolaemia can be detrimental to exercise performance and, more importantly, health.

Key point

Hypervolaemia is an abnormal increase in blood plasma volume which can be caused by overdrinking. Hyponatraemia is an abnormally low blood sodium level, caused by overdrinking and/or large sweat sodium losses.

Increased body water content can occur for many reasons:

- Protein breakdown, which increases both plasma proteins and plasma volume.[30]
- Increased plasma volume due to increased plasma sodium concentration.[31]
- Retention of sodium due to increased activity of aldosterone.[32]
- Increased plasma volume due to increased activity of vasopressin.[33]
- Impairment of renal function due to dehydration.[34]

However, a common cause of increased body water content is, of course, fluid overload via excessive fluid intake. The potential causes of hypervolaemia help to explain why the majority of cases of hypervolaemia during exercise occur during ultra-endurance exercise (for example, running races lasting anything greater than a marathon distance)[35–7] as shorter duration exercise would probably be insufficient to generate any of these potential causes (unless, perhaps, in highly abnormal environmental conditions). However, that is not to say that hypervolaemia is always reported during ultra-endurance exercise.[38] As previously mentioned, hypervolaemia increases a person's BM, which can be detrimental to exercise performance as the person has to transport this increased mass for the duration of the exercise bout. However, a more serious potential consequence of hypervolaemia is the development of hyponatraemia.

The prevalence of hyponatraemia during endurance exercise competitions ranges from approximately 13–29% of participating athletes, much higher than previously thought.[39] Features of hyponatraemia can range from no or minimal symptoms such as weakness, dizziness, headache, nausea, and vomiting, to serious symptoms including fluid accumulation in the brain (cerebral oedema) leading to brain swelling, altered mental function, seizures, fluid accumulation in the lungs (pulmonary oedema), coma, and death.[39] The severity of symptoms is dependent in part on the rate and extent of the drop in extracellular sodium content.[39]

Key point

The prevalence of hyponatraemia during endurance exercise is higher than originally thought. Symptoms of hyponatraemia range from weakness, dizziness, headache, and nausea to fluid accumulation in the brain and lungs, seizures, coma, and death.

There are multiple potential risk factors for development of hyponatraemia during endurance exercise. These include the composition of ingested fluids, low BM index, slower exercise performance/longer exercise time, lack of endurance exercise experience, use of nonsteroidal anti-inflammatory drugs, and female gender[40] (for a discussion of these risk factors, the reader is referred to Rosner & Kirven[39]). However, studies have established that the strongest risk factor for development of hyponatraemia is excessive fluid intake during exercise.[39–41] This highlights a clear link between hypervolaemia and hyponatraemia. It is also important to consider sweat composition as a potential risk factor for hyponatraemia. Production of salty sweat (sweat with a high sodium content) reduces the amount of overdrinking necessary to cause hyponatraemia.[41] Therefore, people who produce salty sweat may be at a relatively greater risk of hyponatraemia than those with more dilute sweat.

Key point

The primary cause of exercise-associated hyponatraemia is overdrinking during exercise. High sweat sodium concentrations can also increase the risk of hyponatraemia, as less fluid intake is required to dilute blood sodium to dangerous levels.

We now know that the primary risk factor for hyponatraemia is over-drinking during exercise, and that sweat sodium content can also influence the risk of developing hyponatraemia. Sweat composition is different between individuals, and appropriate fluid intake during exercise is dependent on many factors such as body size, exercise intensity, sweat rate, and environmental conditions, all of which are individual and/or highly variable between exercise bouts. Therefore, it is easy to see how fluid intake guidelines that encourage athletes to drink as much as is tolerable during exercise, or to drink specific absolute amounts of fluid without reference to individual factors such as sweat rate/composition, exercise intensity, or body size, could place an athlete at significant risk of developing hyponatraemia. These same reasons make it unfeasible to produce universal guidelines for the prevention of hyponatraemia. However, general recommendations have been made, the key one being that athletes should drink according to thirst and no more than 400–800 ml/hour, depending on exertion level (body size, environmental conditions, duration of exercise).[39] This rate of fluid intake is much lower than that shown to produce hyponatraemia (up to 1,500 ml/hour).[39] Implementation of guidelines to restrict excessive fluid intake is associated with reductions in the number of cases of exercise associated hyponatraemia.[42–3]

Key point

Fluid intake guidelines that encourage high rates of fluid ingestion can place athletes at increased risk of developing hyponatraemia. In situations where guidelines to restrict excessive fluid intake have been implemented, cases of hyponatraemia have fallen.

4.5 Hyperthermia

4.5.1 How hot is too hot?

Hyperthermia is an abnormally high core body temperature. Normal core body temperature is between 36.5–37.5°C, however the specific value will differ very slightly (approximately 0.1°C) dependent on the location of measurement (rectal, oesophageal, tympanic, etc). Technically, hyperthermia is therefore a body temperature greater than 37.5°C. However, there are different severities of hyperthermia, depending on the core temperature reached.

Hyperthermia and fever (as part of an illness) both involve an elevated core temperature, but they are not the same thing as they have different causes and are regulated in different ways. A fever occurs when specific immune cells produced in response to infection release substances that stimulate the hypothamalus to raise core temperature. Essentially, normal core temperature is now considered too cold, and the hypothalamus raises core temperature to a new, higher set point. This process is analogous to raising the temperature setting on a thermostat. Conversely, hyperthermia occurs when core body temperature rises without a direct prior stimulation of the temperature control regions in the brain, usually as a result of an imbalance between heat production and heat dissipation (see Section 4.5.2).

Key point

Normal core temperature is between 36.5–37.5°C. Technically, hyperthermia is any core temperature above this range. Hyperthermia can differ in severity dependent on factors including the core temperature reached.

4.5.2 Development of hyperthermia during exercise

Hyperthermia can develop whenever body heat gain exceeds body heat loss. A classic cause of hyperthermia during exercise was described in Section 4.2.3 and Figure 4.2. To briefly recap, exercise can cause a reduction in plasma volume that leads to an increased cardiac and circulatory stress via competition for blood flow between core organs and tissues and the skin. This competition may reduce skin blood flow, impairing the body's ability to lose heat via evaporation and leading to an increase in core body temperature. Fundamentally, core temperature will increase when body heat gain from metabolism, radiation, convection and conduction (if air temperature is higher than skin temperature) is greater than heat loss via the methods of conduction, convection, radiation, and evaporation (by far the most important method of heat loss during exercise). Therefore, it is no surprise that the development of hyperthermia is most common in situations where dissipation of body heat is impaired. This includes exercise in the heat and/or humidity, with insufficient air flow, while wearing excessive clothing, without sufficient shading, or a combination of these factors. The most challenging environment in which to maintain normal body temperature is when it is both hot and humid. Exercise in the heat leads to warmer skin temperatures (Section 4.6.3). While this is beneficial for evaporative heat loss, it reduces the temperature difference between the body core and skin, and between the skin and ambient air, thereby making it more difficult to transfer heat from the core to the skin, and then to the surrounding air, via conduction, convection, and radiation. When humidity is added into the equation, evaporative heat loss is greatly impaired, as sweat on the surface of the skin cannot easily vaporise into the air due to the high ambient moisture level already present (particularly when humidity levels exceed about 60%). Therefore, exercise in hot and humid conditions significantly impairs all body heat loss avenues, increasing the likelihood of body heat gain. Continued exercise in a situation of net body heat gain will lead to a progressive increase in core temperature, potentially exacerbating the above-mentioned cardiac and circulatory stresses.

4.6 Hyperthermia and fatigue: research findings

It is not the purpose of this section to argue that hyperthermia does not impair exercise performance. This would be a flawed argument, as there are countless sporting examples of athletes performing at a lower standard in the heat compared with milder temperatures. What this section will do is highlight the potential role of hyperthermia in impaired exercise performance, discuss the 'critical core temperature hypothesis' (the suggestion that fatigue occurs upon attainment of a specific core temperature), and highlight more recent work that challenges this hypothesis. Hyperthermia can impact on exercise performance in several ways, both peripheral and central (Figure 4.3). These mechanisms will now be discussed.

4.6.1 Peripheral fatigue associated with hyperthermia

Exercising in the heat increases blood flow to the skin to enable heat transfer from the body tissues to the surrounding environment. In a situation of high blood demand by both the working muscle and the skin, the required cardiac output may not be met,[44–45] particularly if cardiac output is already reduced due to an attenuated stroke volume caused by decreased plasma volume.[46]

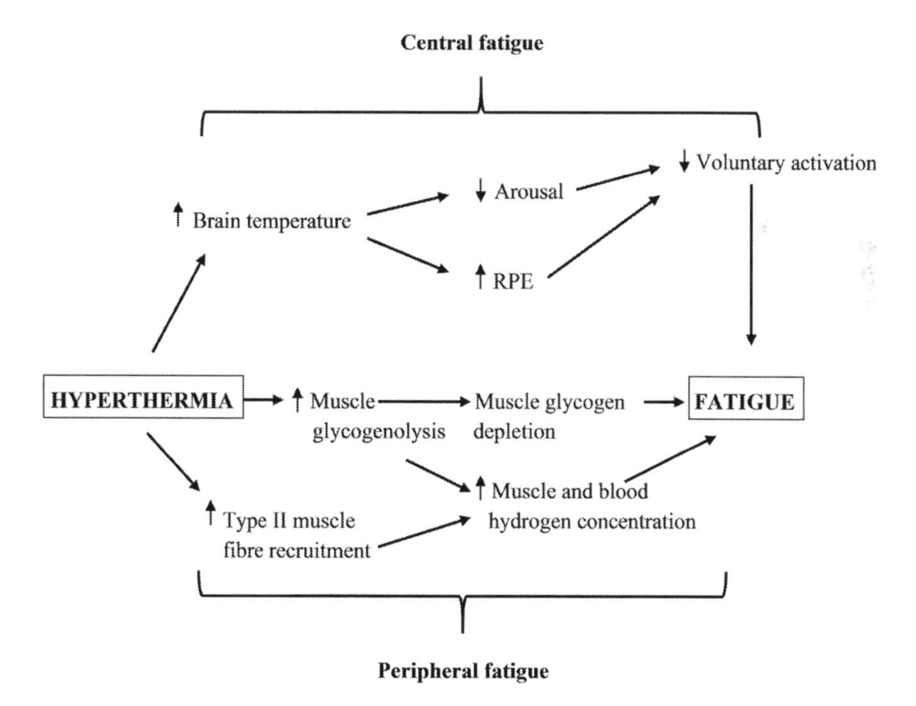

Figure 4.4 Potential causes of hyperthermia-induced fatigue during exercise. The causes of fatigue are characterised as central or peripheral in origin. Adapted from Cheung and Sleivert.[44]

Reduced cardiac function would be even more likely if the athlete were also hypohydrated, as previously discussed (Figure 4.2). Therefore, impaired cardiovascular function is a potential cause of fatigue during exercise in the heat. Indeed, during exercise that requires the athlete to exercise at their maximum rate of oxygen consumption (VO_{2max}), blood flow to the working muscle is reduced, indicating a failure of the cardiovascular system to deliver oxygen at the required rate.[47] However, during prolonged submaximal exercise in the heat, muscle oxygen delivery and uptake remains similar to exercise carried out at the same intensity in a normal temperature, yet exercise performance in the heat is still impaired.[48] Therefore, it appears that altered cardiovascular function may not be the main cause of fatigue during prolonged submaximal exercise in the heat,[49] and that the mechanisms of fatigue associated with hyperthermia may be different depending on the intensity and, perhaps, the duration of exercise.

Although muscle oxygen uptake is maintained during prolonged exercise in the heat, there is still a reduction in blood flow to the working muscle (particularly if hypohydration is also present). The muscle actually maintains oxygen uptake by extracting more oxygen from the blood that is still flowing to it.[50] Reduced muscle blood flow is accompanied by an increase in muscle glycogen use and a reduction in fat metabolism.[51] Therefore, increased muscle glycogen use and, hence, muscle glycogen depletion has been cited as a potential cause of impaired performance during exercise in the heat (see Chapter 2 for more information on muscle glycogen depletion and fatigue). However, it has consistently been shown that muscle glycogen stores are far from depleted at exhaustion when exercising in the heat,[46] so glycogen depletion does not explain fatigue in this situation.[50]

Exercise-induced hyperthermia, up to a core temperature of approximately 41°C and muscle temperature of approximately 42°C, does not impair the ability of muscles to contract.[46] Direct electrical stimulation of the motor neurons (see Section 1.2.1) of skeletal muscles shows that the muscles are able to produce the same amount of force when hyperthermic compared to normal temperature.[48] Overall, it appears that peripheral alterations associated with hyperthermia are not critically important in the development of fatigue, at least during submaximal exercise.

Key point

Potential causes of peripheral fatigue with hyperthermia include impaired cardiovascular function leading to reduced blood flow to working muscle, increased muscle glycogen breakdown, and impaired muscle contraction. However, none of these causes satisfactorily explain fatigue development during submaximal exercise in the heat.

4.6.2 Central fatigue associated with hyperthermia

As mentioned in Section 4.6.1, hyperthermia does not directly impair the ability of muscles to contract. Similarly, hyperthermia does not appear to impair the ability of a person to voluntarily contract their muscle for a short period of time (a few seconds). However, sustained voluntary muscle force production deteriorates significantly when hyperthermia is present (Figure 4.5). This observation of a reduced ability to generate muscle force despite no change in the ability of the muscle itself to produce force suggests that central factors may be important in the development of fatigue with hyperthermia. However, the role of peripheral factors should not be overlooked. Sensory feedback from working muscles and skin (see Section 4.6.3) may modify central alterations in neuromuscular recruitment.[46]

Key point

There is good evidence to show that hyperthermia reduces the ability to produce muscle force despite no change in the ability of the muscle itself to produce force. This suggests that central factors may be more important than peripheral factors in hyperthermia-induced fatigue.

During prolonged exercise in hyperthermia, the metabolic rate of the brain increases but overall brain blood flow decreases.[52] The electrical activity of the brain also slows.[48] These responses are associated with a progressive increase in the perception of exercise difficulty, and a reduction in power output/speed during exercise.[53] Essentially, the athlete finds it harder and harder to maintain a given exercise intensity, and begins to slow down. Therefore, there is a link between hyperthermia, brain blood flow and function, and exercise performance.[54]

As well as reductions in brain blood flow, during exercise in the heat the temperature of blood in the jugular vein (the main vein that brings blood back from the head to the heart) drops slightly, meaning the temperature difference between jugular vein blood and blood in the aorta (the main blood vessel leading away from the heart) is reduced.[46–7] This implies that the brain is storing heat during exercise in hot temperatures. Indeed, average brain temperature increases in line with the aortic blood temperature, remaining at least 0.2°C warmer then core temperature.[47] Brain temperature is becoming recognised as a potentially crucial factor for exercise performance during hyperthermia in humans. This stems from research performed in animals, which showed that increasing brain temperatures without increasing core temperature reduced the ability and willingness of the animals to continue exercising.[55] These behavioural responses are similar to those seen in people during exercise in hyperthermic states. However, it is difficult to confirm that

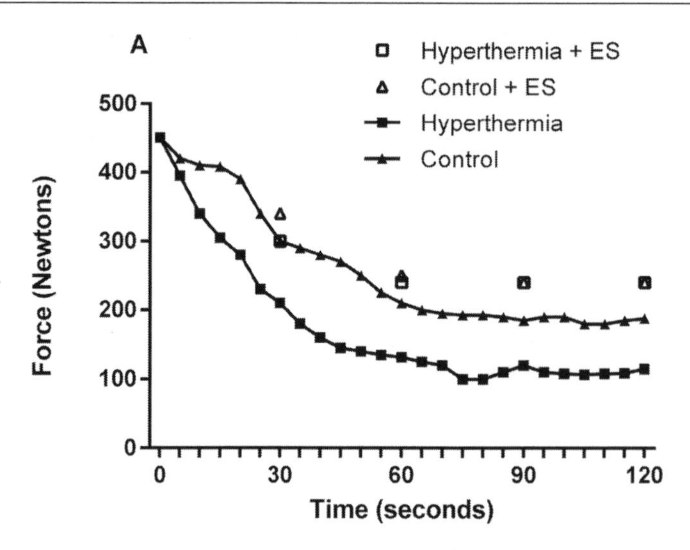

Figure 4.5 Force production from the thigh muscle during a 2 minute maximal knee extension during hyperthermia (core temperature of 40°C) and control (core temperature of 38°C). Participants were asked to make a maximal effort for the entire 2 minutes. Electrical stimulation of the muscle was applied every 30 seconds during the contraction. Electrical stimulation showed that the ability of the muscle to contract was not influenced by hyperthermia. However, participants were not able to voluntarily maintain the level of force production that the muscle was capable of, or that they could maintain in the control trial. This suggests that the causes of reduced force production in the hyperthermia trial were central in origin. From Nybo and Nielsen.[48]

increased brain temperature has the same effect in humans, because it is not feasible to selectively cool or warm a human brain without also altering core temperature.[47] This difficulty is one of the reasons why there is still debate around the role of brain temperature, and the benefits of a 'cooler brain' on human exercise fatigue.[56–7] There is also a potential link between alterations in brain neurotransmitters and the development of central fatigue during exercise in the heat. This is discussed in Section 6.2.1.2.

Key point

During exercise in hyperthermia, brain metabolic rate increases but both blood flow to the brain and brain electrical activity decrease. These changes are associated with a progressive increase in the perception of exercise effort, demonstrating a link between brain blood flow and function, and exercise performance.

Key point

Brain temperature increases during exercise in the heat. Research in animals shows that increasing brain temperature reduces the willingness to exercise, independent of core temperature. Therefore, brain temperature may be a crucial factor for hyperthermic exercise performance in humans. However, this is difficult to confirm, as human brain temperature cannot feasibly be altered without also affecting core temperature.

4.6.3 High core temperature or high skin temperature?

Early research observed that during exercise in the heat, people voluntarily stopped exercise at a very similar core temperature (approximately 40°C), despite the many factors (motivation, training status, heat acclimatisation, hydration etc) that can influence performance in the heat.[51,58–9] Fatigue at, or very close, to this core temperature occurred despite differences in initial core temperature and the rate of heat storage during exercise. Attainment of high core temperature was associated with reduced motor drive from the central nervous system (CNS), leading to the suggestion that core temperature is a safety brake to prevent development of catastrophic hyperthermia, or is perhaps the threshold for a progressive reduction in performance.[46,60–1] This belief, termed the critical core temperature hypothesis, has become the mainstay by which impaired exercise performance in the heat is explained, and has rarely been questioned.[49]

Much of the research that supports the critical core temperature hypothesis used methods that raised not only the core temperature, but also that of the muscle and skin. This is an important point, as raising the temperature of the skin narrows the temperature gradient between the body core and the skin. Narrowing this gradient means that a greater skin blood flow is required to dissipate core body heat. As discussed earlier in this chapter, elevated skin blood flow may impair cardiovascular function via reduced cardiac filling pressure. Increased skin blood flow due to elevated skin temperatures may also reduce brain blood flow and oxygen delivery, [52] although this is unlikely in itself to induce a central fatigue response.[62] Therefore, research that increases core and skin temperature together will find it very difficult to confidently separate and identify the effects of increases in core or skin temperature independently. It is also worth considering that a core temperature of 40°C is much lower than what would be required for cellular damage to occur,[63] and that the CNS appears able to tolerate temperatures of more than 41°C for several hours without damage.[64] This questions the relevance of a critical core temperature of 40°C.

Key point

Most research that identified a 'critical' core temperature limiting performance in the heat used protocols that also caused elevated core and skin temperature. Therefore, the role of increased core temperature in isolation cannot be determined.

Key point

The 'critical' core temperature of approximately 40°C is much lower than the temperature required to cause cellular damage. Therefore, the relevance of this temperature as a limiting factor in exercise performance should be questioned.

Key point

Elevated skin temperature increases skin blood flow requirements, potentially impairing cardiovascular responses to exercise. High skin temperature may also reduce brain blood flow and oxygen delivery.

High skin temperatures alone can impair exercise performance, independent of changes in core temperature. Some studies have shown high skin temperature to cause fatigue at modest core temperatures (approximately 38°C) and with no difference in heart rate response compared to a control trial. Other studies have shown the onset of fatigue with high skin temperatures at core temperatures lower than 38.5°C, but with a higher heart rate relative to exercise intensity, indicating cardiovascular strain (Table 4.2).[65–6] These studies appear to show that high skin temperatures can cause fatigue at core temperatures much lower than those associated with the critical core temperature hypothesis.[49] Furthermore, high skin temperature can exacerbate the negative consequences of hypohydration on exercise performance.[67] Therefore, exercise in the heat, where both hyperthermia and hypohydration are a possibility, could be particularly susceptible to performance decrements from high skin temperature. Indeed, this is the main way in which high skin temperature is thought to impair exercise in the heat: increasing the demand for skin blood flow, reducing central blood volume, cardiac output and, hence, VO_{2max}. As a consequence of reduced VO_{2max},

Table 4.2 Estimated skin blood flow requirements during prolonged high-intensity running at different body core and skin temperatures

Core temp. (°C)	*Skin temp. (°C)*	*Temp. gradient (°C)*	*Skin blood flow (litres per min)*
38	30	8	1.1
38	32	6	1.5
38	34	4	2.2
38	36	2	4.4
39	30	9	1.0
39	32	7	1.3
39	34	5	1.8
39	36	3	2.9

Note: At any given skin temperature, increased core temperature increases the temperature gradient between the core and the skin, and there is a reduction in skin blood flow. At any given core temperature, increasing the skin temperature reduces the temperature gradient between the core and the skin, and there is an increase in skin blood flow.

Source: Sawka *et al.*[49]

relative exercise intensity will increase, making exercise feel harder and eventually causing the cessation of exercise. The change in cardiovascular demand due to increased skin temperature would be exacerbated in the presence of hypohydration, where cardiovascular integrity may already be compromised.

Key point

High skin temperature can impair exercise performance, independent of changes in core temperature.

Further argument against the critical core temperature hypothesis comes from research showing that endurance exercise performance can be maintained despite core temperatures much higher than the 40°C 'cut-off' temperature. Researchers have reported no difference in running speed during an 8km time trial when core temperature was below or above 40°C.[60] Similar findings have been reported over longer distance running, with no association between high core temperature and performance.[68–9] Interestingly, in the studies that found no effect of high core temperature on performance, skin temperatures were only cool to warm.

Key point

Research shows that exercise performance can be maintained with a core temperature greater than the proposed 'critical' temperature of 40°C. This argues for the presence of other factors that limit exercise performance in the heat.

The above discussions clearly demonstrate that potential causes of fatigue during exercise in the heat go a lot further than the attainment of a critically high core temperature. In fact, the critical core temperature hypothesis has received strong challenge in recent years. Current knowledge now identifies a range of potential causes of hyperthermia related fatigue including high core temperature, high skin temperature, reduced brain blood flow and electrical activity, and increased brain temperature. While the field has moved on notably in the last decade, the exact causes of fatigue during exercise in the heat are unknown. This is mainly due to the difficulty in measuring some known factors of hyperthermia associated fatigue, most notably brain temperature, in the exercising human. However, what is now clear is that hyperthermia-induced fatigue is not an all-or-nothing event that occurs upon reaching a critical core temperature, but is instead a progressive, integrated occurrence involving both peripheral feedback and central processes.[47]

Key point

Hyperthermia-induced fatigue is a progressive, integrated occurrence involving both peripheral feedback and central processes. It is not an all-or-nothing event that occurs upon reaching a critical core temperature.

4.7 Summary

- Research investigating hydration and exercise performance is primarily concerned with the concepts of euhydration, hyperhydration, dehydration, and hypohydration.
- Dehydration and hypohydration are not the same. Dehydration is the dynamic process of body water loss, and hypohydration is the end result of this water loss (the extent of body water loss).

- Water is critical for life and for exercise performance, due to its abundance in the body and its involvement in many cellular, tissue, and organ system processes.
- Hydration status is commonly assessed by quantifying body water balance, defined as the balance between water intake and water loss.
- Dehydration can reduce blood plasma volume, meaning less blood enters the heart during each cardiac cycle. This can decrease stroke volume and cardiac output, and increase heart rate. Furthermore, a competition for blood flow between the skin and the core organs may develop, impairing evaporative heat loss and increasing the risk of hyperthermia.
- Dehydration may increase muscle glycogen use at a given exercise intensity, which could contribute to fatigue via glycogen depletion. However, increased muscle glycogen use with dehydration may also depend of the presence of hyperthermia.
- Dehydration may increase effort perception and impair aspects of cognitive function during exercise.
- Early hydration research identified an apparent threshold fluid decrement of 2% of BM, above which aerobic exercise performance appeared to be impaired. However, this research was subject to limitations.
- A number of recent studies that attempted to address the limitations of the earlier research have shown little or no performance decrement, and perhaps a small performance enhancement, during endurance exercise with hypohydration greater than 2% of BM.
- The emerging consensus is that hypohydration (unless severe) does not impair endurance exercise performance, and that drinking to thirst appears the most effective strategy for maximising performance during self-paced exercise.
- Excessive fluid intake during exercise appears to be the most important risk factor for the development of hypervolaemia and hyponatraemia. Strategies to reduce excessive fluid intake are associated with fewer incidences of hyponatraemia.
- Hyperthermia is an abnormally high core temperature (normal core temperature ranges from 36.5–37.5°C).
- Hyperthermia can develop any time body heat gain is greater than body heat dissipation. The most challenging environment for maintenance of body temperature is when it is hot and humid.
- Potential peripheral factors associated with hyperthermia-induced fatigue include reduced blood and oxygen delivery to working muscles due to reduced central blood volume and increased muscle glycogen use. However, there is not good evidence for these factors causing fatigue.
- It appears that central alterations due to hyperthermia (increased core temperature, increased brain temperature, reduced brain blood and oxygen delivery, reduced brain electrical activity, suppression of motor

output) may exert more of an influence on hyperthermia-induced fatigue during exercise.
- The concept of a 'critical' core temperature of approximately 40°C that, once reached, causes fatigue during exercise appears to be false.
- A high skin temperature may be more important than high core temperature in contributing to hyperthermia-induced fatigue during exercise. High skin temperatures require a higher skin blood flow, which may impair cardiac function, reduce VO_{2max}, and increase relative exercise intensity, causing the athlete to fatigue earlier.
- Fatigue during exercise in the heat is a progressive occurrence that likely involves both peripheral feedback and central processes.

To think about . . .

The incidence of major sporting events being hosted in countries with extreme environmental conditions is increasing. An example of this is the 2022 FIFA World Cup, which at the time of writing this book is due to be held in the Arab state of Qatar. During the summer months (when the World Cup is scheduled), temperatures in Qatar can reach up to 42°C with humidity levels up to 90%. In contrast, teams may qualify for the World Cup from countries who are more used to playing football in temperatures no warmer than 20°C, or even in the snow!

What are your thoughts about holding major sporting events in extreme environments? Do you think that it is fair to all nations/teams taking part, or does it favour those from countries that regularly experience this type of weather? Are there any ethical issues (from a sporting, medical, or health perspective) associated with hosting competitions in these conditions? What about the sponsors, employees, and fans of these teams – what thoughts might they have about the situation? And would these thoughts differ based on country location?

Test yourself

Answer the following questions to the best of your ability. Try to understand the information gained from answering these questions before you progress with the book.

1 Define and differentiate between the terms dehydration, hypohydration, and hyperhydration.
2 Briefly explain the 'classical' mechanism of dehydration-induced performance decrement.
3 What are the other ways in which dehydration may impair exercise performance?
4 What are the key limitations with some of the hydration research that has been used to justify the 2% of body mass dehydration threshold?
5 Define and briefly explain the terms hypervolaemia and hyponatraemia.
6 What are the primary possible causes of peripheral and central fatigue associated with hyperthermia?
7 What are the key arguments against the critical core temperature hypothesis?
8 How might high skin temperature contribute to fatigue, independent of changes in core temperature?

References

1 Casa DJ, Armstrong LE, Hillman SK, Montain SJ, Reiff RV, Rich BSE, Roberts WO, Stone JA (2000) National Athletic Trainers Association position statement: fluid replacement for athletes. *J Athl Train* 35: 212–24.
2 Sawka MN, Burke LM, Eichner ER, Maughan RJ, Montain SJ, Stachenfeld NS (2007) American College of Sports Medicine Position Stand: exercise and fluid replacement. *Med Sci Sports Exerc* 39: 377–90.
3 Logan-Sprenger HM, Heigenhauser GJ, Killian KJ, Spreit LL (2012) Effects of dehydration during cycling on skeletal muscle metabolism in females. *Med Sci Sports Exerc* 44: 1949–57.
4 Logan-Sprenger HM, Heigenhauser GJ, Jones GL, Spreit LL (2013) Increase in skeletal-muscle glycogenolysis and perceived exertion with progressive dehydration during cycling in hydrated men. *Int J Sport Nutr Exerc Metab* 23: 220–9.
5 Ganio MS, Armstrong LE, Casa DJ, McDermott BP, Lee EC, Yamamoto LM, Marzano S, Lopez RM, Jimenez L, Bellego L, Chevillotte E, Lieberman HR (2011) Mild dehydration impairs cognitive performance and mood of men. *Br J Nutr* 106; 1535–43.
6 Casa DJ, Clarkson PM, Roberts WO (2005) American College of Sports Medicine roundtable on hydration and physical activity: consensus statements. *Curr Sports Med Rep* 4: 115–27.
7 Cheuvront SN, Carter III R, Sawka MN (2003) Fluid balance and endurance exercise performance. *Curr Sports Med Rep* 2: 202–8.
8 Sawka MN, Noakes TD (2007) Does dehydration impair exercise performance? *Med Sci Sports Exerc* 39: 1209–17.
9 Sawka MN (1992) Physiological consequences of hypohydration: exercise performance and thermoregulation. *Med Sci Sports Exerc* 24: 657–70.
10 Craig FN, Cummings EG (1966) Dehydration and muscular work. *J Appl Physiol* 21: 670–4.
11 Dougherty KA, Baker LB, Chow M, Kenney WL (2006) Two percent dehydration impairs and six percent carbohydrate drink improves boys basketball skills. *Med Sci Sports Exerc* 38: 1650–8.

12 Armstrong LE, Costill DL, Fink WJ (1985) Influence of diuretic-induced dehydration on competitive running performance. *Med Sci Sports Exerc* 17: 456–61.

13 Dugas JP, Oosthuizen V, Tucker R, Noakes TD (2006) Drinking 'ad libitum' optimises performance and physiological function during 80 km indoor cycling trials in hot and humid conditions with appropriate convective cooling. *Med Sci Sports Exerc* 38: S176.

14 Jeukendrup A, Saris WHM, Brouns F, Kester ADM (1996) A new validated endurance performance test. *Med Sci Sports Exerc* 28: 266–70.

15 Mündel T (2011) To drink or not to drink? Explaining 'contradictory findings' in fluid replacement and exercise performance: evidence from a more valid model for real-life competition. *Br J Sports Med* 45: 2.

16 Dion T, Savoie FA, Audrey A, Gariepy C, Goulet EDB (2013) Half-marathon running performance is not improved by a rate of fluid intake above that dictated by thirst sensation in trained distance runners. *Eur J Appl Physiol* 113: 3011–20.

17 Marino FE, Cannon J, Kay D (2011) Neuromuscular responses to hydration in moderate to warm ambient conditions during self-paced high-intensity exercise. *Br J Sports Med* 44: 961–7.

18 Nolte HW, Noakes TD, van Vuuren B (2011) Protection of total body water content and absence of hyperthermia despite 2% body mass loss ('voluntary dehydration') in soldiers drinking ad libitum during prolonged exercise in cool environmental conditions. *Br J Sports Med* 45: 1106–12.

19 Zouhal H, Groussard C, Minter G, Vincent S, Cretual A, Gratas-Delamarche A, Delamarche P, Noakes TD (2011) Inverse relationship between percentage body weight change and finishing time in 643 forty two-kilometre marathon runners. *Br J Sports Med* 45: 1101–5.

20 Aragón-Vargas LF, Wilk B, Timmons BW, Bar-Or O (2013) Body weight changes in child and adolescent athletes during a triathlon competition. *Eur J Appl Physiol* 113: 233–9.

21 Kao WF, Shy CL, Yang XW, Hsu TF, Chen JJ, Kao WC, Polun C, Huang YJ, Kuo FC, Huang CI, Lee CH (2008) Athletic performance and serial weight changes during 12-and 24-hour ultra-marathons. *Clin J Sport Med* 18: 155–8.

22 Rüst CA, Knechtle B, Knechtle P, Wirth A, Rosemann T (2012) Body mass change and ultraendurance performance: a decrease in body mass is associated with an increased running speed in male 100-km ultramarathoners. *J Strength Cond Res* 6: 1505–16.

23 Goulet ED (2013) Effect of exercise-induced dehydration on endurance performance: evaluating the impact of exercise protocols on outcomes using a meta-analytic procedure. *Br J Sports Med* 47: 679–86.

24 Maughan RJ, Shirreffs SM, Leiper JB (2007) Errors in the estimation of hydration status from changes in body mass. *J Sports Sci* 25: 797–804.

25 Zouhal H, Groussard C, Vincent S, Jacob C, Abderrahman AR, Delamarche P, Gratas-Delamarche A (2009) Athletic performance and weight changes during the 'Marathon of Sands' in athletes well-trained in endurance. *Int J Sports Med* 30: 516–21.

26 Dugas JP, Oosthuizen U, Tucker R, Noakes TD (2009) Rates of fluid ingestion alter pacing but not thermoregulatory responses during prolonged exercise in hot and humid conditions with appropriate convective cooling. *Eur J Appl Physiol* 105: 69–80.

27 Gigou PY, Dion T, Asselin A, Berrigan F, Goulet ED (2012) Pre-exercise hyperhydration-induced bodyweight gain does not alter prolonged treadmill running time-trial performance in warm ambient conditions. *Nutrients* 4: 949–66.

28 Goulet EDB (2011) Effect of exercise-induced dehydration on time-trial exercise performance: a meta-analysis. *Br J Sports Med* 45: 1149–56.
29 Convertino VA (1983) Heart rate and sweat rate responses associated with exercise-induced hypervolemia. *Med Sci Sports Exerc* 15: 77–82.
30 Mischler I, Boirie Y, Gachon P, Pialoux V, Mounier R, Rousset P, Coudert J, Fellmann, N (2003) Human albumin synthesis is increased by an ultra-endurance trial. *Med Sci Sports Exerc* 35: 75–81.
31 Leiper JB, McCormick K, Robertson JD, Whiting PH, Maughan RJ (1988) Fluid homeostasis during prolonged low-intensity walking on consecutive days. *Clin Sci (London)* 75: 63–70.
32 Fellmann N, Ritz P, Ribeyre J, Beaufrère B, Delaître M, Coudert J (1999) Intracellular hyperhydration induced by a 7-day endurance race. *Eur J Appl Physiol* 80: 353–9.
33 Fellmann N, Sagnol M, Bedu M, Falgairette G, Van Praagh E, Gaillard G, Jouanel P, Coudert J (1988) Enzymatic and hormonal responses following a 24 h endurance run and a 10 h triathlon race. *Eur J Appl Physiol* 57: 545–53.
34 Skenderi KP, Kavouras SA, Anastasiou CA, Yiannakouris N, Matalas AL (2006) Exertional rhabdomyolysis during a 246-km continuous running race. *Med Sci Sports Exerc* 38: 1054–7.
35 Knechtle B, Duff B, Schulze I, Kohler G (2008) A multi-stage ultra-endurance run over 1,200 km leads to a continuous accumulation of total body water. *J Sports Sci Med* 7: 357–64.
36 Knechtle B, Wirth A, Knechtle P, Rosemann T (2009) Increase of total body water with decrease of body mass while running 100 km nonstop – formation of edema? *Res Quart Exerc Sport* 80: 593–603.
37 Noakes TD, Sharwood K, Collins M, Perkins DR (2004) The dipsomania of great distance: water intoxication in an ironman triathlete. *Br J Sports Med* 38: e16.
38 Knechtle B, Senn O, Imoberdorf R (2011) No fluid overload in male ultra-runners during a 100 km ultra-run. *Res Sports Med* 19: 14–27.
39 Rosner MH, Kirven J (2007) Exercise-associated hyponatremia. *Clin J Am Soc Nephrol* 2: 151–61.
40 Almond CSD, Shin AY, Fortescue EB, Mannix RC, Wypij D, Binstadt BA, Duncan CN, Olson DP, Salerno AE, Newburger JW, Greenes DS (2005) Hyponatraemia among runners in the Boston Marathon. *New Eng J Med* 352: 1550–6.
41 Montain SJ, Cheuvront SN, Sawka MN (2005) Exercise associated hyponatraemia: quantitative analysis to understand the aetiology. *Br J Sports Med* 40: 98–106.
42 Sharwood KA, Collins M, Goedecke JH, Wilson G, Noakes TD (2004) Weight changes, medical complications, and performance during an Ironman triathlon. *Br J Sports Med* 38: 718–24.
43 Noakes TD, Speedy DB (2006) Case proven: exercise associated hyponatraemia is due to overdrinking. So why did it take 20 years before the original evidence was accepted? *Br J Sports Med* 40: 567–72.
44 Cheung SS, Sleivert GG (2004) Multiple triggers for hyperthermic fatigue and exhaustion. *Exerc Sport Sci Rev* 32: 100–6.
45 Maughan RJ (2012) Thermoregulatory aspects of performance. *Exp Physiol* 97: 325–6.
46 Nybo L (2008) Hyperthermia and fatigue. *J Appl Physiol* 104: 871–8.
47 Nybo L (2012) Brain temperature and exercise performance. *Exp Physiol* 97: 333–9.

48 Nybo L, Nielsen B (2001) Hyperthermia and central fatigue during prolonged exercise in humans. *J Appl Physiol* 91: 1055–60.
49 Sawka MN, Cheuvront SN, Kenefick RW (2012) High skin temperature and hypohydration impair aerobic performance. *Exp Physiol* 97: 327–32.
50 González-Alonso J, Calbet JAL, Nielsen B (1998) Muscle blood flow is reduced with dehydration during prolonged exercise in humans. *J Physiol* 513: 895–905.
51 González-Alonso J, Calbet JAL, Nielsen B (1999) Metabolic and thermodynamic responses to dehydration-induced reductions in muscle blood flow in exercising humans. *J Physiol* 520: 577–89.
52 Nybo L, Møller K, Volianitis S, Nielsen B, Secher NH (2002) Effects of hyperthermia on cerebral blood flow and metabolism during prolonged exercise in humans. *J Appl Physiol* 93: 58–64.
53 Tucker R, Marle T, Lambert EV, Noakes TD (2004) Impaired exercise performance in the heat is associated with an anticipatory reduction in skeletal muscle recruitment. *Pflug Arch* 448: 422–30.
54 Rasmussen P, Nielsen J, Overgaard M, Krogh-Madsen R, Gjedde A, Secher NH, Petersen NC (2010) Reduced muscle activation during exercise related to brain oxygenation and metabolism in humans. *J Physiol* 588: 1985–95.
55 Caputa SS, McLellan TM (1986) Effect of brain and trunk temperatures on exercise performance in goats. *Pflug Arch Physiol* 406: 184–9.
56 White MD, Greiner JG, McDonald PLL (2011) Point: Humans do demonstrate selective brain cooling during hyperthermia. *J Appl Physiol* 110: 569–71.
57 Marino FE (2011) The critical limiting temperature and selective brain cooling: neuroprotection during exercise? *Int J Hyperther* 27: 582–90.
58 Nielsen B, Hales JRS, Strange NJ, Christensen NJ, Warberg J, Saltin B (1993) Human circulatory and thermoregulatory adaptations with heat acclimation and exercise in a hot, dry environment. *J Physiol* 460: 467–85.
59 Nielsen B, Savard G, Richter EA, Hargreaves M, Saltin B (1990) Muscle blood flow and muscle metabolism during exercise and heat stress. *J Appl Physiol* 69: 1040–6.
60 Ely BR, Ely MR, Cheuvront SN, Kenefick RW, DeGroot DW, Montain SJ (2009) Evidence against a 40°C core temperature threshold for fatigue in humans. *J Appl Physiol* 107: 1519–25.
61 Nybo L (2007) Exercise and heat stress: cerebral challenges and consequences. *Progress Brain Res* 162: 29–43.
62 Thomas MM, Cheung SS, Elder GC, Sleivert GG (2006) Voluntary muscle activation is impaired by core temperature rather than local muscle temperature. *J Appl Physiol* 100: 1361–9.
63 Hales JRS, Hubbard RW, Gaffin SL (1996) Limitation of heat tolerance. In: *Handbook of Physiology*, edited by Fregley MJ, Blatteis CM. New York: Oxford University Press.
64 Dubois M, Sato S, Lee DE, Bull JM, Smith R, White BG, Moore H, Macnamara TE (1980) Electroencephalographic changes during whole body hyperthermia in humans. *Electroencephalogr Clin Neurophysiol* 50: 486–95.
65 Montain SJ, Sawka MN, Cadarette BS, Quigley MD, McKay JM (1994) Physiological tolerance to uncompensable heat stress: effects of exercise intensity, protective clothing, and climate. *J Appl Physiol* 77: 216–22.
66 Latzka WA, Sawka MN, Montain SJ, Skrinar GS, Fielding RA, Matott RP, Pandolf KB (1998) Hyperhydration: tolerance and cardiovascular effects during uncompensable heat stress. *J Appl Physiol* 84: 1858–64.

67 Kenefick RW, Cheuvront SN, Palombo LJ, Ely BR, Sawka MN (2010) Skin temperature modifies the impact of hypohydration on aerobic performance. *J Appl Physiol* 109: 79–86.
68 Byrne C, Lee JK, Chew SA, Lim CL, Tan EY (2006) Continuous thermoregulatory response to mass-participation distance running in the heat. *Med Sci Sports Exerc* 38: 803–10.
69 Lee JK, Nio AQ, Lim CL, Teo EY, Byrne C (2010) Thermoregulation, pacing and fluid balance during mass participation distance running in a warm and humid environment. *Eur J Appl Physiol* 109: 887–98.

Chapter 5

Potassium and calcium

5.1 Introduction

Technological advances have enabled the development of more sophisticated human measurement and analysis tools. Magnetic resonance imagery (MRI, see Section 1.3.6), transcranial magnetic stimulation (Section 1.3.7), and a host of other complex technology usually found in medical and clinical biochemistry settings is becoming more commonplace within sport and exercise science research.

These technological advances have enabled ever more detailed investigation of the function of the body at a cellular and molecular level during exercise. Consequently, new avenues of knowledge have developed regarding the biochemical processes that control body system functions. Within the context of fatigue during exercise, two substances that have come to light as a result of our improved ability to determine their function during exercise are potassium (chemical symbol K) and calcium (chemical symbol Ca). This chapter will summarise the important functional roles of K and Ca, before discussing how disturbances in some of these functions during exercise could potentially contribute to fatigue. As with the other chapters in this book, the information provided is a summary of current knowledge. Investigation into the roles, if any, of K and Ca in exercise fatigue is ongoing.

5.2 Potassium: description and function

Potassium is a chemical element that is necessary for the function of all living cells. It is one of the most common elements in the body, representing approximately 0.2% of body mass (so a 70 kg person will contain approximately 140 grams of K). Potassium is a mineral, meaning that it is a naturally occurring inorganic solid. Sources of dietary K include orange juice, potatoes, bananas, leafy greens, and salmon.

In its ionic form, K is also an electrolyte, meaning that it carries a small electrical charge and enables electricity to be conducted through the solution it is placed in (this is very important for some of the functional roles that

Key point

Potassium is one of the most abundant elements in the body. Dietary sources of K include orange juice, potatoes, bananas, leafy greens, and salmon.

K plays). The ionic form of K is abbreviated as K^+. The '+' sign in the abbreviation indicates a positively charged ion, known as a cation. In fact, K^+ is the most abundant cation found within cells. The vast majority of the body's K^+ stores are located within nerve, muscle, and blood cells, with a small amount present in blood plasma.

Potassium plays crucial roles in body function. First, K^+, along with another electrolyte, sodium (Na^+), helps to regulate intra- and extracellular water content. Water molecules do not have an electrical charge, and cells cannot move water from intra to extracellular locations directly. However, the components of water, hydrogen and oxygen, do have an electrical charge (hydrogen has a positive charge, and oxygen a negative charge). These charges are attracted to the electrical charges of K^+ and Na^+ ions, meaning that electrolytes 'attract' water molecules to them. If a cell membrane is permeable to water, then water will move across the membrane to the side with the highest concentration of electrolytes, as this is the side that is exerting the greatest 'pull' on the water molecules. This movement of water will continue until the electrolyte concentration on both sides of the cell membrane is equal. The force required to move water across a membrane is called the osmotic pressure. It is in this way that cells regulate body water content.

Movement of K^+ and Na^+ across cell membranes is achieved via specialised protein transport channels. At rest, the inside of a muscle cell has a slightly negative electrical charge compared to the outside of the cell. This negative charge, termed the resting membrane potential, is generated by the relative concentration of Na^+ and K^+ within and outside the cell. There is a greater concentration of Na^+ outside, and a greater concentration of K^+ inside the muscle cell. To initiate muscle contraction, an electrical signal moves along a motor neuron, along the surface of a muscle cell, and then inside the cell. The transport, or propagation, of this electrical signal (termed an action potential) is controlled by movement of Na^+ and K^+ across the cell membrane of the motor neuron and muscle (Figure 5.1). Initial stimulus by the action potential makes the cell membrane permeable to Na^+ via the opening of voltage gated Na^+ channels (Figure 5.1). In this situation, Na^+ quickly enters the muscle cell, making the interior of the cell positively charged (depolarised) and enabling the action potential to continue. Almost immediately following this, Na^+ channels close and voltage gated K^+ channels then open, enabling

K^+ to quickly leave the cell (Figure 5.1). This process repolarises the cell, making the intracellular charge negative once again (therefore, Na^+ movement is excitatory, and K^+ movement is inhibitory). The entire process only takes a few milliseconds, and occurs during every action potential. Upon repolarisation the intracellular charge may be slightly more negative than the resting membrane potential (termed hyperpolarisation). In this situation, the Na^+, K^+ pump (integrated specialised channels within the membrane of excitable cells that transport Na^+ and K^+ across the membrane) will regain

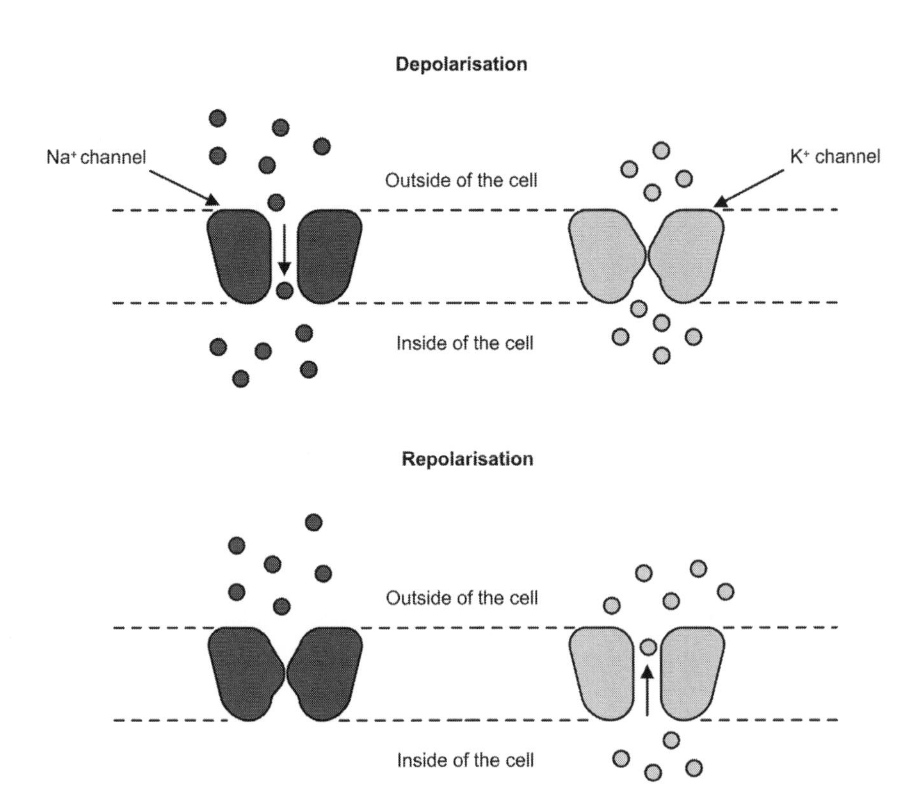

Figure 5.1 At rest, the inside of a nerve or muscle cell has a slightly negative electrical charge compared to the outside of the cell, due in part to the greater concentration of Na^+ outside and greater concentration of K^+ inside the cell. The transport, or propagation, of the electrical signal down a motor neuron and across and into the muscle cell makes the cell membrane permeable to Na^+ via the opening of voltage gated Na^+ channels. Here, Na^+ quickly enters the muscle cell through ion channels present in the cell membrane, depolarising the cell and enabling the action potential to continue. Almost immediately following this, Na^+ channels close and voltage gated K^+ channels open, enabling K^+ to quickly leave the cell. This process repolarises the cell, making the intracellular charge negative once again.

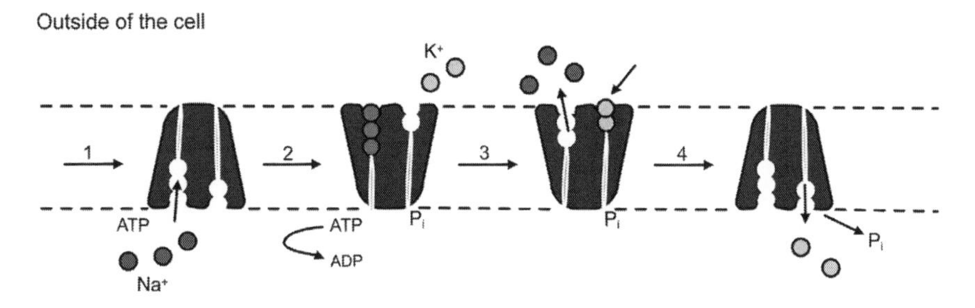

Figure 5.2 The Na^+, K^+ pump. Specialised channels are present within the membrane of excitable cells such as neurons and muscle. Three Na^+ molecules and one ATP molecule bind to the channel (step 1). Hydrolysis of ATP drives a conformational change in the channel, causing it to transport Na^+ across the membrane and out of the cell (step 2). The change also enables two K^+ molecules to bind to the channel on the outside of the cell membrane (step 3). Removal of inorganic phosphate (P_i) returns the channel to its original shape, in doing so bringing K^+ across the membrane into the cell and exposing Na^+ binding sites (step 4). The cycle repeats until resting membrane potential is restored.

and maintain resting membrane potential by actively pumping three Na^+ ions out of the cell for every two K^+ ions that move back into the cell (Figure 5.2). A graphical description of action potential propagation is in Figure 5.3.

Key point

Potassium has key roles to play in a variety of body functions. Some of the most important of these functions include the regulation of body water content, conduction of action potentials along neurons and muscle cells, and aiding in protein synthesis, carbohydrate metabolism, and glycogenesis.

A lesser known role of K^+ is in biochemical reactions. Potassium is important in the synthesis of protein, carbohydrate metabolism, and glycogenesis (conversion of glucose to glycogen for storage in the liver and muscles). The roles of K^+ discussed above highlight the importance of this electrolyte in key processes required for health and function, and also for optimal exercise performance.

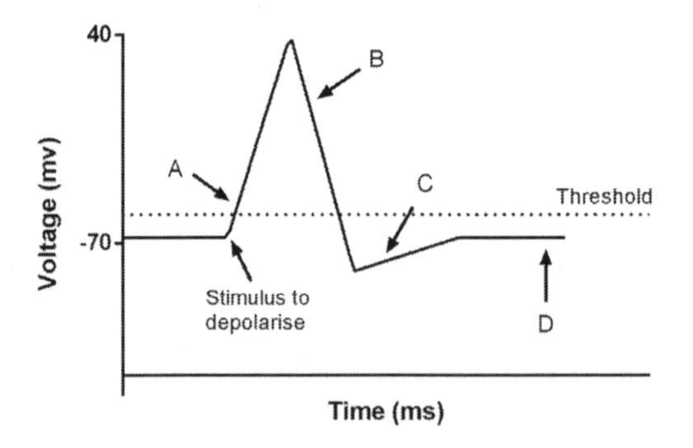

A: Depolarisation

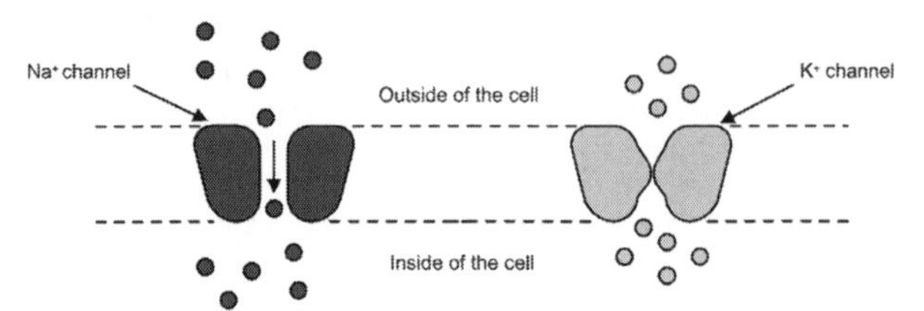

B: Repolarisation and C: Hyperpolarisation

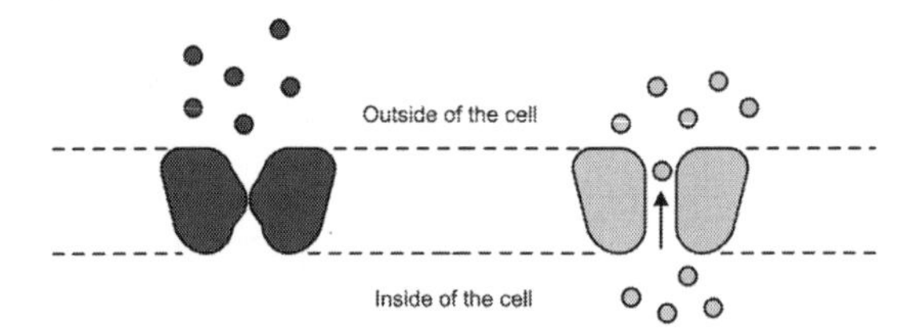

D: Resting potential

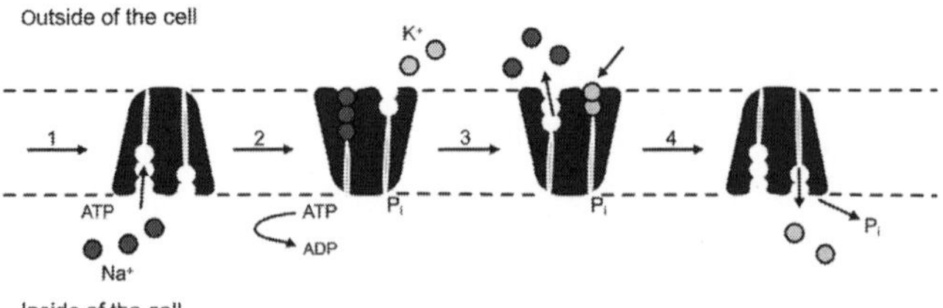

Figure 5.3 A graphical and schematic representation of the depolarisation and repolarisation of a membrane, allowing the propagation of an action potential. The membrane is at a resting potential of –65 to –70 mv. If a depolarising stimulus reaches the required threshold (approximately –50 to –55 mv) then the membrane Na^+ channels open and Na^+ enters the cell, causing depolarisation (A). At the peak of depolarisation, Na^+ channels close and K^+ channels open, allowing K^+ to leave the muscle, thereby causing repolarisation (B). Potassium channels remain open, causing membrane potential to fall below that of the resting potential (hyperpolarisation, C). Potassium channels then close, and the Na^+, K^+ pump restores normal resting membrane potential (D).

5.3 Potassium and exercise fatigue

As discussed in Section 5.2, K^+ plays an important role in conducting the action potential along a motor neuron and muscle fibre. Conduction of this action potential is critical for muscle function, as inadequate electrical stimulation means that insufficient calcium ions (abbreviation Ca^{2+}) may be released from the sarcoplasmic reticulum (SR), which can prevent the muscle from contracting at its optimum rate and/or force (see Section 2.2.3.2.1). Any interference or breakdown in polarisation (a term for the normal functional processes of depolarisation followed by repolarisation) across a muscle cell membrane could significantly impair cell function. Therefore, alterations in the normal membrane transfer of Na^+ or K^+ could contribute to muscle dysfunction and, potentially, fatigue.[1] For example, failure of an action potential can occur due to dysfunction of Na^+ channels as a result of chronic depolarisation (a continued positive change in cell membrane potential), a reduced Na^+ concentration gradient (via a decrease in extracellular Na^+ concentration or an increase in intracellular Na^+ concentration), or permeability of the cell membrane to K^+, as an action potential can only progress if the inward Na^+ current sufficiently exceeds the leak current of K^+.[1,2]

A small amount of K^+ is lost from the muscle with each action potential, meaning that repeated muscle contractions can cause a net loss of K^+ from and a net gain of Na^+ into the muscle cell.[1,3–6] This is particularly prevalent during high-intensity muscle contractions where the muscle remains well perfused (a good blood supply is maintained).[7] The rate of K^+ loss from the muscle occurs quickly following the initiation of contraction, followed by a much slower phase of accumulation.[8] A primary route for K^+ loss from the muscle is via the specialised K^+ channels shown in Figure 5.1.[9–12] It has been suggested that reduced muscle pH during high-intensity exercise causes the K^+ channels to open.[12] However, there is conflicting evidence for this, and it will be discussed later in this section. During high-intensity muscle contractions, the capacity of the Na^+, K^+ pumps to bring K^+ back into the muscle may be exceeded,[3] which could also contribute to the net loss of K^+.

Key point

Alterations in the membrane transport of K^+ could interfere with the normal propagation of action potentials, thereby impairing muscle function.

Key point

Repeated muscle contractions can cause a loss of K^+ from the muscle cell via the specialised K^+ transport channels present in the cell membrane.

5.3.1 Reduced muscle force production and exercise endurance with extracellular potassium accumulation

Potassium loss from the muscle can alter the electrochemical gradient for K^+ across a muscle cell membrane, leading to membrane depolarisation, reduced excitation of the muscle, and reduced force production.[1] Muscle force reduction ranging from 30–80% has been found in animal muscle fibres,[13–14] and rapid force reduction and reduction in action potential activity across the muscle cell membrane has also been reported in humans.[15–16] It appears that the movement of K^+ out of the muscle during contractions cannot always be compensated for by the activity of the Na^+, K^+ pumps.[1] Interestingly, rapid recovery of the action potential and muscle force is seen when the rate of muscle stimulation (and hence the requirement for action potential propagation) is reduced, suggesting that reductions in muscle force may be due to reduced muscle excitation as a result of transmembrane K^+ concentration changes and membrane depolarisation.[1] It also suggests that extracellular K^+ accumulation is dependent, in part, on exercise intensity and the size of the exercising muscle mass.[17] Imbalance in the concentrations of Na^+ and K^+ ions within a muscle cell, in particular K^+ accumulation in the T system (the network of t-tubules that conduct the action potential throughout the fibre so that it can stimulate Ca^{2+} release; see Section 2.2.3.2.1 and Figure 5.4), may prevent the action potential from propagating through the T system, thereby impairing Ca^{2+} release into the muscle.[1] However, despite the suggestion that the largest increases in extracellular K^+ accumulation take place in the T system,[18] there is disagreement as to the role of K^+ accumulation in the T system on Ca^{2+} release, as impairments in Ca^{2+} release may depend on factors including the rate of stimulation and muscle length.[19–21]

A potential role of extracellular K^+ accumulation on fatigue is highlighted by observations of a reduced time to fatigue during exercise when extracellular K^+ accumulation occurs at a faster rate.[12,22] Fatigue has also been shown to occur at the same extracellular K^+ concentration, despite differences in exercise mode, time to fatigue, and training status;[23–4] however, this has not been consistently found.[12,25] Interestingly, high-intensity exercise training has been shown to reduce the extracellular accumulation of K^+ (likely via increased Na^+, K^+ pump activity) and delay fatigue.[24] This training adaptation supports the suggestion that extracellular K^+ accumulation is involved in fatigue development during exercise.

Key point

Reduced membrane depolarisation, muscle excitation, and force production with muscle K^+ loss has been reported in animals and humans. It appears that the rate of K^+ loss cannot always be compensated for by activity of the Na^+, K^+ pump.

Key point

Observations of fatigue occurring at the same extracellular K^+ concentration, and high-intensity training reducing the rate of extracellular K^+ accumulation, provide support for a role of extracellular K^+ accumulation in exercise fatigue.

The influence of extracellular K^+ accumulation on exercise fatigue may not be limited to changes in muscle membrane excitability. Extracellular K^+ accumulation may stimulate type III and IV muscle afferents, which could contribute to the muscle discomfort commonly felt during intense and/or prolonged exercise (also see Section 3.3.1). Stimulation of these muscle afferents by extracellular K^+ accumulation can also inhibit central motor drive, which may contribute to the development of central fatigue during exercise (see Section 6.2.1.1). However, further research is needed to confirm both of these suggestions.

Key point

Extracellular K^+ accumulation may stimulate type III and IV muscle afferents, which could contribute to the development of central fatigue. However, research on this topic is conflicting.

5.4 Evidence against extracellular potassium accumulation as a cause of exercise fatigue

This section will present some of the arguments against extracellular K^+ accumulation as a cause of fatigue during exercise. A level of detail appropriate for this text will be provided, and the reader is referred to the excellent review of Allen *et al.*[1] for further information.

As discussed in Section 5.3, alterations in K^+ movement across a muscle membrane can reduce muscle cell excitability, and this has been associated in some research with the onset of fatigue. However, there are numerous other studies that have failed to show reduced muscle excitability at the point of fatigue during exercise,[16,26–30] even with notable extracellular K^+ accumulation.[29–30] Other studies also show an ability of muscle to produce near maximal force in the face of significant extracellular K^+ accumulation.[8] It may be confusing to read this, particularly after the discussion in Section 5.3 that linked extracellular K^+ accumulation with impaired fatigue resistance during exercise in humans. However, the body has many mechanisms that work to prevent losses in muscle excitability, and in order to do that these mechanisms can work to reduce the influence of extracellular K^+ accumulation on muscle membrane excitability.[1] Some of these mechanisms will now be discussed.

5.4.1 Motor unit recruitment

When a muscle is contracting submaximally, the central nervous system (CNS) is able to vary the specific motor units (a motor unit is a motor neuron and all of the muscle fibres that neuron innervates) used to contract the muscle in order to 'spread the load' across the different motor units.[1,31–2] Varying the use of motor units to achieve a muscle contraction has the effect of reducing the number of action potentials that a particular muscle fibre has to undergo. As discussed in Section 5.3, K^+ loss from a muscle fibre occurs as a result of the depolarisation of the muscle fibre during an action potential. Reducing the number of action potentials could reduce the amount of K^+ that is lost from that particular muscle fibre, thereby reducing extracellular K^+ accumulation.

5.4.2 Alterations to motor neuron firing rate

Motor units function in a way that is extremely well matched to the characteristics of the motor unit itself. Motor units function at a firing rate (i.e. the rate of delivery of action potentials) that is just enough to enable maximum force production. In doing so, the number of action potentials that are required to contract a muscle fibre are kept to a minimum. As discussed in Section 5.4.1, this economy of action potentials would minimise the efflux of K^+ from the muscle fibre.

Similarly, the firing rate of motor neurons decreases during sustained contractions, with this decrease closely matched to the slowing of fibre relaxation that occurs during muscle action.[1] Therefore, the rate of stimulation is just enough to allow the muscle to produce the most force possible at any given time.[33] Appropriately, this intelligent economy of resources is sometimes referred to as 'muscle wisdom'.[34] The delivery of action potentials also represents an economical approach to muscle activation. Action potentials often begin as groups of closely spaced potentials which allow a given force production with less fatigue,[35] and a more effective force production for a given number of action potentials.[1] Again, this minimises the number of action potentials required.

5.4.3 Action potential changes

Depolarisation of a muscle fibre by repeated activation can slow the propagation, reduce the size, and increase the duration of an action potential.[1,36–7]

However, the action potential remains sufficient to propagate into the T system and stimulate Ca^{2+} release. Therefore, these changes to the action potential probably do not contribute to reduced muscle force or fatigue.[33]

5.4.4 The sodium–potassium pump

The Na^+, K^+ pump is critical for lowering extracellular K^+ concentration, particularly in the T system.[1] When muscle excitability is reduced due to high extracellular K^+ or low extracellular Na^+, stimulation of the Na^+, K^+ pump leads to considerable force recovery.[38] Similarly, when the capacity of the Na^+, K^+ pump is reduced, muscle force decline is greater and force recovery is considerably slower.[38] The Na^+, K^+ pump therefore appears to play a significant role in second to second restoration and maintenance of excitability in exercising skeletal muscle,[8,38] in contrast to previous thoughts that the pump was only predominantly active to restore resting membrane potential following contraction.

5.4.5 Chloride channels

Chloride (Cl^-) is another ion present in skeletal muscle that can exert a significant effect on K^+. The T system has a higher permeability to Cl^- than to K^+ (permeability refers to the extent that a membrane allows particles to pass through it), and quite a large concentration of Cl^- is present in the T system. In fact, the membrane potential is weighted towards the Cl^- equilibrium potential (a balance between the movement of an ion in one direction due to its concentration gradient and the movement in the opposite direction due to its electrical potential difference, resulting in no movement of ions across the cell membrane, i.e. an equilibrium). The large amount of Cl^- in the T system and the relatively large amount of Cl^- movement into the cell that would be required to change the intracellular Cl^- concentration means that any inward movement of Cl^- during repolarisation will have much less effect on membrane potential than would a matched outward movement of K^+.[1] The Cl^- conductance (conductance means that an electrical charge can move easily across a membrane; for ions, permeability and conductance occur simultaneously) across the T system membrane means that if enough K^+ moved out of the muscle cell and into the T system, then the membrane potential across the T system will be more negative than the K^+ equilibrium potential.[39] In this situation, K^+ would be 'driven' down its electrochemical gradient back into the muscle fibre through inward rectifier channels (a group of K^+-specific ion channels found in cell membranes).[1] This would assist in returning the cell to its resting membrane potential. Therefore, Cl^- may reduce the rate of K^+ accumulation and help the recovery of K^+ back into the muscle fibre. In support of this, muscles with no Cl^- conductance are unable to maintain a muscle contraction, and complete failure of muscle action potentials are seen.[1,8,40]

5.4.6 Metabolic acidosis

Reduced muscle pH may increase the activity of pH sensitive K^+ channels within the muscle membrane, leading to a greater loss of K^+ from muscle.[41–2] This would suggest that any role of extracellular K^+ accumulation on muscle fatigue would be exacerbated during high-intensity exercise, where reduced muscle pH is more likely. Several studies have shown an association between reductions in exercising muscle pH and increased K^+ loss from the muscle.[12,25,41–2] However, this relationship has been questioned by other work that appears to show a protective effect of reduced muscle pH on force production in muscles that have lost notable amounts of K^+.[43–7] Increased muscle acidosis can reduce the Cl^- conductance across the muscle membrane. This is important because reducing the inhibitory Cl^- shifts the balance between inhibitory Cl^- currents and excitatory Na^+ currents in favour of the excitatory current, meaning that less Na^+ is required to enter the muscle in order to propagate an action potential.[47] This would counteract the depressive effect of increased extracellular K^+ levels on membrane excitability. However, studies reporting a protective effect of pH on muscle force were *in vitro* studies, meaning that they used isolated muscle fibres or groups of fibres to study the relationship between reduced pH and K^+, rather than an intact animal or person (*in vivo* research). As a result, many of the studies used muscle fibres that did not have an active Na^+, K^+ pump, which caused a larger membrane depolarisation than would occur during normal muscle activity.[44] Furthermore, some of the studies incubated the muscle preparations in lactic acid, lowering extracellular pH more than intracellular pH, which would not occur when muscles are stimulated to fatigue *in vivo*.[44] This may explain why a protective effect of reduced pH on K^+-depressed muscle force is absent during repeated *in vivo* muscle contractions.[44]

Key point

Many studies have shown no reduction in muscle excitability at the point of fatigue during exercise. The body has many mechanisms that work to prevent losses in muscle excitability. Therefore, these mechanisms can also work to reduce the influence of extracellular K^+ accumulation on muscle excitability.

Key point

The protective effect of acidosis on the force production of K^+ depressed muscle has been shown using *in vitro* research. This research may not be able to accurately replicate the full functionality of *in vivo* muscle tissue, which could explain the absence of a protective effect of acidosis on muscle force in K^+-depressed muscle *in vivo*.

5.5 Is extracellular potassium accumulation a significant cause of exercise fatigue?

There is evidence for a role of extracellular K^+ accumulation in the development of exercise fatigue (Section 5.3). However, much of this support stems from *in vitro* research. As was touched upon in Section 5.4.6, it is possible that results from *in vitro* research are confined to those specific experimental conditions, which involve placing muscle preparations in situations and stimulating muscle function in ways that do not reflect a fully functioning *in vivo* muscle.[48] This is further highlighted by the discussions in Section 5.4 detailing some of the many ways in which intact muscle function can be altered and modified to reduce the influence of factors such as extracellular K^+ accumulation on membrane depolarisation and muscle function. For these reasons, we should be cautious about accepting K^+ loss from muscle as a significant cause of exercise fatigue until the time that more compelling *in vivo* research suggests otherwise.[1,48]

Key point

On balance, current research suggests that extracellular K^+ accumulation is not a significant cause of exercise fatigue. However, further work is warranted to confirm this position, and to fully understand the *in vivo* responses to extracellular K^+ accumulation.

5.6 Calcium: description and function

Like K, Ca is a mineral. Calcium is the most abundant mineral in the body. Milk, yoghurt, and cheese are rich sources of dietary Ca, along with kale, broccoli, sardines, and salmon. While spinach is commonly (and correctly) known to contain a lot of Ca, it is not a particularly good source of dietary

Ca as its bioavailability is poor (bioavailability is the fraction of an ingested substance that reaches the systemic circulation). Ninety-nine per cent of body Ca stores are located in the skeleton (including the teeth), about 1% is located in intracellular fluid, and about 0.1% in extracellular fluid. The cationic form of calcium (Ca^{2+}) is, like K^+, an electrolyte that carries a small positive electrical charge.

Key point

Calcium is the most abundant mineral in the body. Dietary sources of Ca include milk, yoghurt, cheese, kale, broccoli, sardines, and salmon.

Calcium plays important roles in a number of physiological and biochemical processes. These include:

- Acting as a second messenger in signal transduction pathways. Signal transduction is a cascade of processes beginning with an extracellular signaller (a hormone or neurotransmitter) interacting with a receptor on a cell surface, which causes a change in the action of an intracellular messenger which in turn alters the function of the cell. For example, the extracellular signal generated by neurotransmission of an action potential into a muscle fibre stimulates release of Ca^{2+} into the myoplasm where it can then enable the process of muscle contraction to occur (this is discussed later in the chapter).
- Neurotransmitter release from neurons. Neuronal synapses contain Ca^{2+} channels that open when depolarised, allowing Ca^{2+} to flow through the presynaptic membrane and increase internal Ca^{2+} concentration. This activates Ca^{2+}-sensitive proteins attached to vesicles which contain a neurotransmitter. The proteins change shape, allowing the vesicles to open and transfer their neurotransmitter across the synaptic cleft (the narrow space between the pre- and postsynaptic cells).
- A cofactor (a non-protein molecule that assists in biochemical reactions) for enzymes such as those of the blood clotting cascade.
- Cell membrane excitability, particularly in the heart and neurons.
- Bone formation and maintenance of bone mineral density.
- Vasodilation of endothelial tissue (the thin layer of cells coating the inside of blood and lymph vessels).

While the above is not an exhaustive list of the roles of Ca, there is one role that stands out. That is the role of Ca (or more specifically, Ca^{2+}) in muscle contraction. This role will be the focus of discussion for the rest of the chapter (the reader is recommended to consult a general anatomy and physiology text for an overview of the role of Ca^{2+} in muscle contraction).

Key point

Calcium plays important roles in signal transduction cascades, neurotransmitter release, as a cofactor for enzyme function, in cell membrane excitability, bone formation and density, endothelial tissue vasodilation, and muscle contraction.

5.7 Calcium and exercise fatigue

The release of appropriate amounts of Ca^{2+} from its storage site within muscle, the SR, is critical for muscle contraction and appropriate force development (Figure 5.4). If the amount of Ca^{2+} in the SR drops substantially below its normal level, the amount of Ca^{2+} released in each action potential is reduced and muscle force production drops.[49–50] Interestingly, reduced muscle force will still occur even if the amount of Ca^{2+} in the SR drops but is still sufficient to fully saturate binding sites on troponin C,[49] and increasing SR Ca^{2+} content above that normally found does not increase the amount of Ca^{2+} release during an action potential.[50] Therefore, impairments in SR Ca^{2+} kinetics (the coordinated movement of Ca^{2+} into and out of the SR and the myoplasm) can reduce muscle force and may contribute to fatigue development (Figure 5.4). The obvious question is: what can cause impaired SR Ca^{2+} kinetics?

Key point

Release of appropriate amounts of Ca^{2+} from the SR is crucial for muscle force production. If insufficient Ca^{2+} is released, muscle force will decline.

Key point

Alterations in Ca^{2+} kinetics can reduce muscle force and may contribute to fatigue development.

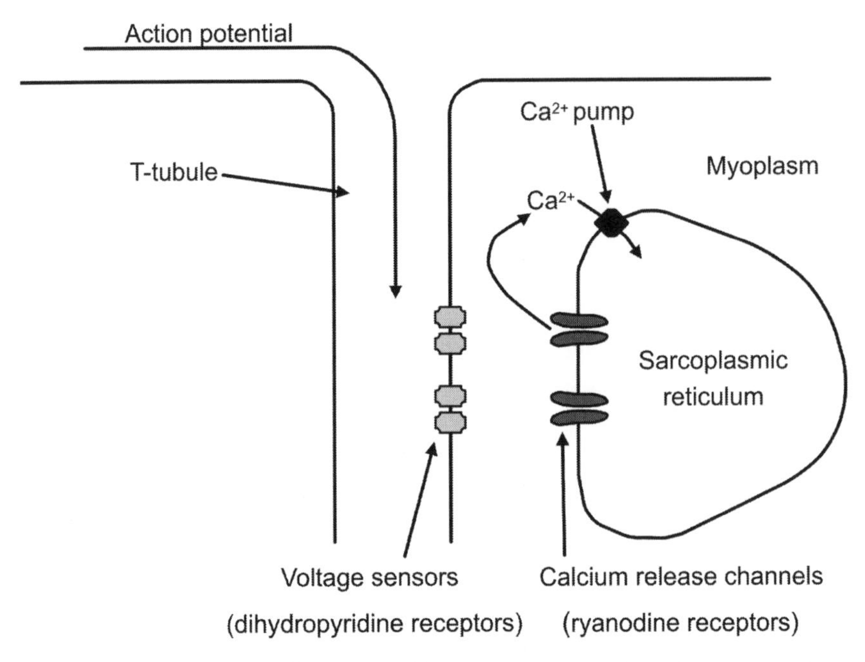

Figure 5.4 The release of Ca^{2+} from the SR. An action potential conducted along the sarcolemma and into the t-tubule stimulates voltage sensors on the t-tubular membrane. These voltage sensors in turn stimulate Ca^{2+} release channels to open, allowing Ca^{2+} to enter the myoplasm. Calcium is sequestered back into the SR via the Ca^{2+} pump.

Source: Allen *et al.*[84]

5.7.1 *Impaired calcium kinetics due to glycogen depletion and acidosis*

Chapter 2 discussed how the link between muscle glycogen depletion and muscle force reduction is not fully understood. However, studies have established an apparent association between muscle glycogen depletion and impaired Ca^{2+} kinetics.[51–5] Calcium kinetics regulates the amount of free Ca^{2+} that is present in the myoplasm, and is therefore crucial for optimal muscle force production. Regulation of Ca^{2+} kinetics is controlled by the opening of Ca^{2+} release channels (which control the release of Ca^{2+} from the SR), and by activity of the SR Ca^{2+} pump (similar to the Na^+, K^+ pump discussed in Section 5.2) which moves Ca^{2+} back into the SR (Figure 5.4). Impaired Ca^{2+} release from the SR could contribute to fatigue by reducing the amount of Ca^{2+} that is available to bind to troponin C, thereby impairing the excitation–contraction coupling process, and reduced Ca^{2+} uptake into the SR can slow the rate of relaxation of a muscle and indirectly cause reduced force production.

There is limited research into the influence of exercise on SR responses in humans. However, existing studies have identified that prolonged exercise can cause disturbances in Ca^{2+} uptake and release.[52–3,56–7] Interestingly, Ca^{2+} release is impaired in a low glycogen state, but this impairment is delayed when sufficient carbohydrate is consumed to modify muscle glycogen stores.[52] Despite this knowledge, the specific role of low muscle glycogen in impaired Ca^{2+} kinetics is still under debate. It is plausible that muscles contracting with depleted glycogen stores experience a reduced ability to regenerate ATP, leading to ATP depletion in specific areas of the cell that could affect both SR Ca^{2+} release and uptake (this was also touched upon in Section 2.2.3.2.1).[58–9] There is also some evidence to suggest the presence of a 'complex' of enzymes associated with glycogen synthesis and breakdown in close association with the SR.[53,60–1] Depletion of glycogen stores could impair the function of this enzyme complex, which in turn could impact on energy availability in important areas of the SR (for example the Ca^{2+} pump and Ca^{2+} release channels). Therefore, glycogen could impair Ca^{2+} kinetics due to its role as an energy source.

Interestingly, there is some evidence to suggest that the influence of glycogen content on Ca^{2+} kinetics is *not* related to its role as a fuel source. Some studies have shown that the ability of a muscle to respond to depolarisations of the t-tubular system is dependent on muscle glycogen concentration even when other sources of fuel are available, such as ATP and PCr. It may be that glycogen depletion locally to the SR could cause structural changes in the SR itself, which may impair SR function.[53,55] Whatever the specific mechanism(s), it does appear that adequate muscle glycogen is important for optimal SR Ca^{2+} kinetics. This further reinforces the potential importance of glycogen in the fatigue process (Chapter 2).

Key point

Calcium release from the SR is delayed in a low muscle glycogen state, which may be related to localised ATP depletion. However, impaired Ca^{2+} kinetics are seen in a low glycogen state despite the availability of other fuel sources, suggesting the role of glycogen in impaired Ca^{2+} handling may not be related to its role as a fuel source.

The role of acidosis in SR Ca^{2+} release and binding to troponin C was discussed in Section 3.3.2.1, and the reader is referred to this section. To briefly summarise, it appears that acidosis does not impair the normal process of Ca^{2+} release from the SR, not does it significantly impact on the contractile process once Ca^{2+} has been released from the SR.

Key point

Under normal physiological conditions, acidosis causes little inhibitory effects on Ca^{2+} release from the SR or on the contractile process once Ca^{2+} has been released.

5.7.2 Inorganic phosphate

When energy demand for muscle contraction is high, ATP concentration will remain constant for a very short time but phosphocreatine (PCr) will be broken down to creatine and inorganic phosphate (P_i).[1] As a result, P_i can accumulate within the muscle (P_i is also produced by the hydrolysis of ATP, as summarised in equation 2.1). Inorganic phosphate plays very important roles in a number of biochemical and biological processes, including energy metabolism. However, as we shall see in this section, accumulation of P_i outside of normal physiological concentrations can be a problem.

Elevated P_i concentration can directly impair muscle force by inhibiting the ability of the contractile proteins actin and myosin to enter a high force state.[1] The reduction in muscle force attributed to P_i-induced interference with cross bridging occurs early on in the fatigue process, at least in type II muscle fibres. However, it is important to note that a lot of the research showing reduced force production via direct influence of P_i on contractile proteins was *in vitro* work conducted at much lower temperatures than are found inside the body. In fact, the inhibition of cross-bridge force production by P_i is greatly reduced as the muscle temperature rises.[62] The extent of the decrease in cross-bridge force production as a result of P_i accumulation is probably only about 10% of maximum force production at normal physiological muscle temperature.[1]

Key point

Accumulation of P_i can prevent actin-myosin cross-bridges from entering a high force state, thereby reducing muscle force. This occurs early in the fatigue process, at least in type II fibres.

Key point

The inhibition of cross-bridge force production by P_i is greatly reduced as muscle temperature rises, and is only equivalent to about 10% of maximal force production at normal physiological temperature.

Although the direct influence of P_i on actin-myosin cross bridging may be comparatively minor, any changes in cross-bridge function can also influence the relationship between intracellular Ca^{2+} concentration and muscle force.[1] Specifically, increased P_i concentration may reduce the contractile response (and hence force production) of the muscle fibre to a given Ca^{2+} concentration.[63–5] This is termed a reduction in Ca^{2+} sensitivity.[63] Interestingly, the reduction in Ca^{2+} sensitivity due to P_i accumulation appears to be greater as muscle temperature gets nearer to normal physiological temperature. This is the opposite response to the inhibition of cross-bridge force by P_i, which decreases as the temperature rises. Therefore, impaired Ca^{2+} sensitivity due to P_i accumulation may play a much more important role than cross-bridge inhibition in muscle fatigue, particularly in the later stages of fatigue when intracellular Ca^{2+} concentration decreases (discussed below).[1]

Key point

Accumulation of P_i can reduce Ca^{2+} sensitivity (the amount of force produced for a given myoplasmic Ca^{2+} concentration). Calcium sensitivity is further reduced as muscle reaches normal physiological temperature, which is the opposite response to cross-bridge inhibition. Therefore, reduced Ca^{2+} sensitivity may be important in the later stages of fatigue when myoplasmic Ca^{2+} concentration decreases.

Continuation of the fatigue process is associated with a reduced myoplasmic Ca^{2+} concentration which, along with reduced Ca^{2+} sensitivity, is thought to account largely for the rapid reduction in muscle force that usually precedes exercise termination.[1] Reduced myoplasmic Ca^{2+} concentration suggests that the amount of Ca^{2+} being released from the SR is also reduced. There are two main ways in which reduced SR Ca^{2+} release may occur: one is inhibition of the SR Ca^{2+} release channels by P_i, and the other is Ca^{2+} and P_i precipitation in the SR.

Key point

The later stages of the fatigue process are associated with reduced myoplasmic Ca^{2+} concentration. Along with reduced Ca^{2+} sensitivity, this is thought to account largely for the rapid reduction in muscle force that usually precedes exercise termination.

Key point

Two main ways in which reduced SR Ca^{2+} release may occur are inhibition of the SR Ca^{2+} release channels by P_i, and Ca^{2+} and P_i precipitation in the SR.

As summarised in Section 5.7 and Figure 5.4, Ca^{2+} leaves the SR via specialised release channels. In the early stages of muscle fatigue, P_i appears to act on the SR Ca^{2+} release channel in such a way that myoplasmic Ca^{2+} concentration increases. However, in the later stages of fatigue this is reversed, and P_i accumulation contributes to a reduction in myoplasmic Ca^{2+} concentration, probably by affecting the sarcoplasmic Ca^{2+} release mechanism.[1,66] The inhibition of SR Ca^{2+} release by P_i depends on changes in myoplasmic magnesium (Mg^{2+}) concentration (Section 5.7.3), with the inhibitory effect of P_i larger at greater Mg^{2+} concentrations.[67] Magnesium also binds to many of the same intramuscular sites as Ca^{2+}, and it is this competitive binding that allows Mg^{2+} to exert many of its inhibitory effects.

Key point

In the early stages of fatigue, P_i appears to act on the SR release channel in a way that increases myoplasmic Ca^{2+} concentration. In the later stages of fatigue this is reversed, and P_i contributes to reduced myoplasmic Ca^{2+} concentration, perhaps by affecting SR Ca^{2+} release.

Key point

Inhibition of SR Ca^{2+} release by P_i is greater when myoplasmic Mg^{2+} concentration is higher.

A second way by which P_i may reduce SR Ca^{2+} release is via Ca^{2+}–P_i precipitation in the SR. When P_i accumulates in the myoplasm, some P_i may enter the SR and combine with free Ca^{2+} to form a Ca^{2+}–P_i solid (termed a precipitate). This has the effect of reducing the concentration of free Ca^{2+} in the SR, and therefore the amount of Ca^{2+} that is able to be released into the myoplasm with each action potential.

Key point

Accumulation of P_i may cause it to enter the SR and combine with Ca^{2+} to form a Ca^{2+}–P_i precipitate. This would reduce the amount of free Ca^{2+} in the SR, and therefore the amount that is able to be released into the myoplasm.

The existence of a phosphate permeable channel in the SR was discovered in 2001,[68] providing further support for the theory of Ca^{2+}–P_i precipitation in the SR. Despite this, it is interesting and important to note that Ca^{2+}–P_i precipitation has not been conclusively demonstrated in a research setting.[69] However, there is evidence to suggest that precipitation does occur. *In vitro* studies have shown reduced resting myoplasmic Ca^{2+} concentration and faster Ca^{2+} reuptake into the SR following injections of P_i, which points to a reduced SR Ca^{2+} concentration.[70–1] Furthermore, substances that stimulate SR Ca^{2+} release, such as caffeine, stimulate less Ca^{2+} release in fatigued muscle, which is suggestive of a reduced SR Ca^{2+} availability.[72] Sarcoplasmic reticulum Ca^{2+} concentration has also been shown to decrease during fatiguing contractions stimulated by agents such as caffeine or via t-tubular action potentials, with Ca^{2+} leakage/loss from the muscle cells unable to account for this reduction.[73] Finally, the theory of Ca^{2+}–P_i precipitation is strengthened by the fact that reduced myoplasmic Ca^{2+} concentration (suggestive of reduced SR Ca^{2+} concentration/release) is lessened or delayed in mice that do not have the enzyme creatine kinase.[74] This means that the mice are unable to effectively break down PCr; therefore, the normal fatigue-induced rise in P_i concentration is greatly reduced.

Key point

The precipitation of Ca^{2+} and P_i in the SR has not conclusively been demonstrated. However, there is evidence to suggest that precipitation does occur.

It appears that Ca^{2+}–P_i precipitation has research support, and should be considered a candidate for causing reduced muscle force production during exercise fatigue. However, as always, it is not quite that simple! As mentioned above, the accumulation of P_i in the myoplasm occurs quite early on in the fatigue process (via breakdown of PCr), but reductions in myoplasmic Ca^{2+} concentration occur later in the process. If reduced Ca^{2+} release from the SR is caused by P_i entering the SR, why is there a delay between P_i appearance and reduced Ca^{2+} release from the SR? Also, there appears to be an association between reduced myoplasmic Ca^{2+} concentration and myoplasmic Mg^{2+} concentration, which is likely associated with ATP breakdown.[1,75] Some of the SR membrane channels that may transport P_i into the SR open more readily in the face of low ATP levels, meaning that P_i movement into the SR may be inhibited by ATP.[76] This may also explain delayed entry of P_i into the SR, as some of the channels through which P_i enters the SR are blocked at normal ATP levels and may only open during the final stages of fatigue when local ATP depletion can occur. However, not all research agrees with this suggestion.[66] Finally, the amount of Ca^{2+} and P_i required to cause precipitation may be greater in the SR than in the relatively simple experimental solutions used in *in vitro* research. This is because Mg^{2+} and ATP both inhibit precipitation of Ca^{2+} and P_i, and Mg^{2+} and ATP are often omitted from experimental solutions.[66] As a result, *in vitro* research may overestimate the potential for Ca^{2+}–P_i precipitation *in vivo*. Presently, there remains insufficient direct evidence to confirm that Ca^{2+}–P_i precipitation has a significant role to play in altered Ca^{2+} kinetics and exercise fatigue in humans.

Key point

Some research findings cannot be easily reconciled with the theory of Ca^{2+}–P_i accumulation in the SR. Currently, there is not enough evidence to conclusively say that Ca^{2+}–P_i precipitation alters Ca^{2+} cycling and contributes to fatigue in exercising humans.

5.7.3 ATP depletion and Magnesium accumulation

During intense exercise ATP concentration may fall (particularly in localised areas) and PCr concentration can be significantly reduced (Sections 2.2.1 and 2.2.2). Adenosine diphosphate (ADP) and Mg^{2+} concentrations can also increase (Mg^{2+} is bound to ATP, and the hydrolysis of ATP produces Mg^{2+} as a by-product as ADP, adenosine monophosphate (AMP) and inosine monophosphate (IMP), which all can be produced via ATP hydrolysis, have a lower affinity for Mg^{2+} than does ATP).[1] There is little direct influence of ATP depletion (unless to very low levels) or Mg^{2+} accumulation on the contractile apparatus, but elevated Mg^{2+} reduces Ca^{2+} sensitivity.[1,77]

Key point

There is little direct influence of ATP depletion (unless to very low levels) or Mg^{2+} accumulation on the contractile apparatus in muscle. However, high Mg^{2+} levels reduce Ca^{2+} sensitivity.

Sarcoplasmic reticulum Ca^{2+} pumps play a crucial role in Ca^{2+} kinetics, as they transport Ca^{2+} back into the SR to ensure an appropriate rate of muscle relaxation following contraction (Figure 5.4). If ATP concentration at the sites of the SR pumps is reduced (SR pump activity is ATP dependent) then Ca^{2+} reuptake into the SR is also reduced. Simply put, less Ca^{2+} is pumped into the SR for a given amount of ATP hydrolysis, meaning the process has become less energy efficient.[1] Increased ADP concentration (which is, of course, associated with greater ATP depletion) also reduces SR Ca^{2+} pump rate and increases leakage of Ca^{2+} back through the pumps into the myoplasm.[1,78] However, this issue appears to be prevalent only in type II muscle fibres.[79] As for the role of Mg^{2+} in SR Ca^{2+} pump activity? Raised Mg^{2+} concentration seems to have little to no effect on the rate of SR Ca^{2+} uptake.[80]

Key point

ATP depletion at the site of the SR Ca^{2+} pumps can reduced Ca^{2+} reuptake into the SR. Accumulation of ADP also reduces Ca^{2+} pump rate. Raised Mg^{2+} concentration has little effect on the rate of SR Ca^{2+} uptake.

The SR Ca^{2+} release channels (Figure 5.4) are stimulated by ATP in a similar way to the SR Ca^{2+} pump. When ATP concentration falls, voltage-sensor-stimulated Ca^{2+} release from the SR is reduced.[1] The presence of Mg^{2+} is a strong inhibitor of SR Ca^{2+} release channels,[81] and has been shown to reduce SR Ca^{2+} release by up to 40%.[82] When localised ATP depletion and Mg^{2+} accumulation occur at the same time, the reduction in Ca^{2+} release is even greater.[1] As a result, reduced ATP concentration and increased Mg^{2+} concentration are probably at least partly responsible for the reduced myoplasmic Ca^{2+} concentration that is observed during high-intensity muscle contraction.[1,83] This reduction in myoplasmic Ca^{2+} content may be a protective response from the muscle in the face of reduced ATP concentration. Reduced SR Ca^{2+} release would reduce the amount of Ca^{2+} available to take part in the cross-bridge process and the amount that would be needed to be pumped back into the SR. Both these processes (cross bridging and SR Ca^{2+} reuptake) require ATP, so by reducing their activity the cell is conserving remaining ATP stores, albeit at the expense of muscle force.[1]

Key point

ATP depletion and Mg^{2+} accumulation both inhibit Ca^{2+} release from the SR, and this reduction is greater when ATP depletion and Mg^{2+} accumulation occur together.

5.8 Are altered calcium kinetics a significant cause of exercise fatigue?

There is a large amount of research to suggest that changes in muscle Ca^{2+} kinetics play a significant role in muscle fatigue during exercise. Reductions in muscle force production during the early phase of fatigue may be due to direct impairment of cross-bridge function due to P_i accumulation, with the later stages of fatigue associated with reduced Ca^{2+} sensitivity of contractile proteins and impaired release and reuptake of Ca^{2+} from/to the SR.[1] However, there is still debate about the relative importance of the mechanisms of change in muscle Ca^{2+} levels during contraction.[69] It should be considered that much of our knowledge of alterations in Ca^{2+} kinetics during exercise has come from *in vitro* studies on isolated animal muscle fibres.[1] The experimental models used in this form of research do not always accurately reflect the highly complex and dynamic intramuscular environment of intact human muscle. Our acceptance and application of the findings should be tempered with this awareness.

5.9 Summary

- Potassium is one of the most common chemical elements in the body, and plays important roles in processes such as cellular water balance, many biochemical reactions, and changing of the electrical potential across cell membranes that allows the propagation of action potentials.
- Appropriate action potential propagation is crucial for muscle function, and disturbances could lead to impaired function.
- Repeated muscle contractions cause a net loss of K^+ from the muscle, and an accumulation of K^+ in the extracellular space. This K^+ loss occurs mainly through specialised K^+ channels in the muscle membrane.
- Accumulation of extracellular K^+ has been associated with reduced muscle excitation and force production, perhaps due to the altered electrochemical gradient and reduced membrane depolarisation associated with extracellular K^+ accumulation.
- Recovery of the action potential and muscle force occurs when the rate of muscle stimulation is reduced, which suggests that reduced muscle force is due to reduced muscle cell excitation caused by membrane depolarisation. It also suggests that the influence of extracellular K^+ accumulation is dependent in part on exercise intensity.
- Reduced time to fatigue, and the occurrence of fatigue at the same extracellular K^+ concentration, provides further support for the role of extracellular K^+ accumulation in the fatigue process.
- There is contrasting evidence on the influence of extracellular K^+ accumulation on muscle function, with some studies showing no impairment of muscle membrane excitability at fatigue, even with notable extracellular K^+ accumulation.

- The body has many mechanisms that work in concert to prevent or minimise losses in membrane excitability, such as alterations to motor unit recruitment, motor neuron firing rate, action potential firing rate, activation of the Na^+, K^+ pump, and the importance of Cl^- on the membrane potential and movement of K^+ across the muscle membrane.
- These mechanisms suggest that intact muscle responses can be altered and modified to minimise the potential impact of extracellular K^+ accumulation on muscle function. For these reasons, findings from *in vitro* work into K^+ and muscle function should be interpreted with caution.
- Potassium accumulation may contribute to muscle soreness and discomfort, and the development of central fatigue, via stimulation of type III and IV muscle afferents.
- Calcium is the most abundant mineral in the body, and plays important roles in signal transduction, neurotransmitter release, enzyme function, membrane excitability, bone formation and density, endothelial tissue vasodilation, and muscle contraction.
- The release of appropriate amounts of Ca^{2+} into the SR and the adequate reuptake of Ca^{2+} back into the SR is crucial for optimal muscle function.
- If the amount of Ca^{2+} in the SR drops substantially, less Ca^{2+} is released from the SR with each action potential, and muscle force declines.
- Muscle glycogen appears to have a regulatory role in Ca^{2+} release and/or reuptake. This role could relate to glycogen as a source of ATP resynthesis (i.e. a fuel source), or it may be independent of this and instead be due to structural changes in the SR caused by low muscle glycogen content.
- Under normal physiological conditions, acidosis does not appear to impair SR Ca^{2+} release or the role of Ca^{2+} in the contractile process itself.
- Accumulation of P_i could directly impair the ability of actin and myosin to enter high force states, reducing muscle force. However, this mechanism is thought to be minor, at least at physiological temperatures.
- Inorganic phosphate can also reduce the contractile response to a given amount of Ca^{2+} (Ca^{2+} sensitivity), and reduce the amount of Ca^{2+} released from the SR by inhibiting the activity of SR release channels and by precipitating with Ca^{2+} in the SR.
- Calcium-P_i precipitation is supported by indirect experimental evidence, however other findings make precipitation difficult to justify. As a result, the specific extent of precipitation, and any role it may play in Ca^{2+} kinetics and muscle fatigue, remains under debate.
- Depletion of ATP and accumulation of Mg^{2+} can, individually and in combination, reduce Ca^{2+} release from and reuptake into the SR, although Mg^{2+} does not appear to have much influence on the rate of SR Ca^{2+} uptake.

To think about . . .

As we develop the ability to study the function of the body in ever more detail, the importance of the complex interplay between so many organ systems, metabolic pathways, hormones, compounds, molecules, and elements and how this influences function and performance becomes more pronounced. Clearly, this benefits our understanding of human exercise physiology. However, it may also open up new avenues of human function that could be unfairly exploited in order to gain a competitive advantage in sport.

What are your thoughts on this? What benefits do you see in studying the molecular control of exercise performance? And what are the risks/negatives? Do you think that the benefits outweigh the risks?

Test yourself

Answer the following questions to the best of your ability. Try to understand the information gained from answering these questions before you progress with the book.

1. What are the primary dietary sources of K?
2. What are the main roles that K^+ plays in body function?
3. Describe the process of action potential propagation, with reference to the movement of Na^+ and K^+ across the neuron and muscle membranes.
4. How might accumulation of extracellular K^+ contribute to muscle dysfunction?
5. List and briefly describe the six mechanisms that can help to minimise the influence of extracellular K^+ accumulation on muscle membrane depolarisation.
6. What are the primary dietary sources of Ca?
7. What are the main roles that Ca plays in body function?
8. What is meant by the term Ca^{2+} kinetics?
9. What are the two ways in which reduced muscle glycogen is thought to impair Ca^{2+} kinetics?
10. List the four ways in which P_i accumulation may impair Ca^{2+} kinetics.
11. What is the main impact of ATP depletion and Mg^{2+} accumulation, alone and in combination, on SR Ca^{2+} release and reuptake?

References

1 Allen DG, Lamb GD, Westerblad H (2008) Skeletal muscle fatigue: cellular mechanisms. *Physiol Rev* 88: 287–332.
2 Stephenson D (2006) Tubular system excitability: an essential component of excitation-contraction coupling in fast twitch fibres of vertebrate skeletal muscle. *J Muscle Res Cell Motil* 27: 259–74.
3 Clausen T, Nielsen OB, Harrison AP, Flatman JA, Overgaard K (1998) The Na^+, K^+ pump and muscle excitability. *Acta Physiol Scand* 162: 183–90.
4 Clausen T (2008) Role of Na^+, K^+ pumps and transmembrane Na+, K^+ distribution in muscle function. *Acta Physiol* 192: 339–49.
5 McKenna MJ, Bangsbo J, Renaud JM (2008) Muscle K^+, Na^+, and Cl^- disturbances and Na+, K^+ pump inactivation: implications for fatigue. *J Appl Physiol* 104: 288–95.
6 Pedersen KK, Nielsen OB, Overgaard K (2013) Effects of high-frequency stimulation and doublets on dynamic contractions in rat soleus muscle exposed to normal and high extracellular [K^+]. *Physiol Rep* 1: 1–11.
7 Sejersted OM, Sjøgaard G (2000) Dynamics and consequences of K^+ shifts in skeletal muscle and heart during exercise. *Physiol Rev* 80: 1411–81.
8 Clausen T (2011) In isolated skeletal muscle, excitation may increase extracellular K^+ 10-fold; how can contractility be maintained? *Exp Physiol* 96: 356–68.
9 Davies NW (1990) Modulation of ATP-sensitive K^+ channels in skeletal muscle by intracellular protons. *Nature* 343: 375.
10 Fitts RH, Balog EM (1996) Effect of intracellular and extracellular ion changes on E-C coupling and skeletal muscle fatigue. *Acta Physiol Scand* 156: 169–81.
11 Medbø JI, Sejersted OM (1990) Plasma potassium changes with high intensity exercise. *J Physiol* 421: 105–22.
12 Nordsborg N, Mohr M, Pedersen LD, Nielsen JJ, Langberg H, Bangsbo J (2003) Muscle interstitial K^+ kinetics during intensity exhaustive exercise: effect of previous arm exercise. *Am J Physiol Regul Integr Comp Physiol* 285: R143–8.
13 Balog EM, Fitts RH (1996) Effects of fatiguing stimulation on intracellular Na^+ and K^+ in frog skeletal muscle. *J Appl Physiol* 81: 679–85.
14 Juel C (1986) K^+ and sodium shifts during *in vitro* isometric muscle contraction, the time course of the ion-gradient recovery. *Pflugers Arch* 406: 458–63.
15 Jones DA, Bigland-Ritchie B, Edwards RHT (1979) Excitation frequency and muscle fatigue: mechanical responses during voluntary and stimulated contractions. *Exp Neurol* 64: 414–27.
16 Bigland-Ritchie B, Jones DA, Woods JJ (1979) Excitation frequency and muscle fatigue: electrical responses during human voluntary and stimulated contractions. *Exp Neurol* 64: 414–27.
17 Nielsen OB, de Paoli FV (2007) Regulation of Na^+–K^+ homeostasis and excitability in contracting muscles: implications for fatigue. *Appl Physiol Nutr Metab* 32: 974–84.
18 Clausen T (2003) Na^+, K^+ pump regulation and skeletal muscle contractility. *Physiol Rev* 83: 1269–324.
19 Cairns SP, Dulhunty AF (1995) High-frequency fatigue in rat skeletal muscle: role of extracellular ion concentrations. *Muscle Nerve* 18: 890–8.
20 Dutka TL, Lamb GD (2007) Transverse tubular system depolarisation reduces tetanic force in rat skeletal muscle fibres by impairing action potential repriming. *Am J Physiol Cell Physiol* 292: C2112–21.
21 Thompson LV, Balog EM, Riley DA, Fitts RH (1992) Muscle fatigue in frog semitendinosus: alterations in contractile function. *Am J Physiol Cell Physiol* 262: C1500–6.

22 Bangsbo J, Madsen K, Kiens B, Richter EA (1996) Effect of muscle acidity on muscle metabolism and fatigue during intensity exercise in man. *J Physiol* 495: 587–96.
23 Bangsbo J, Graham T, Johansen L, Strange S, Christensen C, Saltin B (1992) Elevated muscle acidity and energy production during exhaustive exercise in humans. *Am J Physiol Regul Integr Comp Physiol* 263: R891–9.
24 Nielsen JJ, Mohr M, Klarskov C, Kristensen M, Krustrup P, Juel C, Bangsbo J (2004) Effects of high-intensity intermittent training on potassium kinetics and performance in human skeletal muscle. *J Physiol* 554: 857–70.
25 Mohr M, Nordsborg N, Nielsen JJ, Pedersen LD, Fischer C, Krustrup P, Bangsbo J (2004) Potassium kinetics in human muscle interstitium during repeated intense exercise in relation to fatigue. *Pflugers Arch* 448: 452–6.
26 Bigland-Ritchie B, Cafarelli E, Vøllestad NK (1986) Fatigue of submaximal static contractions. *Acta Physiol Scand Suppl* 556: 137–48.
27 Bigland-Ritchie B, Furbush F, Woods JJ (1986) Fatigue of intermittent submaximal voluntary contractions: central and peripheral factors. *J Appl Physiol* 61: 421–9.
28 Bigland-Ritchie B, Johansson R, Lippold OC, Woods JJ (1983) Contractile speed and EMG changes during fatigue of sustained maximal voluntary contractions. *J Neurophysiol* 50: 313–24.
29 Sandiford SD, Green HJ, Duhamel TA, Schertzer JD, Perco JD, Ouyang J (2005) Muscle Na-K-pump and fatigue responses to progressive exercise in normoxia and hypoxia. *Am J Physiol Regul Integr Comp Physiol* 289: R441–9.
30 West W, Hicks A, Mckelvie R, O'Brien J (1996) The relationship between plasma K^+, muscle membrane excitability and force following quadriceps fatigue. *Pflugers Arch* 432: 43–9.
31 Enoka RM, Stuart DG (1992) Neurobiology of muscle fatigue. *J Appl Physiol* 72: 1631–48.
32 Bigland-Ritchie B, Woods JJ (1984) Changes in muscle contractile properties and neural control during human muscular fatigue. *Muscle Nerve* 7: 691–9.
33 Balog EM, Thompson LV, Fitts RH (1994) Role of sarcolemma action potentials and excitability in muscle fatigue. *J Appl Physiol* 76: 2157–62.
34 Gandevia SC (2001) Spinal and supraspinal factors in human muscle fatigue. *Physiol Rev* 81: 1725–89.
35 Bigland-Ritchie B, Zijdewind I, Thomas CK (2000) Muscle fatigue induced by stimulation with and without doublets. *Muscle Nerve* 23: 1348–55.
36 Juel C (1988) Muscle action potential propagation velocity changes during activity. *Muscle Nerve* 11: 714–9.
37 Lännergren J, Westerblad H (1986) Force and membrane potential during and after fatiguing, continuous high-frequency stimulation of single *Xenopus* muscle fibres. *Acta Physiol Scand* 128: 359–68.
38 Clausen T, Nielsen OB, Harrison AP, Flatman JA, Overgaard K (1998) The Na^+, K^+ pump and muscle excitability. *Acta Physiol Scand* 162: 183–90.
39 Wallinga W, Meijer SL, Alberink MJ, Vliek M, Wienk ED, Ypey DL (1999) Modelling action potentials and membrane currents of mammalian skeletal muscle fibres in coherence with potassium concentration changes in the T-tubular system. *Eur Biophys J* 28: 317–29.
40 Van Beekvelt MC, Drost G, Rongen G, Stegeman DF, Van Engelen BG, Zwarts MJ (2006) Na^+-K^+-ATPase is not involved in the warming-up phenomenon in generalized myotonia. *Muscle Nerve* 33: 514–23.
41 Davies NW, Standen NB, Stanfield PR (1992) The effect of intracellular pH on ATP-dependent potassium channels of frog skeletal muscle. *J Physiol* 445: 549–68.
42 Davies NW, Standen NB, Stanfield PR (1991) ATP-dependent potassium channels of muscle cells: their properties, regulation and possible function. *J Bioenerg Biomembr* 23: 509–23.

43 Hansen AK, Clausen T, Nielsen OB (2005) Effects of lactic acid and catecholamines on contractility in fast twitch muscles exposed to hyperkalemia. *Am J Physiol Cell Physiol* 289: C104–12.
44 Kristensen M, Albertsen J, Rentsch M, Juel C (2005) Lactate and force production in skeletal muscle. *J Physiol* 562: 521–6.
45 Overgaard K, Højfeldt G, Nielsen O (2010) Effects of acidification and increased extracellular potassium on dynamic muscle contractions in isolated rat muscles. *J Physiol* 588: 5065–76.
46 Pedersen TH, Nielsen OB, Lamb GD, Stephenson DG (2004) Intracellular acidosis enhances the excitability of working muscle. *Science* 305: 1144–7.
47 Pedersen TH, de Paoli F, Nielsen OB (2005) Increased excitability of acidified skeletal muscle: role of chloride conductance. *J Gen Physiol* 125: 237–46.
48 Place N (2008) Is interstitial K^+ accumulation a key factor in the fatigue process under physiological conditions? *J Physiol* 586: 1207–8.
49 Dutka TL, Cole L, Lamb GD (2005) Ca^{2+} phosphate precipitation in the sarcoplasmic reticulum reduces action potential-mediated Ca^{2+} release in mammalian skeletal muscle. *Am J Physiol Cell Physiol* 289: C1502–12.
50 Posterino GS, Lamb GD (2003) Effect of sarcoplasmic reticulum Ca^{2+} content on action potential-induced Ca^{2+} release in rat skeletal muscle fibres. *J Physiol* 551: 219–37.
51 Chin ER, Allen DG (1997) Effects of reduced muscle glycogen concentration on force, Ca^{2+} release and contractile protein function in intact mouse skeletal muscle. *J Physiol* 498: 17–29.
52 Duhamel TA, Perco JG, Green HJ (2006) Manipulation of dietary carbohydrates after prolonged effort modifies muscle sarcoplasmic reticulum responses in exercising males. *Am J Physiol Regul Integr Comp Physiol* 291: R1100–10.
53 Duhamel TA, Green HJ, Stewart RD, Foley KP, Smith IC, Ouyang J (2007) Muscle metabolic, SR Ca^{2+}-cycling responses to prolonged cycling, with and without glucose supplementation. *J Appl Physiol* 103: 1986–98.
54 Helander I, Westerblad H, Katz A (2002) Effects of glucose on contractile function, $[Ca^{2+}]_i$ and glycogen in isolated mouse skeletal muscle. *Am J Physiol Cell Physiol* 282: C1306–12.
55 Lees SJ, Franks PD, Spangenburg EE, Williams JH (2001) Glycogen and glycogen phosphorylase associated with sarcoplasmic reticulum: effects of fatiguing activity. *J Appl Physiol* 91: 1638–44.
56 Duhamel TA, Green HJ, Perco JD, Sandiford SD, Ouyang J (2004) Human muscle sarcoplasmic reticulum function during submaximal exercise in normoxia and hypoxia. *J Appl Physiol* 97: 180–7.
57 Duhamel TA, Green HJ, Sandiford SD, Perco JG, Ouyang J (2004) Effects of progressive exercise and hypoxia on human muscle sarcoplasmic reticulum function. *J Appl Physiol* 97: 188–96.
58 Favero TG (1999) Sarcoplasmic reticulum Ca^{2+} release and muscle fatigue. *J Appl Physiol* 87: 471–83.
59 Korge P (1998) Factors limiting ATPase activity in skeletal muscle. In: *Biochemistry of Exercise* X, edited by Hargreaves M and Thompson M. Champaign, IL: Human Kinetics: 125–34.
60 Ørtenblad N, Westerblad H, Nielsen J (2013) Muscle glycogen stores and fatigue. *J Physiol* 591: 4405–13.
61 Xu K, Zweier J, Becker L (1995) Functional coupling between glycolysis and sarcoplasmic reticulum Ca^{2+} transport. *Circ Res* 77: 88–97.
62 Coupland ME, Puchert E, Ranatunga KW (2001) Temperature dependence of active tension in mammalian (rabbit psoas) muscle fibres: effect of inorganic phosphate. *J Physiol* 36: 879–91.

63 Varian KD, Raman S, Janssen PML (2006) Measurement of myofilament calcium sensitivity at physiological temperature in intact cardiac trabeculae. *Am J Physiol* 290: H2092–7.
64 Martyn DA, Gordon AM (1992) Force and stiffness in glycerinated rabbit psoas fibers: Effects of calcium and elevated phosphate. *J Gen Physiol* 99: 795–816.
65 Millar NC, Homsher E (1990) The effect of phosphate and calcium on force generation in glycerinated rabbit skeletal muscle fibers: a steady-state and transient kinetic study. *J Biol Chem* 265: 20234–40.
66 Steele DS, Duke AM (2003) Metabolic factors contributing to altered Ca^{2+} regulation in skeletal muscle fatigue. *Acta Physiol Scand* 179: 39–48.
67 Jahnen-Dechent W, Ketteler M (2012) Magnesium basics. *Clin Kidney J* 5: 3–14.
68 Laver DR, Lenz GKE, Dulhunty AF (2001) Phosphate ion channels in the sarcoplasmic reticulum of rabbit skeletal muscle. *J Physiol* 537: 763–78.
69 Allen DG, Trajanovska S (2012) The multiple roles of phosphate in muscle fatigue. *Front Physiol* 3: 1–8.
70 Allen DG, Clugston E, Petersen Y, Röder V, Chapman B, Rudolf R (2011) Interactions between intracellular calcium and phosphate in intact mouse muscle during fatigue. *J Appl Physiol* 111: 358–66.
71 Westerblad H, Allen DG (1996) The effects of intracellular injections of phosphate on intracellular calcium and force in single fibres of mouse skeletal muscle. *Pflügers Arch* 431: 964–70.
72 Westerblad H, Allen DG (1991) Changes of myoplasmic calcium concentration during fatigue in single mouse muscle fibers. *J Gen Physiol* 98: 615–35.
73 Kabbara AA, Allen DG (2001) The use of fluo-5N to measure sarcoplasmic reticulum calcium in single muscle fibres of the cane toad. *J Physiol* 534: 87–97.
74 Dahlstedt AJ, Westerblad H (2001) Inhibition of creatine kinase reduces the fatigue-induced decrease of tetanic $[Ca^{2+}]i$ in mouse skeletal muscle. *J Physiol* 533: 639–49.
75 Westerblad H, Allen DG (1992) Myoplasmic free Mg^{2+} concentration during repetitive stimulation of single fibres from mouse skeletal muscle. *J Physiol* 453: 413–34.
76 Posterino GS, Fryer MW (1998) Mechanisms underlying phosphate induced failure of Ca^{2+} release in single skinned skeletal muscle fibres of the rat. *J Physiol* 512: 97–108.
77 Blazev R, Lamb GD (1999) Low [ATP] and elevated $[Mg^{2+}]$ reduce depolarization-induced Ca^{2+} release in mammalian skeletal muscle. *J Physiol* 520: 203–15.
78 MacDonald WA, Stephenson DG (2001) Effects of ADP on sarcoplasmic reticulum function in mechanically skinned skeletal muscle fibres of the rat. *J Physiol* 532: 499–508.
79 MacDonald WA, Stephenson DG (2006) Effect of ADP on slow-twitch muscle fibres of the rat: implications for muscle fatigue. *J Physiol* 573: 187–98.
80 Kabbara AA, Stephenson DG (1994) Effects of Mg^{2+} on Ca^{2+} handling by the sarcoplasmic reticulum in skinned skeletal and cardiac muscle fibres. *Pflügers Arch* 428: 331–9.
81 Laver DR, O'Neill ER, Lamb GD (2004) Luminal Ca^{2+}-regulated Mg^{2+} inhibition of skeletal RyRs reconstituted as isolated channels or coupled clusters. *J Gen Physiol* 124: 741–58.
82 Dutka TL, Lamb GD (2004) Effect of low cytoplasmic [ATP] on excitation-contraction coupling in fast-twitch muscle fibres of the rat. *J Physiol* 560: 451–68.
83 Dahlstedt AJ, Katz A, Wieringa B, Westerblad H (2000) Is creatine kinase responsible for fatigue? Studies of isolated skeletal muscle deficient in creatine kinase. *FASEB J* 14: 982–90.
84 Allen DG, Lamb GD, Westerblad H (2008) Impaired calcium release during fatigue. *J Appl Physiol* 104: 296–305.

Chapter 6

Central fatigue and central regulation of performance

6.1 Introduction

In Chapter 1, two prevalent fatigue theories were introduced: peripheral fatigue and central fatigue (Section 1.1). Briefly, peripheral fatigue refers to causes of fatigue that are outside of the central nervous system (CNS), through processes distal to the neuromuscular junction. Central fatigue refers to causes of fatigue located within the CNS, with loss of contractile force occurring through processes proximal to the neuromuscular junction (within the brain, spinal nerves, and motor neurons). Up to now, Part II of this book has discussed potential causes of exercise fatigue that are more peripheral in origin (although the interactive effect of peripheral and central processes should be considered). Historically, fatigue research tended to focus exclusively on central or peripheral fatigue, with minimal crossover or investigation into the combined influence of these mechanisms. This may have been due to the fundamental difficulties in studying fatigue, in particular central fatigue.

Despite the development of numerous hypotheses (mainly related to peripheral fatigue) over the decades in an attempt to explain exercise fatigue, including those discussed in previous chapters, no clear and consistent link has been established between any single hypothesis and fatigue during exercise. Perhaps in response to this lack of consensus, there has been a resurgence in research over the last two decades investigating the role of central processes in the regulation of exercise performance. This research is offering new insights, and raising new debates, into fatigue during exercise. This chapter will begin by discussing some of the potential causes of central fatigue during exercise, before addressing a related concept, the central regulation of exercise performance.

6.2 Central fatigue

6.2.1 Potential 'causes' of central fatigue

Central fatigue does not have a model as clearly defined as that of peripheral fatigue. Reduced CNS drive to the motor neurons can be caused by a reduction in corticospinal impulses reaching the motor neuron (descending) and/or neurally-mediated afferent feedback from muscle (ascending).[1] The development of central fatigue was addressed in Chapter 4 with regard to hyperthermia. However, there are other hypotheses of how central fatigue may develop, and these are discussed in the following sections.

6.2.1.1 Sensory feedback from muscle afferents

Observation of a concurrent reduction in force, contraction relaxation rate and motor neuron discharge rate during maximal voluntary contractions and electrically stimulated contractions led to a 'sensory feedback hypothesis' which states that inhibition of neuronal firing rates is due to a reflex mediated by feedback from group III and IV muscle afferents. These muscle afferents can be stimulated by mechanical and chemical stimuli such as H^+ and K^+ production, both of which can accumulate in and around the muscle during exercise (Sections 3.3.2 and 5.3.1). Stimulation of group III and IV afferents inhibit central motor drive during exercise, which would reduce the extent of muscle activation and therefore generate a central fatigue response.[2] The stimulation of these muscle afferents by substances such as H^+ and K^+ provides an example of how peripheral changes may influence central responses, highlighting a link between peripheral and central fatigue. It is possible that stimulation of group III and IV muscle afferents may increase sensations of pain and discomfort from the exercising muscles, which could increase the perception of effort during exercise and contribute to impaired exercise performance and/or tolerance (Sections 3.3.1 and 5.3.1).

Interestingly, group III and IV afferent stimulation is also involved in the attenuation of peripheral fatigue, as they provide feedback to brain centres that control cardiovascular and ventilatory responses to exercise.[3–5] Research has shown that when group III and IV muscle afferent feedback is blocked by the use of local anaesthetics during exercise, blood circulation and ventilation are significantly impaired, causing arterial hypoxemia (abnormally low arterial blood oxygen levels) and increased metabolic acidosis.[2]

Key point

Stimulation of group III and IV muscle afferents by mechanical and chemical stimuli during exercise can inhibit central motor drive, reducing muscle activation and generating a central fatigue response.

6.2.1.2 Brain neurotransmitters

Newsholme *et al.*[6] developed the first hypothesis to implicate changes in central neurotransmission with the development of fatigue, termed the 'central fatigue hypothesis'. These authors suggested that during prolonged exercise the production and metabolism of key monoamines (compounds with a single amine group, in particular neurotransmitters) was altered, and that this influenced central function during exercise. Of particular interest was the brain neurotransmitter serotonin. The serotinergic system is an important modulator of mood, sleep, emotion and appetite.[7] Simply put, increased production of serotonin increases feelings of lethargy and tiredness. Serotonin is synthesised within the brain, as it is unable to cross the blood–brain barrier (BBB). A key precursor for the synthesis of serotonin is the essential amino acid tryptophan (TRP). Tryptophan transport across the BBB is the rate-limiting step in serotonin synthesis within the brain,[7] meaning that the more TRP that crosses the BBB into the brain, the more brain serotonin is synthesised. At rest, most (80–90%) available TRP is transported in the blood bound to a binding protein called albumin, with the rest circulating freely in plasma (free TRP, or f-TRP). However, during exercise an increase in blood free fatty acid (FFA) concentration occurs. These FFA compete with TRP for binding to albumin, meaning that during prolonged exercise (when blood FFA may increase the most due to lower glycogen availability), a significant increase in f-TRP can occur. A strong positive relationship has been found between the proportion of f-TRP in blood and brain TRP concentrations,[8] suggesting that TRP crosses the BBB more easily when it is present in its free form. As mentioned before, increased concentrations of brain TRP lead to increased brain serotonin production, and it is this exercise-induced brain TRP uptake that was originally proposed to cause the sensations of tiredness, lethargy, and lack of motivation to continue exercise characteristic of central fatigue.[6]

Tryptophan utilises the same BBB transport proteins as the amino acids leucine, isoleucine, and valine. These three amino acids are commonly referred to as branched chain amino acids (BCAAs), as their structures contain side-chains composed of carbon atoms. The greater the plasma concentration of BCAAs, the more competition there will be between TRP and BCAAs for entry into the brain, and less TRP will make it to the brain. During prolonged exercise, plasma BCAA concentration remains stable or falls.[9] This, combined with the exercise-induced increase in plasma f-TRP concentration, would further increase brain TRP uptake and, therefore, serotonin synthesis. A logical assumption would be that reducing the plasma concentration ratio of f-TRP to BCAA via ingestion of BCAA during prolonged exercise would reduce brain TRP uptake, serotonin production and, hence, central fatigue.[7] While initial field-based research did find support for the use of BCAA's in improving physical and mental performance during prolonged exercise,[10] much subsequent laboratory work has not corroborated these findings.[11–16] Therefore, the evidence supporting BCAA supplementation for improving prolonged exercise performance is limited and, at best, circumstantial.[7] There is some evidence to support the use of BCAA supplementation for improving mental/cognitive performance during prolonged exercise. Wisnik *et al.*[17] found that BCAA ingestion improved multiple-choice reaction time during a treadmill-based simulated soccer protocol by ~10% compared to a placebo.

The complexity of brain function makes it unlikely that a single neurotransmitter is responsible for central fatigue, and this is further supported by the contradictory and largely negative results from studies that have manipulated only serotonergic activity.[7] Dopamine and noradrenaline are catecholaminergic neurotransmitters that have been implicated in enhancing prolonged exercise performance,[18–19] potentially via inhibition of serotonin synthesis and direct activation of central motor pathways.[1] Dopamine has been implicated in increased arousal, motivation and cognition, and the control of motor behaviour.[20] However, in humans exercising in mild ambient temperatures it has been consistently reported that supplementation with dopamine precursors (substances that are required for the synthesis of dopamine) and re-uptake inhibitors (substances that block the removal of dopamine from its synaptic targets and its return to its pre-synaptic neuron) fails to improve prolonged exercise performance.[21–3] This may be because the influence of dopamine is not strong enough in normal environmental temperatures.[24]

Similarly to dopamine, noradrenaline is involved in the regulation of arousal, consciousness, and brain reward centres. Less well researched than dopamine, the use of noradrenaline re-uptake inhibitors has failed to find significant improvements in endurance exercise performance.[25] In fact, noradrenaline re-uptake inhibitors are associated with reduced endurance exercise performance of ~5–10%. This may be due to the stimulatory effect of noradrenaline neurons on the serotinergic system.[26] Interestingly, the use of a dopamine re-uptake inhibitor that also inhibits the re-uptake of noradrenaline has been demonstrated to improve prolonged exercise only when performed in the heat.[23] Both dopamine and noradrenaline have been linked to thermoregulation, and this may explain why manipulations that increase their concentration seem to improve performance during exercise in the heat, as they may work to extend the 'safe' limits of hyperthermia.[27]

The influence of brain neurotransmitters on central fatigue during prolonged exercise in humans is still being investigated. While it does appear that serotonin and dopamine are involved in central fatigue, they do not seem able to significantly influence fatigue individually.[26] Noradrenaline negatively effects exercise performance in a temperate environment. During exercise in the heat, dopamine and noradrenaline in combination appear to have a greater effect on performance than serotonin. The apparent difficulty in altering exercise performance in thermoneutral environments by manipulation of neurotransmitters suggests other potential causes of central fatigue should be investigated.

Key point

Any potential role of central neurotransmitters on fatigue is likely to involve a combination of the key neurotransmitters serotonin, dopamine, and noradrenaline. The exact influence, if any, may also depend on the exercise duration and environmental temperature.

6.2.1.3 Brain ammonia accumulation

Ammonia is a natural by-product of the metabolism of nitrogenous (nitrogen containing) compounds, such as proteins and amino acids. It is crucial that ammonia is metabolised as excess accumulation can result in significant cellular and organ dysfunction and can be life threatening. In humans, ammonia is metabolised to urea via the urea cycle in the liver. This urea is then excreted in urine.

Ammonia is produced in the body in several ways. At rest, most ammonia is produced from the gastrointestinal tract via the breakdown of the amino acid glutamine and urea.[28] Ammonia is also produced in the brain, kidneys, and skeletal muscle. Within skeletal muscle, ammonia is produced via the deamination (removal of an amine group) of adenosine monophosphate (AMP) as part of the purine nucleotide cycle (Figure 6.1). This indicates that skeletal muscle ammonia production will increase during intense muscle contraction. Indeed, at exercise intensities below 50–60% VO_{2max} very little ammonia accumulation occurs, but accumulation rapidly increases as intensity rises above this level.[29] During exercise, skeletal muscle oxidation of BCAA's can increase ~4 fold over resting rates. If exercise is prolonged, BCAA oxidation increases further due to the depletion of glycogen stores.[30] Greater oxidation of BCAA's can also significantly increase ammonia production. Anything from 75–90% of the ammonia produced in muscle during exercise is retained in the muscle until completion of exercise, where it is gradually released and metabolised.[31] This is beneficial, as rapid release from muscle could raise blood ammonia concentrations to levels that could cause significant health risks.

Key point

During exercise, ammonia is produced in muscle through the breakdown, in separate reactions, of adenosine monophosphate and branched chain amino acids.

$$1.\ AMP + H_2O + H^+ \xrightarrow{AMPD} IMP + NH_4^+$$

$$2.\ IMP + GTP + Aspartate \xrightarrow{AS} Adenylosuccinate + GDP + P_i$$

$$3.\ Adenylosuccinate \xrightarrow{AL} AMP + Fumarate$$

Figure 6.1 The three interlinked reactions that compose the purine nucleotide cycle. This metabolic pathway acts to increase the concentration of Krebs cycle metabolites via the production of fumarate, an intermediate of the Krebs cycle. Note the production of ammonium ($NH4^+$, protonated ammonia) as a result of the deamination of AMP (reaction 1). During intense exercise, accumulation of IMP inhibits reactions 2 and 3 of the cycle. This prevents the reamination of AMP, promoting the accumulation of IMP and ammonia. AMP = adenosine monophosphate; AMPD = AMP deaminase, IMP = inosine monophosphate; GTP = guanosine-5'-triphosphate; AS = adenylosuccinate synthetase, GDP = guanosine diphosphate; AL = adenylosuccinate lyase.

Ammonia influences brain function positively at low concentrations, by providing substrate for neuron metabolism and neurotransmission, and negatively at high concentrations, by impairing normal cellular function.[32] These negative influences manifest in symptoms including impaired brain mitochondrial function[33] and inhibition of locomotor activity via ammonia-stimulated glutamate production in brain regions controlling motor activity.[32] Performing fatiguing, intense exercise has been shown to produce systemic ammonia concentrations similar to those observed in patients with liver disorders. The influence of ammonia accumulation in the periphery, even during severe exercise, appears inconsequential with regard to fatigue development,[34] and as a result, the role of ammonia in exercise-induced fatigue fell somewhat out of favour as a research topic.[32] However, research investigating the influence of ammonia production on central function during exercise has revealed some interesting findings. It appears that peripheral ammonia production, as occurs during hard and/or exhaustive exercise, may lead to an increase in ammonia transport across the BBB and into the cerebral tissues.[32] Once in the brain, ammonia may act negatively on central function, as summarised above. Indeed, research has now demonstrated a significant uptake and accumulation of ammonia in the cerebral tissue during long duration (2–3 hrs cycling)[33] and shorter exhaustive exercise (arm and leg, 9–16 mins duration).[35] However, it is not yet clear whether this accumulation is significant enough to contribute to cellular and neurotransmitter dysfunction.[32]

Ammonia appears to accumulate and exert effects mainly in brain areas associated with learning, memory, and motor activity.[36] It is unlikely that this accumulation will exert any negative effects during short duration exercise, regardless of the intensity.[35] Impairments in cognitive function of diseased patients can take 2–3 hrs after the onset of hyperammonaemia.[37] During prolonged exercise, uptake of ammonia across the BBB can exceed its rate of detoxification, leading to an accumulation that could have negative consequences.[33] Therefore, any contribution of ammonia to fatigue during exercise is likely to occur during prolonged exercise, and manifest as negative alterations in cognitive function. However, more research is required that directly tests and evidences this theory.[32]

Key point

The influence of ammonia accumulation on fatigue development during exercise would probably be limited to cognitive disturbances during prolonged exercise only.

6.2.1.4 Cytokines

Cytokines are intercellular signalling proteins produced by numerous cells throughout the body, including skeletal muscle. They play a key role in intercellular communication and are intimately involved in the immune system response to illness. For example, pro-inflammatory cytokines (those involved in generating a systemic inflammatory response) are thought to induce the feelings of fatigue, lethargy, and sluggishness characteristic of many common transient and more chronic illnesses.

It is this fatigue-inducing role of cytokines during illness that lead to the hypothesis that cytokine production elicits sensations of fatigue during and after exercise.[38] During exercise, skeletal muscle production of the pro-inflammatory cytokine interleukin 6 (IL-6) can reach 50 times that at rest.[38] This is likely stimulated by an energy crisis in the working muscles (Figure 6.2),[39] suggesting IL-6 production is greater during prolonged exercise. Interleukin-6 may also be produced post-exercise in the inflammatory response to exercise-induced muscle damage.[40] The combined effect of IL-6 production and of the inflammatory response to muscle damage causes increased production of the cytokines interleukin 1 (IL-1) and tumour necrosis factor (TNF). Both IL-1 and IL-6 induce sleep-promoting effects on the CNS, and all three of these cytokines have pyrogenic (fever-inducing) capabilities.[41–2] Therefore, they may produce sensations of fatigue during exercise. This is reinforced by research demonstrating increased sensations of fatigue and reduced exercise performance with acute administration of IL-6.[42]

Further evidence for a role of cytokine production on central fatigue comes from research in people with chronic diseases that have a strong inflammatory component, such as rheumatoid arthritis and cancer. In these conditions, lethargy, tiredness, and lack of motivation have been associated with pro-inflammatory cytokine production.[43] Furthermore, cytokine production can influence central neurotransmission by altering the availability of amino acid precursors of brain neurotransmitters including dopamine and serotonin, and the function of the neurotransmitters themselves (highlighting a potential link between cytokine production and the brain neurotransmitter hypothesis discussed in Section 6.2.1.2).[43] However, the relevance of this in an acute exercise situation has not been studied. While cytokine production may correlate with loss of muscle function, or at least reduced exercise performance,[42] the causal relationship between their production and fatigue still needs to be clearly demonstrated.[44]

Key point

Cytokines are small intercellular signalling proteins. Skeletal muscle produces cytokines during exercise that may be involved in generating fatigue-inducing sensations in the CNS.

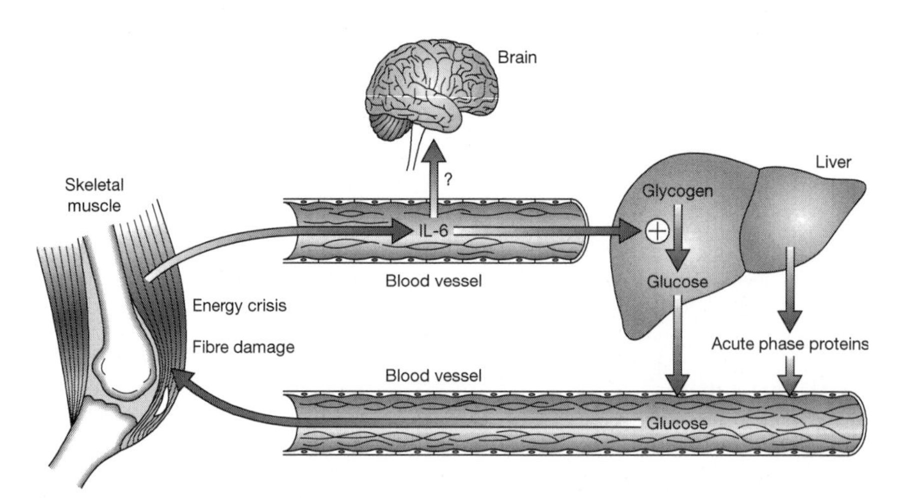

Figure 6.2 Energy crisis within working skeletal muscle, most likely glycogen depletion, increases the skeletal muscle production of IL-6. This increases the systemic concentration of IL-6, which acts to promote liver glycogenolysis, lipolysis, and production of acute-phase proteins. Interleukin 6 may also influence the development of central fatigue, individually and in combination with IL-1 and TNF, both of which are produced partly as a result of IL-6 production. Adapted from Gleeson.[39]

6.2.1.5 *Summary*

Central fatigue has multiple hypotheses for its development. Each hypothesis has research that both supports and refutes it, in a similar vein to the peripheral fatigue hypotheses discussed in earlier chapters. The difficulty in identifying a specific cause(s) for the onset of central fatigue probably relates to the complexity behind the central control of exercise performance, the multitude of factors that can influence this control, and the difficulty in establishing experimental designs that can accurately and reliably measure parameters associated with central fatigue hypotheses.

6.3 Central regulation of exercise performance

The inability of peripheral and central fatigue processes to conclusively explain sport and exercise fatigue has required exercise scientists to widen their view in an attempt to solve the fatigue 'riddle'. An interesting perspective that has arisen, or more accurately been revived, over the last decade is the concept of the brain acting as a central 'master regulator' of exercise performance.

6.3.1 Origins of the role of the brain in exercise regulation

Figure 6.3 is an overview of the cardiovascular/anaerobic/catastrophic model of exercise performance, originally proposed by Hill and colleagues in the 1920s. You may remember that this figure was also included in the introduction to peripheral fatigue (Section 1.1.1). The figure has been included in this section for an important reason. In the top left corner of the figure is an image of the brain with the words 'governor in the brain or the heart causing a "slowing of the circulation"'. Hill suggested the presence of a 'governor' either in the heart or brain that was responsible for reducing the pumping capacity of the heart, thereby protecting it from damage due to the myocardial ischaemia that, it was thought at the time, was the cause of fatigue during exercise (Section 1.1.1).[45] Therefore, Hill and colleagues' model of fatigue, traditionally thought of as a purely peripheral model, actually included a central component, which was also alluded to in the even earlier work by Mosso[46] (Chapter 1, Part I).

Key point

The peripheral catastrophe model of exercise fatigue described by Hill and colleagues in the 1920s is traditionally considered a purely peripheral model of fatigue. However, the original model actually referred to a 'central governor' that was hypothesised to protect the heart from ischaemic damage.

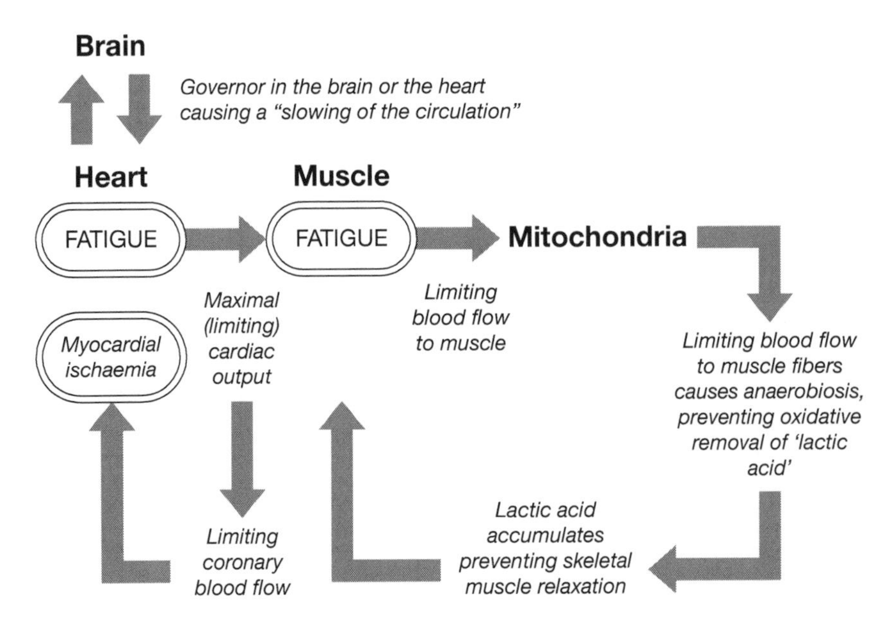

Figure 6.3 Overview of the cardiovascular/anaerobic/catastrophic model of exercise performance originally proposed by Hill and colleagues in the 1920s. From Noakes.[47]

As discussed by Noakes,[47] the 'governor' component of Hill's peripheral model of exercise fatigue was omitted in subsequent generations of academic teaching. This may be at least partly because research established that the healthy heart does not become ischaemic during even maximal exercise, thereby discrediting the role of this 'governor' as proposed by Hill *et al.* Rather than using the absence of myocardial ischaemia as stimulus to challenge Hill's model, it appears that the 'governor' component was ignored/forgotten, and the peripheral catastrophe model of exercise fatigue went on to dominate teaching and research (Section 1.1.1).

Key point

The 'central governor' component of Hill's peripheral fatigue model was omitted in subsequent generations of teaching, perhaps due to the finding that the healthy heart does not become ischaemic during even the most severe exercise.

6.3.2 Reintroduction of the role of the brain in exercise regulation

Ulmer[48] re-introduced the concept of a central programmer or governor that regulates muscle metabolic activity and performance through afferent peripheral feedback. Ulmer[48] suggested that this central programmer takes into account the finishing point of an exercise bout by using previous exercise experience and training, and knowledge of the current exercise bout, and regulates metabolic demand from the onset of exercise to achieve successful completion of exercise without catastrophic physiological failure. This maintenance of an 'appropriate' metabolic demand by the brain is termed teleoanticipation.

In a series of articles the central governor was developed further,[49–53] culminating in a full description of a model termed the 'anticipatory feedback model' of exercise regulation by Tucker.[54] The model is summarised in Figure 6.4, and a more detailed description of each phase of the model is in Table 6.1, which should be read with reference to Figure 6.4. To briefly summarise, the model states that self-paced exercise is regulated from the outset by previous exercise experience, knowledge of the expected distance or duration of the current exercise bout, and afferent physiological feedback regarding variables such as muscle glycogen levels, skin and core body temperature. The synthesis of this information allows the brain to 'predict' the most appropriate exercise intensity that will enable optimal performance without causing severe disruption to homeostasis. This prediction manifests as a rating of perceived exertion (RPE) 'template' whereby RPE will progressively rise from the beginning of exercise and reach its maximum at the predicted termination of exercise. Physical, mechanical, and biochemical variables during exercise are continuously monitored by the brain, and this afferent feedback is used to generate the athletes conscious RPE, which is continually compared to the 'template' RPE. Exercise intensity is modulated if actual RPE deviates too much (either lower or higher) from the template RPE. This modulation of exercise intensity continues until the conscious RPE returns to an acceptable level that the brain interprets can be tolerated until the end of exercise. The anticipatory feedback model therefore holds that fatigue, rather than a physical state, is in-fact a conscious sensation generated from interpretation of subconscious regulatory processes.[52,55] It also suggests that RPE, rather than simply a direct manifestation of afferent physiological feedback, plays a significant role in preventing excessive exercise duration / intensity by acting as the motivator behind an athlete's decision to stop exercise or to adjust intensity to ensure exercise completion without significant physical damage.[54] In essence, the model states that the brain protects us from ourselves.

It is important to note that the anticipatory feedback model described in Figure 6.4 and Table 6.1 relates to self-paced exercise, where the athlete is able to voluntarily alter exercise intensity. During fixed intensity exercise to

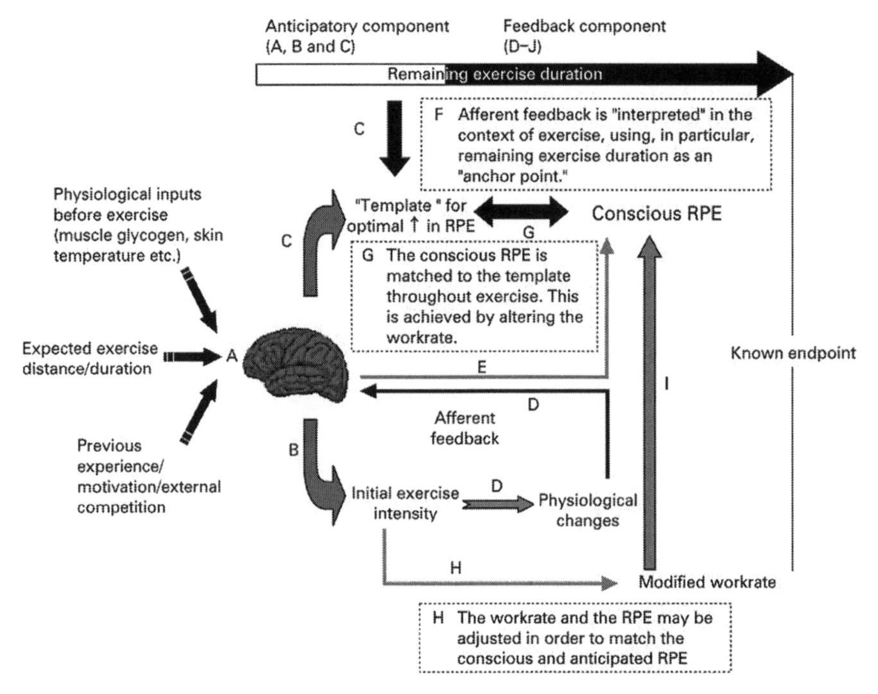

Figure 6.4 The anticipatory feedback model of exercise regulation. This proposes that afferent information from a variety of sources allows the brain to develop an ideal template RPE and, therefore, exercise intensity for a given exercise bout that will enable optimal performance while preventing significant homeostatic disruption. From the onset of exercise, actual RPE is measured against this template, and work rate is modulated to ensure that the actual exercise intensity does not deviate significantly from the template. Continued regulation is enabled by afferent monitoring of physiological changes and knowledge of the remaining duration of the exercise bout. Adapted from Tucker.[54]

Key point

The concept of a central governor that regulates exercise performance was reintroduced in the 1990s. Subsequent research developed the model into the anticipatory regulation model of exercise performance.

exhaustion (for example, running on a treadmill at 75% VO_{2max} for as long as possible), it is proposed that RPE is set by the brain at the onset of exercise as described above, and that the rate of rise of RPE is influenced by afferent feedback and the duration of exercise completed. However, the expected

Table 6.1 Summary of each phase of the proposed anticipatory feedback model of exercise regulation. The descriptions in the table should be read with continued reference to Figure 6.4 to aid clarity

Phase	*Description*
A	Afferent information from physiological variables, knowledge of the expected exercise duration, previous experience, and level of motivation/competition enables the brain to forecast the most appropriate exercise intensity (and RPE) for the upcoming exercise bout.
B	Using the information derived from phase A, the athlete selects the most appropriate exercise intensity at the onset of exercise.
C	In conjunction with phase B, a template for optimal rate of rise in RPE is developed, with the goal of reaching maximal RPE at exercise termination and not before. Conscious (i.e. actual) RPE is continually compared to this 'ideal' RPE throughout exercise.
D	Changes in physiological variables that occur during exercise are constantly relayed back to the brain.
E	These signals are interpreted by the brain, and conscious RPE is developed and modulated depending on the nature of these afferent physiological signals.
F	The remaining exercise duration is a key anchor that afferent physiological data is compared against, and thereby influences conscious RPE.
G	Conscious RPE is continually compared with the anticipated ideal rate of rise in RPE, to determine if the current, conscious RPE is acceptable based on the brains initial projections made in phases A and B.
H	Exercising work rate is adjusted, if necessary, to ensure that the conscious RPE and the template RPE remain closely matched.
I	Work rate is continually adjusted until conscious RPE returns to an acceptable level that the brain interprets can be sustained until the end of the exercise bout.

Source: information in the table is based on descriptions by Tucker.[54]

Key point

The anticipatory regulation model of exercise performance states that the brain 'predicts' the appropriate intensity of an exercise bout based on prior experience, knowledge of the exercise duration/distance, and physiological status before exercise. During exercise, continual physiological afferent feedback and knowledge of remaining exercise duration/distance generates the conscious perception of effort (RPE) which is compared to the template RPE, and exercise intensity is modified to keep the template and conscious RPE as similar as possible.

exercise duration/distance cannot be used to modify RPE as there is no known duration/distance. Also, the athlete is unable to modify exercise intensity based on changes in RPE. As a result, time to fatigue is determined by the rate at which RPE rises to the maximal level that can be tolerated.[54] A slower rate of rise in RPE would facilitate a longer time to fatigue; a higher rate of rise in RPE would mean a shorter time to fatigue.

6.4 Support for the anticipatory regulation model of exercise performance

6.4.1 Anecdotal support

Anecdotal support for a hypothesis (particularly one as complex as the anticipatory regulation model) is, of course, the weakest type of support. However, it is still worth touching on. Exercise, regardless of the type, intensity, or duration, is almost always voluntarily ended by the individual before they encounter serious physical damage to any body systems (physical damage through exercise as a result of underlying health problems is not considered here). Absence of physical damage regardless of how motivated a person may be to push themselves to their 'maximum' is interesting. If exercise termination were due to the peripheral catastrophe suggested by Hill and colleagues, whereby the exercise intensity immediately preceding exercise termination represented maximal recruitment of all available motor units and an exertion on the heart so great that the heart was near failure, then it would be reasonable to expect a greater prevalence of negative health consequences during hard/maximal exercise.

Key point

Regardless of type, duration, or intensity, exercise is almost always voluntarily ended without serious physical damage, regardless of the motivation of the individual to push themselves to their 'maximum'. If exercise termination is due to the occurrences predicted in the peripheral catastrophe model of fatigue, the prevalence of physical damage and health consequences could perhaps be expected to be greater.

6.4.2 The end-spurt phenomenon

Look back at the 'to think about' case study at the end of Chapter 1. The case study discussed the great Ethiopian runner Kenenisa Bekele setting the word record for the 10,000 metres of 26 minutes 17 seconds. Bekele ran the first 9 km of the race at an average pace of 2:38 per km, yet ran the final km in 2:32, 6 secs faster than the average speed for 90% of the race. You could of course suggest that Bekele made a pacing error, suddenly realising that he had taken the first 9 km too easy and having to pick up his pace over the final km – highly unlikely for an athlete of his calibre during a world record run! More likely is that Bekele displayed an end-spurt – a phenomenon that is actually quite commonplace in endurance exercise. The end-spurt phenomenon is characterised by a significant increase in exercise intensity near the end of a race, regardless of how hard the athlete was pushing throughout the event. Important questions are: 1. What causes, or more accurately enables, the end-spurt phenomenon to occur? 2. How does the existence of an end-spurt fit in with current theories of exercise fatigue such as those discussed in this book up to now?

Key point

The end-spurt phenomenon is characterised by a significant increase in exercise intensity near the end of a race, regardless of how hard the athlete was pushing during exercise.

The anticipatory regulation model states that exercise demand is continually monitored by the brain through afferent feedback, and this monitoring is used to influence the RPE in order for the athlete to achieve the optimal rate of rise in RPE that maximises exercise performance. Logically, the model states that knowledge of the end-point of exercise (both expected duration from the onset of the exercise bout and the duration of exercise remaining at any point during the exercise bout) is a crucial part of the calculations made by the brain in determining the appropriate exercise intensity to maintain (Figure 6.4 and phase A in Table 6.1). However, during exercise there is often a degree of uncertainty about the precise end-point of the exercise bout, and the type of effort that will need to be expended (particularly with longer duration exercise). This would be particularly true of competition events, where the final exercise time (i.e. the end-point of exercise) and the required exercise demand throughout the event would be partly dependent on the tactics and pace employed by an athlete's competitors. These factors would influence the pace of the athlete at any given time, and could necessitate alterations to pace that could not be anticipated prior to the exercise bout. As the proposed purpose of the anticipatory regulatory role of the brain is to prevent the occurrence of catastrophic changes in homeostasis,[54] this uncertainty may result in the maintenance of a motor unit and metabolic 'reserve' throughout exercise.[54] Simply put, the athlete cannot be certain of what may occur in the remainder of the exercise bout, so they (subconsciously) hold something back to enable them to respond to any potential physical challenges, and to complete the exercise bout without significant homeostatic disruption. As the end-point of exercise draws nearer, the athlete's uncertainty may decrease to the point where this 'reserve' is no longer required, and the athlete is 'allowed' to significantly increase metabolic demand and speed / power output.[54] Hence, the occurrence of the end-spurt.

Key point

Uncertainty regarding the end-point of exercise may cause a subconscious maintenance of a motor unit/metabolic 'reserve' to allow the athlete to respond to any potential physical challenges and finish exercise without significant homeostatic disruption. As the end of exercise draws nearer, uncertainty may decrease to the point where this 'reserve' is no longer required, and the athlete is 'allowed' to increase speed/power output.

The end-spurt phenomenon is not just anecdotal. Schabort *et al.*[56] asked participants to complete a 100-km cycle time trial (TT), comprising four 1-km and four 4-km maximal sprints at regular intervals, to be completed as quickly as possible. Power output decreased in each successive 1-km and 4-km sprint. However, power output increased significantly in the last 5 km of the TT compared to the first 5 km. Put another way, the participants were cycling harder from 95–100 km than they were from 0–5 km. Similarly, Kay et al.[57] asked participants to complete a 60-min self-paced cycle TT in warm, humid conditions, with six 1-min sprints interspersed throughout the TT. The authors reported that average power output, as a percentage of initial sprint power output, and quadriceps electromyography (EMG; Section 1.3.2) during the sprints fell from sprints 2–5. However, during the final sprint, power output and quadriceps EMG recovered to 94% and 90% of sprint 1 values, respectively. These findings demonstrate that neuromuscular activity declines early in exercise despite a conscious effort by participants to maintain maximal power output.[58] The EMG data suggests that the CNS reduces the amount of muscle mass recruited during exercise, even in the presence of a large muscle reserve, perhaps in order to prevent a significant metabolic crisis from occurring during the exercise bout.[53] This metabolic/neuromuscular reserve is emphasised by St Clair Gibson *et al.*,[58] who found that muscle force production during a 100 km TT declines from very early on in the time trial, despite recruitment of only about 20% of available muscle mass.

It also appears that the end-spurt phenomenon is not limited to prolonged exercise. Marcora and Staiano[59] measured participants' peak power output during a 5-second cycle sprint. On a separate occasion the participants cycled

Key point

Research has shown reductions in power output and EMG activity from the early stages of prolonged exercise, followed by an increase in these measures to levels similar to those at the beginning of exercise. This provides support for the suggestion that a metabolic and neuromuscular reserve is maintained during exercise, which the athlete is subsequently able to access near the end of the exercise bout.

at a resistance equal to 80% of their peak aerobic power until they could no longer maintain that power output (i.e. they became 'fatigued'). At this time, participants immediately completed another 5-second cycle sprint. While peak power was lower following the exhaustive exercise, it was still on average three times greater than power output at 80% of peak aerobic power which the participants had been unable to maintain just a few seconds earlier. Therefore, participants must have been physiologically able to continue exercise at 80% of peak aerobic power for longer than they did. So why did they stop? Marcora and Staiano[59] suggest that the known short duration of the peak power test (5 seconds) motivated the participants to exert a greater effort in comparison to the submaximal cycle to exhaustion, which had an unknown exercise duration. The authors also stated that their findings are evidence that fatigue (at least during the type of exercise used in their study) is not caused by an inability of the muscle to produce force, i.e. 'muscle fatigue'. The findings also agree to some extent with the anticipatory feedback model; if exercise duration is unknown, then the brain cannot accurately reconcile the physiological status of the body with the remaining exercise duration, and exercise may be stopped with a notable physiological and neuromuscular reserve, which was found by Marcora and Staiano.[59] Further support comes from research that shows people only exert their true peak power if the expected exercise duration is less than 30 seconds.[60]

Key point

The end-spurt phenomenon is not limited to prolonged exercise. Research has shown an ability to produce very high power output immediately following a cycle to voluntary 'fatigue'.

The end-spurt phenomenon has been characterised by an increase in EMG activity to working muscle.[57] This suggests that the end-spurt is central in origin (i.e. it is driven by the CNS), as EMG is a measure of the electrical signal arriving at the muscle from the motor neurons. The presence of an end-spurt ability refutes the peripheral catastrophe model of fatigue on at least two counts. First, the linear catastrophe model states that fatigue is a catastrophic failure of muscle force production that occurs when all motor units and hence muscle fibres have been fully activated. However, it has been clearly demonstrated that all motor units are not simultaneously recruited during exercise (in fact, far from it), even when subjects are required to perform maximally.[58] Second, the catastrophic nature of the peripheral fatigue model implies complete failure of force production due to factors including intramuscular substrate depletion or metabolite accumulation. If this were the case then an athlete would be unable to increase muscle force towards the end of exercise when they would be most 'fatigued', as energy depletion/metabolite accumulation would not allow it.[3] Simply put, according to the peripheral fatigue model, an end-spurt response to exercise is impossible.[3] Indeed, most of our current definitions of fatigue (Table 1.1) quantify it as an inability to maintain the required work rate. However, the display of an end-spurt at the point when an athlete should be most tired means that the athlete cannot be fatigued according to these prevalent definitions. A contrast between exercise regulation according to the peripheral catastrophe and the anticipatory regulation models is in Figure 6.5.

Key point

The end-spurt phenomenon refutes the peripheral catastrophe model of fatigue on at least two counts: 1. Not all motor units are recruited at fatigue. 2. Substrate depletion or metabolite accumulation at fatigue would render a person unable to increase their exercise intensity. Simply put, according to the peripheral fatigue model, an end-spurt exercise response is impossible.

6.4.3 Pacing strategies

The concept of pacing strategies is not exclusive to exercise; it applies to all situations where effort must be distributed in some fashion to accomplish a task.[61] With regard to sport and exercise, pacing has been defined as 'the goal directed distribution and management of effort across the duration of an exercise bout'.[61] As has been discussed previously in this book, during exercise in healthy people no physiological system demonstrates catastrophic failure,[58] and no single physiological variable accurately predicts performance or the development of fatigue in all situations.[47,62] Therefore, the concept of pacing in sport and exercise cannot be investigated from a purely physiological

A. Peripheral catastrophe model of exercise regulation

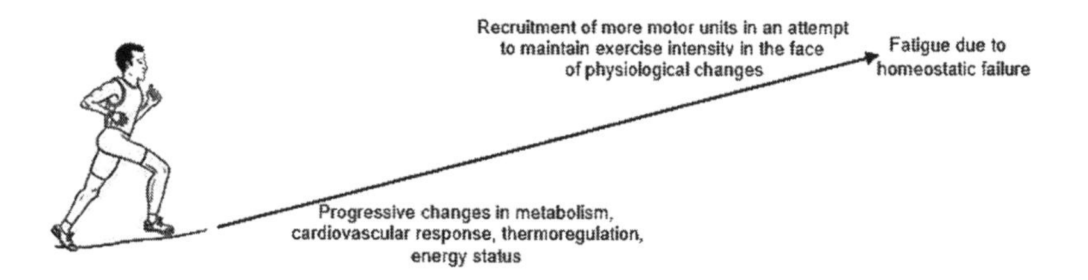

B. Anticipatory regulation model of exercise regulation

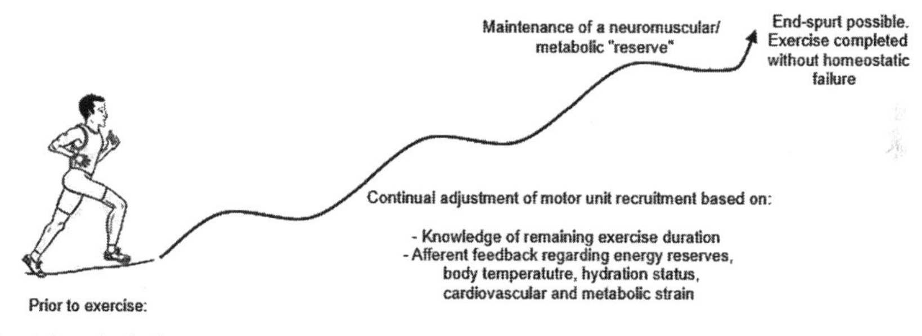

Figure 6.5 A summary of exercise regulation as explained by the peripheral catastrophe model (A) and the anticipatory regulation model (B). The peripheral catastrophe model describes a linear, progressive change in various cardiovascular, metabolic, and thermoregulatory parameters that would increasingly challenge the athlete's ability to maintain exercise intensity. In response to these changes, more motor units are recruitment in an effort to maintain intensity, until all motor units are fully recruited and fatigue occurs due to a failure in homeostasis. In contrast, the anticipatory regulation model states that an initial exercise intensity is set prior to exercise, based on knowledge of exercise duration, experience, and afferent physiological feedback. During exercise, continual afferent feedback and awareness of remaining exercise duration allows a continued adjustment of motor unit recruitment and exercise intensity, allowing the athlete to maintain a neuromuscular and/or metabolic reserve that can be accessed in the final stages of exercise. Access to this reserve enables the end-spurt phenomenon to occur, and allows the athlete to complete exercise without significant homeostatic failure.

perspective.[61] Consequently, the role of central processes must be considered in the development of a pacing strategy and how this strategy is carried out.

Five common pacing strategies used in sport and exercise are shown in Figure 6.6. The presence of pacing strategies such as these during self-paced exercises are important from the perspective of the proposed anticipatory regulation model of exercise performance. People perform exercise less well when the exercise is unfamiliar to them and the demands of the exercise are unclear.[63] Furthermore, people voluntarily reduce their exercise intensity when confronted with factors such as high ambient temperature or humidity (which could potentially impair performance), but this reduction in intensity is in advance of any actual physical need to do so (e.g. before significant increases in body heat storage), and before impairment of performance occurs as a result of any physiological system failure.[64–5] In fact, alterations in exercise intensity during endurance exercise have been reported in the first few minutes of exercise, before any peripheral physiological 'cause' of fatigue could be present.[66] These findings all suggest that the modification of exercise intensity (i.e. pacing) during self-paced exercise is conducted in anticipation of, rather than as a result of, physiological system stress/failure.[61,67]

Key point

Research shows that people voluntarily reduce exercise intensity in challenging environments and situations before there is a physical need to do so, indicating an anticipatory aspect to pacing.

As discussed in Section 6.3.2, Figure 6.4, and Table 6.1, the athlete's prior knowledge/experience of the exercise that is about to be completed may be important information that the brain uses to select an appropriate initial exercise intensity. Research into the use of pacing strategies in exercise has confirmed that the ability to pace accurately is improved with training and experience.[68–9] As Edwards and Polman[61] state, if pacing strategies are used as a way of enabling successful exercise completion without physical damage, then previous experience along with accurate knowledge of exercise demands is critical (the importance of knowledge of exercise demands in discussed in Section 6.4.4).

Key point

Prior experience improves the ability to pace effectively during exercise. This validates one aspect of the anticipatory regulation model of exercise performance.

The above paragraphs demonstrate how the use of pacing strategies in sport and exercise may provide support for aspects of the anticipatory feedback model. However, use of pacing strategies also refutes aspects of the peripheral linear catastrophe model. For example, during exercise that begins in hot conditions athletes will initiate pacing almost from the onset of exercise,[70–1] demonstrating a lower exercise intensity than would be seen at the onset of the same exercise bout in a thermoneutral environment. This pacing strategy is implemented despite fully functioning thermoregulatory systems.[70] If this exercise scenario were described by the peripheral linear catastrophe model of exercise regulation, then fatigue would occur gradually and inexorably due to a failing physiological system (in this case, thermoregulation) which would culminate in complete thermoregulatory failure and a state of exhaustion.[61] However, this scenario does not occur when an athlete can self-regulate their own performance (of course some people do suffer heat exhaustion during exercise in severe environments; however, the peripheral fatigue model states that everyone taking part in exercise in the heat would experience this. Clearly, that is not the case). Instead, during self-paced exercise a pacing strategy is observed that is dependent on the environment, exercise demands and goals, and afferent physiological feedback, which is in line with the anticipatory regulation model.[61]

Key point

The peripheral linear catastrophe model predicts that an exercising person would show a gradual and inexorable decline in pace due to a failing physiological system, before total failure of that system renders the athlete exhausted. However, this is rarely seen in a person who is free to self-regulate their exercise performance.

If an athlete's pacing strategy is determined by the accumulation of metabolic by-products, or depletion of energy stores, as predicted by the peripheral linear catastrophe model, then athletes would always begin exercise at an unsustainable pace and then gradually slow as the negative effect of the particular peripheral variables took hold.[47] In other words, the peripheral linear catastrophe model states that the only pacing strategy it is possible to follow in sport and exercise is akin to the positive strategy depicted in Figure 6.6A. The model simply does not allow for the existence of the other strategies in Figure 6.6. Yet, evidence for these other strategies is plentiful.

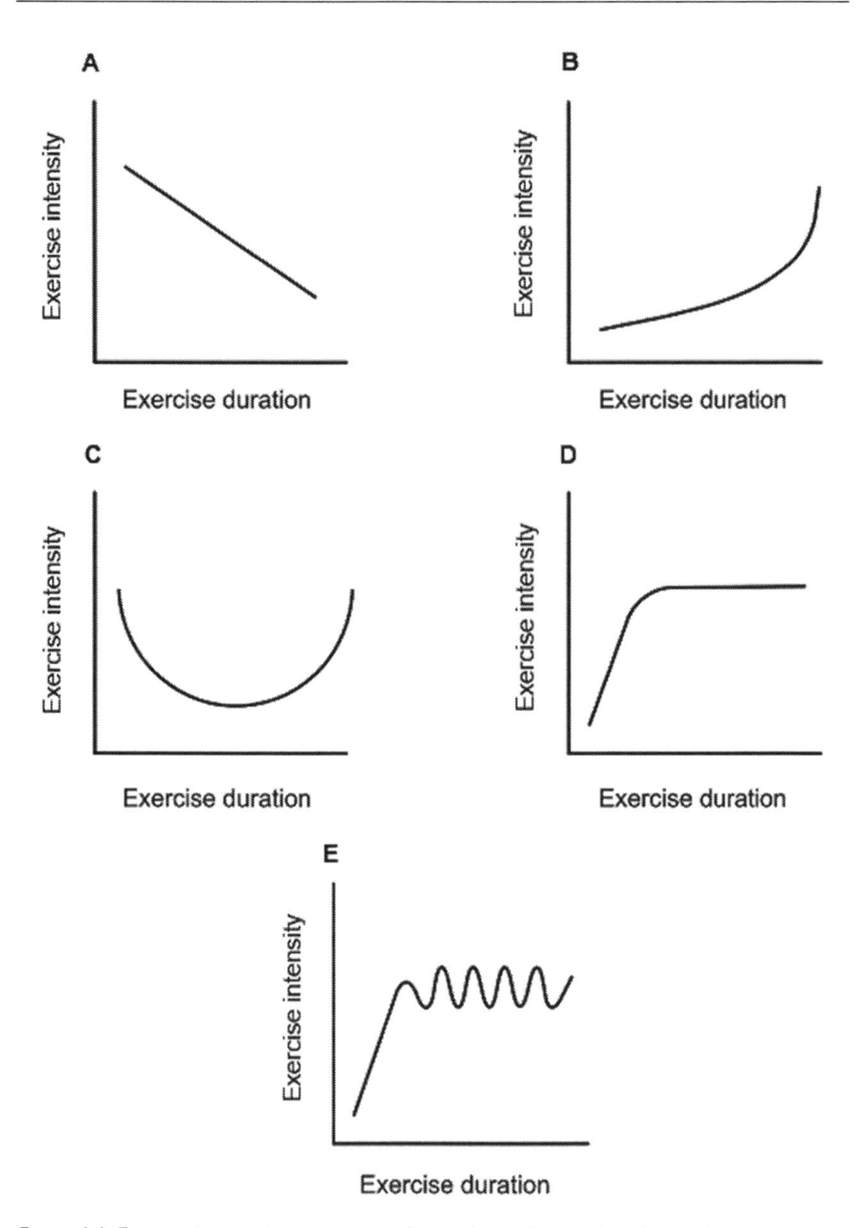

Figure 6.6 Five pacing strategies commonly employed in sport and exercise. A = positive strategy; B = negative strategy; C = parabolic strategy; D = even strategy; E = variable strategy.

Key point

The peripheral linear catastrophe model does not allow for the existence of the varied pacing strategies that have been clearly documented in the sport and exercise literature.

6.4.4 Deception studies

The importance of knowledge of exercise duration as a regulator of exercise performance is perhaps most clear when deception is employed in research studies. Commonly, participants in these studies believe they are exercising for a given period of time, but almost at completion of this time are asked to continue exercising for longer. A good example of this research model is the study of Baden *et al.*[72] These authors asked participants to run on a treadmill at 75% of their peak speed. On one occasion, they were asked to run for 20 minutes and were stopped at 20 minutes. On a second occasion, they were asked to run for 10 minutes, but at 10 minutes were asked to run for a further 10 minutes. On a third occasion, they were asked to run but were not told for how long (they were stopped after 20 minutes). The important thing to remember is that all three trials were conducted at the same running speed, and all lasted for 20 minutes. However, participants' RPE increased significantly between 10 and 11 minutes in the 10-minute deception trial, which was immediately after the deception was revealed that the participants were required to continue exercising. Correspondingly, participants affect score (a measure of how pleasurable exercise is) decreased significantly at the same time point. These changes to the perception of effort and pleasure occurred despite no changes in running speed or physiological responses to the exercise bout. The significant increase in RPE when participants are required to exercise for longer than originally thought has also been found by other researchers using very similar protocols.[73] In the study of Eston *et al.*,[73] affect also increased in the last few minutes of exercise, perhaps due to the participants being aware that the exercise was almost over. This finding relates back to the end-spurt phenomenon discussed in Section 6.4.2; an increase in pleasurable feelings towards the end of exercise may play a role in 'allowing' the end-spurt to occur. Perhaps unsurprisingly, Eston *et al.*[73] found no increase in affect in the trial where participants did not know how long they were to exercise for; in fact, affect continued to decrease throughout this trial. It therefore seems that knowledge of exercise duration is crucial for appropriate regulation of exercise performance, as suggested in the anticipatory feedback model (Figure 6.4). The increase in RPE when deception is revealed may reflect a disruption to the feed-forward/feedback mechanism (of which RPE is crucial) also suggested by the model (Figure 6.4 and Table 6.1).

Key point

When people are asked to continue exercising for longer than they anticipated, RPE can increase and affect decrease, despite no difference in exercise intensity or physiological responses to exercise.

An interesting point to raise is that Eston *et al.*[73] reported a significant increase in RPE immediately following participants being asked to continue running for longer than they thought they would have to, but this increase in RPE was not seen when participants were asked to continue cycling for longer than they thought. This finding suggests that exercise mode may influence the perceptual regulation of exercise. Eston *et al.*[73] suggested that the absence of an increase in RPE during deceived cycling exercise may be due to the lower relative exercise intensity used in the cycling compared with running trials (that the requirement to complete an additional 10-minutes of seated cycling was not considered to be as challenging as completing 10 more minutes of running), or related to the way in which RPE was collected. Eston *et al.*[73] asked participants to rate their overall (whole body) RPE; however, during cycle exercise the perceptual signals arising from the leg muscles are greater than the overall perception of exertion.[74] Therefore, overall RPE may not have been sensitive enough to reflect sudden changes in RPE arising from the legs as a result of the deception of cycling exercise duration.[73]

As well as a significant increase in RPE accompanying deception of exercise duration, it has also been shown that both RPE and physiological responses (VO_2, heart rate) are lower during exercise with an unknown duration compared to a known duration, despite no difference in the exercise intensity.[72–3] These responses may reflect a subconscious improvement in exercise economy in an effort to conserve energy due to the unknown duration of the exercise bout. This again highlights that knowledge of the end point of exercise plays a large role in the perceptual and physiological responses to that exercise bout.[75] This is further evidenced by the observation that RPE responses to exercise are robust when the exercise duration is known, even

Key point

When people are required to exercise for an unknown duration, both RPE and physiological responses such as VO_2 and heart rate may be lower compared to exercise at the same intensity for a known duration. This may reflect a subconscious improvement in exercise economy in order to conserve energy due to the unknown exercise duration.

when no information is provided to the participant about how much distance has been covered or duration is remaining.[76]

Some research has also investigated the influence of deception during repeated sprint exercise. Billaut *et al.*[77] asked participants to perform 10 × 6-second cycle sprints interspersed with 24 seconds recovery. On a second occasion, they told the participants that they would be performing 5 × 6-second sprints, but immediately after the fifth sprint participants were asked to complete a further five sprints. In a third trial, participants were asked to perform repeated 6-second sprints, but were not told how many they were going to do (they did 10). Interestingly, while RPE was not different between the three trials, more work was done in the first five sprints of the deception trial compared to the control and unknown trials. Also, the work completed in all sprints in the unknown trial was significantly lower than in the other two trials. This suggests that participants were 'holding something back' in the control and unknown trials, despite being asked to perform the sprints maximally. These findings show that pacing also occurs during short, repeated sprint exercise, and that this pacing is related to the anticipated number of sprints to be completed.

Key point

Pacing in anticipation of exercise duration also occurs during short, repeated sprint exercise. It appears that the pacing during this type of exercise is related to anticipation of the number of sprints to be performed.

Research findings from deception studies provide further evidence for some process by which people can hold back a physiological reserve during exercise of an uncertain duration.[73] These findings also provide support for a key role of the CNS in the regulation of exercise performance,[73] perhaps to ensure the maintenance of homeostasis and the presence of an emergency 'reserve' of energy/physical ability.[73,78]

6.4.4.1 The relationship between rate of rise in RPE and performance

During constant intensity exercise that continues until the individual reaches exhaustion, RPE increases linearly across a variety of intensities and environmental conditions[55] and time to fatigue is inversely related to the rate of rise in RPE.[55,79] These findings indicate that time to fatigue can essentially be 'predicted' within the first few moments of exercise.[55] Crewe *et al.*[55] suggested that the subconscious brain predicts exercise duration (perhaps through feedback from the information suggested in Figure 6.4 and Table

6.1) and sets both the early-exercise RPE and its rate of increase. This was evident in the fact that the rate of rise in RPE was set at a faster rate from the start of exercise when cycling at higher exercise intensities and in higher ambient temperatures. The findings suggest that the brain is able to sense both the increased intensity and hotter conditions, and rapidly factor these variables into its prediction of how exercise should best be regulated.

Key point

During constant load exercise to exhaustion, RPE increases linearly across a range of exercise intensities and environmental conditions, and time to fatigue is inversely related to the rate of rise in RPE. Therefore, the rate of rise in RPE can be used to predict exercise duration.

Tucker *et al.*[80] conducted a novel study in which they asked participants to cycle at a pre-determined RPE. Participants were free to vary the exercise intensity they were cycling at in order to maintain this RPE. A protocol such as this enables investigation of the influence of physiological changes on RPE and exercise performance. Participants cycled in three different ambient temperatures (15°C, 25°C, and 35°C). The authors found that after only a few minutes of exercise in the hot trial (35°C), cycling power output began to decrease more rapidly than in the other two temperatures. In other words, participants were having to reduce their exercise intensity in order to maintain the pre-determined RPE. Importantly, this lowering of exercise intensity (i.e. alteration in pacing strategy) occurred despite the absence of a higher core temperature or heart rate in the hot trial compared with the other two trials. By lowering the exercise intensity, participants slowed their rate of body heat storage so that heat storage was similar between all three trials after 20 min, and remained so for the rest of the exercise (exercise to exhaustion lasting about 35–50 minutes, depending on the environmental temperature). Tucker *et al.*[80] concluded that exercise intensity in the heat is regulated by afferent feedback related to the rate of body heat storage in the first few minutes of exercise, and that this is used to regulate intensity and, hence, rate of heat storage, for the remainder of exercise. The observation of a change in exercise intensity within the first few minutes of exercise in the heat, no difference in body heat storage between ambient temperatures, and that a critically high core temperature was not reached in any trial, suggests that the alteration in exercise intensity was made in an anticipatory fashion, driven through changes in RPE, to prevent the occurrence of a homeostatic crisis (in this case, an excessively high core body temperature).

Studies showing a relationship between changes in RPE during exercise and exercise duration shed further light on the anticipatory regulation model, as they suggest that RPE is a crucial regulator of exercise performance. Also, the suggestion that RPE can be modified from the onset of exercise by changes in ambient temperature and exercise intensity, in advance of actual physiological changes, and that this change in RPE also alters exercise intensity, provides support for a role of RPE in the *anticipatory* regulation of exercise. This also leads to the suggestion that RPE may not be a direct reflection of an exercising person's physiological state, but may instead be an anticipatory sensory regulator of exercise performance. Put another way, RPE may change during exercise in anticipation of physiological changes occurring, not as a result of those physiological changes. This suggestion also requires us to consider the nature of fatigue itself. As Baden *et al.*[72] state, fatigue may be an emotional construct as opposed to a physical process, and this emotion may be driven by expectations about the nature of the exercise that is to be completed.

Key point

It appears that RPE changes during exercise in anticipation of physiological changes occurring, not as a result of those physiological changes. This provides support for the importance of RPE in the anticipatory regulation of exercise. It also poses the suggestion that fatigue may be an emotion rather than an actual physical process.

6.4.5 Support from other research areas

Further indirect support for the anticipatory feedback model can be found by looking at the wider base of exercise fatigue research, such as that reviewed in earlier chapters. As we have already discussed, the peripheral linear catastrophe model of exercise performance states that homeostatic failure will occur at the point of fatigue. This perspective implies that fatigue is a developing characteristic of exercising to a point of exhaustion where it becomes of critical physiological importance to stop exercising immediately.[61] However, skeletal muscle is never fully recruited, even during maximal intensity exercise,[58,81] as discussed earlier in this chapter. Second, muscle ATP concentration is not fully depleted during exercise (Section 2.2.1). Therefore, the presence of an 'energy crisis' in working muscle cannot be the homeostatic failure that the peripheral linear catastrophe model states has to occur in order to 'cause' fatigue. In line with this, the intramuscular fuel sources phosphocreatine (PCr) and glycogen can be significantly depleted during prolonged and/or intense exercise, but they are not fully depleted in all muscle fibres (Sections 2.2.2 and 2.2.3). Along with the use of fat, this means that ATP resynthesis is always possible. Finally, exercise termination can occur without accumulation of metabolites such as lactate, H^+, or extracellular K^+, without disturbances to muscle Ca^{2+} kinetics,[61,82] and without attainment of an abnormally high core temperature or significant hypohydration (Chapters 3–5). All of these observations contradict the prediction of the peripheral linear catastrophe model that some form of homeostatic failure has to occur in order to 'cause' fatigue. While these observations may contradict the peripheral linear catastrophe model, and thereby provide indirect support for alternative models of fatigue, they do not provide focused support for the anticipatory feedback model, hence why the support is indirect.

Key point

Indirect support for the anticipatory regulation model comes from the wider base of exercise fatigue research discussed in previous chapters. This includes the absence of full skeletal muscle recruitment, lack of complete ATP, PCr, and muscle glycogen depletion, and termination of exercise in the absence of metabolite accumulation, a critically high core temperature, or hypohydration.

6.5 Criticism of the anticipatory feedback model

The above findings seem to confirm that fatigue during self-paced exercise is mediated by central alterations in perception of effort and neuromuscular activation, not peripheral failure of the contractile mechanism. However, there is criticism of the central governor/anticipatory feedback model that should be presented to provide a balanced perspective.

Some authors have argued that the central governor/anticipatory feedback model is unnecessarily complicated. For example, Marcora[83] speculated that the model is 'internally inconsistent, unnecessarily complex, and biologically implausible.' Some of the reasons given for this suggestion are as follows. The anticipatory feedback model states that a central regulator in the brain holds subconscious control over skeletal muscle recruitment during exercise, in order to prevent the recruitment of sufficient muscle mass that would allow the individual to exercise to the point of physical damage. However, the presence of a single region of the brain that is dedicated to regulating exercise performance is highly unlikely, as the suggestion goes against all we know of how the brain functions, namely as an incredibly complex integrated organ where each region contributes to overall brain function.[61] This may also explain why the specific brain regions thought to be the central governor have not been located.

The model also states that the perception of effort is crucial in deterring the individual from continuing on to dangerous levels of exercise. However, Marcora[83] points out that if a subconscious central regulator has control over skeletal muscle recruitment, then the conscious perception of effort is, in theory, redundant, as the subconscious regulator will stop the individual from exercising to a dangerous level regardless of how much motivation there is to continue. The argument, essentially, is that the anticipatory feedback model could exist without inclusion of effort perception (hence the issues with consistency and complexity).

Marcora[83] proposed an alternative, simplified model to explain some of the findings attributed to the anticipatory feedback model. This model states that exercise termination occurs when the effort required to continue exercise is equal to the maximum effort that the individual is willing to provide, or when the individual believes that they have provided a true maximal effort and therefore perceive the continuation of exercise to be impossible.[83] Increasing the effort that the individual is willing to put into exercise (for example, by giving verbal encouragement), will improve exercise tolerance provided it does not exceed what the individual perceives to be their maximal effort.[83] Therefore, effort perception remains important, but the existence of a central governor in the brain is not required.

It has also been suggested that the progressive increase in RPE over time and at different rates in response to changes in exercise intensity and ambient temperature (Section 6.4.4.1) can be explained by factors other than a central regulator that uses effort perception as a 'safety brake'. The anticipatory feedback model states that afferent feedback from different physiological and metabolic systems during exercise is interpreted by the brain and used to generate the conscious RPE (Figure 6.4; Table 6.1). However, other authors claim that RPE actually arises from *efferent* sensory signals.[83–4] This claim has partly arisen from research that has attempted to quantify RPE while controlling for, or removing afferent feedback that is commonly thought to regulate RPE. For example, studies using drugs that induce muscle weakness have shown significant increases in RPE during exercise without a corresponding increase in measures of metabolic stress, such as blood lactate concentration.[85] Similar studies have examined RPE responses to exercise with spinal blockade, which greatly reduces sensory afferent feedback from skeletal muscles.[86–7] If afferent feedback from skeletal muscle is important for perception of effort during exercise, it would be expected that RPE would be reduced when exercising with spinal blockade. However, these studies have found that RPE is either unchanged or actually increases during exercise with spinal blockade.[84]

Similar findings have been reported regarding the influence of afferent feedback from the heart and lungs on RPE during exercise. In experiments where heart rate is reduced by methods such as blocking the stimulating effect of adrenaline on heart rate, the RPE response to exercise is unchanged.[88] It also appears that people who have had a heart transplant, and do not have the same afferent sensory links between the heart and CNS, show a normal effort perception during exercise.[89] Similarly, the sensations of difficult or laboured breathing experienced during exercise are due to central motor commands being sent to the respiratory muscles, as opposed to afferent feedback from those muscles.[84,90]

If sensory afferent feedback to the CNS is not responsible for generating RPE, what is? Marcora[83] contends that it is moment-to-moment increases in central motor command to working muscles (both skeletal and respiratory) that are needed to compensate for reductions in motor neuron and muscle responsiveness during prolonged submaximal exercise that explains the increase in RPE over time. The fundamental suggestion is that RPE is generated via signals leaving the CNS, rather than by signals arriving into the CNS. However, in this explanation, Marcora[83] specifically referred to 'prolonged submaximal exercise at a constant workload'. What about other forms of exercise, such as the self-paced, variable intensity exercise commonly seen in team games or many other forms of competitive sport? This is highlighted in a rebuttal to the paper of Marcora[83] by Noakes and Tucker.[91] Noakes and Tucker[91] discuss that RPE has been shown to alter almost from the onset of exercise, as a result of differences in exercise intensity and ambient temperature,[55] and that this finding is not well explained by Marcora's[83] suggestion that RPE increases due to requirement for a progressive increase in CNS discharge. Also, Noakes and Tucker[91] argue that if the CNS is being required to increase its motor commands to the working muscles, and this is responsible for the increase in RPE, then the CNS must be receiving some information from the working muscles which 'tells' it that these increased motor commands are needed. In essence, increased motor commands from the CNS could not happen without some form of afferent feedback. Therefore, the argument is that the model proposed by Marcora[83] cannot work without afferent sensory feedback, which makes it fundamentally similar to the anticipatory feedback model.[91]

Key point

Some authors have suggested that RPE during exercise is generated by increased efferent signals from the CNS, rather than peripheral afferent feedback. Support for this comes from observation of a normal RPE response when various afferent signals are blocked. However, counter arguments suggest that some afferent feedback must still be required to stimulate the increased efferent signals from the CNS.

The above discussion highlights the difficulties and debates surrounding the anticipatory feedback model of exercise performance. Whether to accept or reject this model is hampered by the fact that the nature of perceived exertion, primarily how it is generated during exercise, is still unknown. This uncertainty was highlighted in a recent review,[92] where the author suggested that generation of effort perception during exercise is likely centrally generated, with peripheral feedback playing an unimportant role (agreeing with Marcora[83]). However, it was also stated that ultimately, regulation of performance is likely due to sense of effort (centrally generated) and specific sensations such as temperature, pain, and other muscular sensations (from afferent sensory feedback).[92] As RPE is a central tenet of the anticipatory feedback model, it is likely that the model will remain a source of debate until the mechanisms behind the sensation of effort during exercise are better understood.

Key point

There is ongoing debate surrounding the origins of RPE during exercise. As RPE is a central tenet of the anticipatory feedback model, it is likely that the validity of this model will continue to be argued until exercising RPE is better understood.

Shephard[93] published an article commenting on many components of the anticipatory feedback model. The author argued that the presence of a central governor that regulates physical performance was, from an evolutionary perspective, unnecessary, and was unlikely to have developed in humans. The ability of the anticipatory regulator to protect the body from critical damage during exercise was also questioned. Shephard[93] supported this argument with data on the prevalence of death from heat stroke in American football players, and the approximate 50-fold increase in the risk of sudden cardiac death as a result of vigorous exercise. However, these arguments were followed by statements that reduced their strength. For example, discussion of the approximate 50-fold increase in the risk of sudden cardiac death during vigorous exercise was qualified by the statement that many of those contributing to the statistic might have had existing cardiac or vascular disease. Shephard[93] also argues that technical issues associated with measuring equipment could be responsible for some of the data that supports the central governor/anticipatory feedback model. However, no specific examples of such technical issues were provided.

The fundamental argument of Shephard[93] is that the anticipatory feedback model should be treated with scepticism as there is a lack of experimental evidence for its existence. However, the model is exceedingly complex, and poses significant challenges to researchers who attempt to experimentally investigate it.[94] Furthermore, much of the evidence that argues against the model comes from studies on isolated component physiological systems.

Caution should be used when interpreting this research as evidence against the model, as investigating isolated component systems disregards the complex physiological, psychological, and neurological interplay proposed by the anticipatory feedback model.[94] Therefore, this research is not a sufficiently rigorous test of the model.[94] The proposed complexity of the model poses a great difficulty in studying it, or quantifying its existence.[94]

This complexity may be one of the key reasons behind much of the criticism of the central governor/anticipatory feedback model. The available research supporting the model, while generally well conducted, cannot conclusively state that the observations made are a result of the existence of an anticipatory regulating system that 'oversees' the balance between exercise demand and athlete ability in real-time. The combined integration of numerous physiological, metabolic, neurological, psychological, and environmental factors (as well as the self-regulation of most of these factors in isolation) means that fully controlling and accounting for the influence of all within a centrally governed network has not yet been achieved within a research design. Indeed, this may not currently be possible. Furthermore, arguing for the existence of the model is hampered by the inability to clearly identify the 'location' of the central governor/regulator, or which specific central / brain processes are involved, or compose, the governor or the development of RPE. More extensive research focusing on, among other things, the relationships and influences between physiological/metabolic factors, central brain and motor function, and the conscious perception of effort, is required to more clearly address the question of whether or not the anticipatory feedback model exists in its proposed form.

Key point

The existence of the anticipatory feedback model is refuted by some based on a lack of experimental evidence. However, the complex nature of the model hampers the ability to experimentally test it. Also, some experimental research used to refute the model does not reflect the complexity of the model to be a sufficiently valid test of its existence.

Key point

Debate into the existence of the anticipatory feedback model will likely continue until a sufficiently complex and rigorous research methodology can be developed to experimentally test the model in its full proposed complexity.

6.6 Summary

- Stimulation of group III and IV muscle afferents by mechanical and chemical stimuli during exercise can inhibit central motor drive, and may contribute to increased effort perception by increasing sensations of muscular pain/discomfort.
- Alterations in central neurotransmitters, particularly serotonin, dopamine, and noradrenaline, are likely involved in central fatigue, but in a synergistic fashion. The relative influence of central neurotransmitters is probably influenced by factors including exercise duration and environmental temperature. The exact role of central neurotransmitter disturbances on central fatigue is still being investigated.
- Ammonia produced during exercise can cross the blood–brain barrier and accumulate in the cerebral tissues, impairing cognitive function and potentially motor activity. Any contribution of ammonia to fatigue during exercise is likely to occur during prolonged exercise.
- Pro-inflammatory cytokines may induce feelings of fatigue, lethargy, and sluggishness characteristic of many illnesses, and increased cytokine production during exercise could encourage similar sensations. Cytokine production can also influence central neurotransmitter production and function. The causal relationship between cytokine production and fatigue still needs to be better demonstrated.
- Central regulation of exercise performance is not a new concept. Some form of central regulation of performance has been speculated upon for over 100 years.
- Central regulation of exercise was reintroduced in the mid-1990s with the concept of a central programmer or governor that uses information about the finishing point of an exercise bout and regulates metabolic demand to achieve this end-point without catastrophic physiological failure (teleoanticipation).
- This concept was developed further, culminating in the anticipatory feedback model of exercise performance.
- The anticipatory feedback model states that exercise is regulated from the outset by previous exercise experience, knowledge of the expected distance or duration of the current exercise bout, and afferent physiological feedback. The synthesis of this information allows the brain to 'predict' the most appropriate exercise intensity that will enable optimal performance without causing severe homeostatic disruption.
- Central to the anticipatory feedback model is the RPE. The model states that a 'template' RPE is developed that will enable RPE to reach its maximum at the predicted termination of exercise. Afferent physiological feedback is continuously monitored by the brain and used to generate conscious RPE. If the conscious RPE and 'template' RPE deviate too much, exercise intensity is altered as appropriate to correct the imbalance.

- The anticipatory feedback model holds that fatigue is a conscious sensation rather than a physical state, and that RPE plays a crucial role in preventing excessive exercise duration/intensity by acting as the motivator to stop exercise or adjust exercise intensity to ensure exercise is completed at an intensity that allows optimal performance without significant physical damage.
- Support for the anticipatory feedback model is anecdotal (exercise is almost always voluntarily ended before serious physical damage occurs) and evidence-based (the end-spurt phenomenon, the use of varied pacing strategies, the physiological and psychological responses to deception of exercise intensity or duration, the relationship between RPE and exercise at different durations, intensities, and conditions, and the frequent occurrence of fatigue despite the absence of a direct physiological or metabolic cause).
- Criticism of the anticipatory feedback model includes the questioning of whether a central regulator in the brain is necessary for central exercise regulation to occur, the requirement for conscious RPE to be such a significant part of the model, and the nature of RPE generation during exercise (whether it is generated from afferent feedback of efferent signals).
- One of the consistent criticisms of the model is that it has not been sufficiently tested experimentally. However, the complexity of the model, along with the separate debate concerning components of the model such as RPE, make its integrated testing extremely difficult, perhaps even impossible.

To think about . . .

It is becoming ever more clear that the brain plays a very important role in exercise performance. This role can be related to our fundamental desire to exercise (or not!), the will to keep going when exercise gets difficult, and more complex potential roles such as the potential regulation of exercise discussed in this chapter. Also mentioned in this chapter is the difficulty in investigating and determining the exact roles of the brain during exercise. Due to these difficulties, most research infers the role of the brain by collecting measures that allow exclusion of the role of peripheral factors, by asking participants about their thoughts and feelings during exercise, and designing studies that may show alterations in these thought processes and emotions. The lack of objective measures focused on brain function itself is clearly a hindrance to this form of research.

Consider the information in Chapters 2–6 of this book. Based on this information, do you feel that the body of knowledge is sufficient to state that a brain-regulated model of exercise performance is the most logical explanation for exercise regulation? Or do we still need to wait for that one study that finally gives us the conclusive 'proof' of this? Is it ever sufficient to use a process of elimination and anecdotal support to accept a hypothesis or model? When you are considering these questions, look for some literature outside of the sport and exercise sciences that discusses how the brain regulates things such as our emotions and motivation. This information may shed more light on the above questions.

Test yourself

Answer the following questions to the best of your ability. Try to understand the information gained from answering these questions before you progress with the book.

1. Summarise the key proposed mechanisms behind the development of central fatigue during exercise.
2. In your own words, briefly explain the central governor model of exercise regulation.
3. In your own words, briefly explain the anticipatory feedback model of exercise regulation.
4. Explain the proposed importance of RPE in the anticipatory feedback model.
5. What are the four main areas of support for the anticipatory feedback model?
6. Briefly explain how each of the areas you noted in question 5 supports the existence of the anticipatory feedback model.
7. What are the main arguments that have been put forwards against the anticipatory feedback model?
8. Summarise the main differences between the anticipatory feedback model and the alternative model presented by Marcora.[83]
9. What are the main research findings that indicate RPE may be generated due to efferent signals rather than afferent peripheral feedback?
10. What are the key factors that make it extremely difficult for the anticipatory feedback model to be appropriately tested in a research setting?

References

1 Davis JM, Bailey SP (1997) Possible mechanisms of central nervous system fatigue during exercise. *Med Sci Sports Exerc* 29 (1): 45–57.
2 Amann M (2012) Significance of group III and IV muscle afferents for the endurance exercising human. *Proc Austral Physiol Soc* 43: 1–7
3 Amann M, Blain GM, Proctor LT, *et al.* (2011) Implications of group III and IV muscle afferents for high intensity endurance exercise performance in humans. *J Physiol* 589 (21): 5299–309.
4 Martin PG, Weerakkody N, Gandevia SC, *et al.* (2008) Group III and IV muscle afferents differentially affect the motor cortex and motor neurons in humans. *J Physiol* 586: 1277–89.
5 Enoka RM, Stuart DG (1992) Neurobiology of muscle fatigue. *J Appl Physiol* 72: 1631–48.
6 Newsholme EA, Acworth I, Blomstrand E (1987) Amino acids, brain neurotransmitters and a function link between muscle and brain that is important in sustained exercise. In: Benzi G (ed.) *Advances in Myochemistry*. London: John Libbey Eurotext: 127–33.
7 Meeusen R, Watson P, Hasegawa H, *et al.* (2006) Central fatigue: the serotonin hypothesis and beyond. *Sports Med* 36 (10): 881–909.
8 Chaouloff F, Kennett GA, Serrurrier B, *et al.* (1986) Amino acid analysis demonstrates that increased plasma free tryptophan causes the increase of brain tryptophan during exercise in the rat. *J Neurochem* 46 (5): 1647–50.
9 MacLean DA, Graham TE, Saltin B (1994) Branched-chain amino acids augment ammonia metabolism while attenuating protein breakdown during exercise. *Am J Physiol* 267 (6 Pt 1): E1010–22.
10 Blomstrand E, Hassmen P, Ekblom B, *et al.* (1991) Administration of branched-chain amino acids during sustained exercise-effects on performance and on plasma concentration of some amino acids. *Eur J Appl Physiol* 63 (2): 83–8.
11 Blomstrand E, Andersson S, Hassmen P, *et al.* (1995) Effect of branched-chain amino acid and carbohydrate supplementation on the exercise-induced change in plasma and muscle concentration of amino acids in human subjects. *Acta Physiol Scand* 153 (2): 87–96.
12 Blomstrand E, Hassmen P, Ek S, *et al.* (1997) Influence of ingesting a solution of branched-chain amino acids on perceived exertion during exercise. *Acta Physiol Scand* 159 (1): 41–9.
13 Davis JM, Welsh RS, De Volve KL, *et al.* (1999) Effects of branched-chain amino acids and carbohydrate on fatigue during intermittent, high-intensity running. *Int J Sports Med* 20 (5): 309–14.
14 Greer BK, White J, Arguello EM, *et al.* (2011) Branched-chain amino acid supplementation lowers perceived exertion but does not affect performance in untrained males. *J Strength Cond Res* 25 (2): 539–44.
15 Madsen K, MacLean DA, Kiens B, *et al.* (1996) Effects of glucose, glucose plus branched-chain amino acids, or placebo on bike performance over 100 km. *J Appl Physiol* 81 (6): 2644–50.
16 Struder HK, Hollmann W, Platen P, *et al.* (1998) Influence of paroxetine, branched-chain amino acids and tyrosine on neuroendocrine system responses and fatigue in humans. *Horm Metab Res* 30 (4): 188–94.
17 Wisnik P, Chmura J, Ziemba AW, *et al.* (2011) The effect of branched chain amino acids on psychomotor performance during treadmill exercise of changing intensity simulating a soccer game. *Appl Physiol, Nutr Metab* 36 (6): 856–62.
18 Heyes MP, Garnett ES, Coates G (1986) Central dopaminergic activity influences rats ability to exercise. *Life Sci* 36 (7): 671–7.

19 Gerald MC (1978) Effects of (+)-amphetamine on the treadmill endurance performance of rats. *Neuropharmacol* 17 (9): 703–4.
20 Nestler EJ, Hyman SE, Malenka RC (2001) *Molecular Neuro-pharmacology: A Foundation for Clinical Neuroscience*. New York: McGraw-Hill.
21 Meeusen R, Roeykens J, Magnus L, *et al.* (1997) Endurance performance in humans: the effect of a dopamine precursor or a specific serotonin (5-HT2A/2C) antagonist. *Int J Sports Med* 18 (8): 571–7.
22 Piacentini MF, Meeusen R, Buyse L, *et al.* (2004) Hormonal responses during prolonged exercise are influenced by a selective DA/NA reuptake inhibitor. *Br J Sports Med* 38 (2): 129–33.
23 Watson P, Hasegawa H, Roelands B, *et al.* (2005) Acute dopamine/noradrenaline reuptake inhibition enhances human exercise performance in warm, but not temperate conditions. *J Physiol* 565 (Pt 3): 873–83.
24 Roelands B, Watson P, Cordery P, *et al.* (2012) A dopamine/noradrenaline reuptake inhibitor improves performance in the heat, but only at the maximum therapeutic dose. *Scand J Med Sci Sports* 22 (5): e93–8.
25 Piacentini MF, Meeusen R, Buyse L, *et al.* (2002) No effect of a noradrenergic reuptake inhibitor on performance in trained cyclists. *Med Sci Sports Exerc* 34 (7): 1189–93.
26 Roelands B, Meeusen R (2010) Alterations in central fatigue by pharmacological manipulations of neurotransmitters in normal and high ambient temperature. *Sports Med* 40 (3): 229–46.
27 Coimbra CC, Soares DD, Leite LHR (2012) The involvement of brain monoamines in the onset of hyperthermic central fatigue. In: Zaslav KR (ed.) *An International Perspective on Topics in Sports Medicine and Sports Injury*. ISBN: 978–953–51–0005–8. Available from: www.intechopen.com/books/an-international-perspective-on-topics-in-sports-medicine-and-sports-injury/.
28 Romero-Gomez M, Jover M, Galan JJ, *et al.* (2009) Gut ammonia production and its modulation. *Metabol Brain Dis* 24: 147–57.
29 Buono MJ, Clancy TR, Cook JR (1984) Blood lactate and ammonium ion accumulation during graded exercise in humans. *J Appl Physiol* 57: 135–9.
30 Wagenmakers AJ, Coakley JH, Edwards RH (1990) Metabolism of branched-chain amino acids and ammonia during exercise: clues from McArdle's disease. *Int J Sports Med* 11 (Suppl. 2): S101–13.
31 Graham TE, Rush JWE, MacLean DA (1995) Skeletal muscle amino acid metabolism and ammonia production during exercise. In: Hargreaves M (ed.) *Exercise Metabolism*. Champaign, IL: Human Kinetics: 131–75.
32 Wilkinson DJ, Smeeton NJ, Watt PW (2010) Ammonia metabolism, the brain and fatigue; revisiting the link. *Prog Neurobiol* 91: 200–19.
33 Nybo L, Dalsgaard MK, Steensberg A, *et al.* (2005) Cerebral ammonia uptake and accumulation during prolonged exercise in humans. *J Physiol* 563: 285–90.
34 Shaney RA, Coast JR (2002) Effect of ammonia on in vitro diaphragmatic contractility, fatigue and recovery. *Resp* 69: 534–41.
35 Dalsgaard MK, Ott P, Dela F, *et al.* (2004) The CSF and arterial to jugular venous hormonal differences during exercise in humans. *Exp Physiol* 89: 271–7.
36 Monfort P, Cauli O, Montoliu C, *et al.* (2009) Mechanisms of cognitive alterations in hyperammonemia and hepatic encephalopathy: therapeutical implications. *Neurochem Int* 55: 106–12.
37 Shawcross DL, Balata S, Olde Damink SWM, *et al.* (2004) Low myoinositol and high glutamine levels in brain are associated with neuropsychological deterioration after induced hyperammonemia. *Am J Physiol* 287: 503–9.
38 Pedersen BK, Hoffman-Goetz L (2000) Exercise and the immune system: regulation, integration and adaptation. *Physiol Rev* 80: 1055–81.

39 Gleeson M (2000) Interleukins and exercise. *J Physiol* 529: 1.
40 Clarkson PM, Hubal MJ (2002) Exercise-induced muscle damage in humans. *Am J Phys Med Rehab* 81 (Suppl. 11): S52–69.
41 Kapsimalis F, Richardson G, Opp MR, *et al.* (2005) Cytokines and normal sleep. *Curr Opin Pulm Med* 11: 481–4.
42 Robson-Ansley PJ, de Milander L, Collins M, *et al.* (2004) Acute interleukin-6 administration impairs athletic performance in healthy, trained male runners. *Can J Appl Physiol* 29: 411–8.
43 Dantzer R, Heijnen CJ, Kavelaars A, Laye S, Capuron L (2014) The neuroimmune basis of fatigue. *Trends Neurosci* 37: 39–46.
44 Finsterer J (2012) Biomarkers of peripheral muscle fatigue during exercise. *BMC Musculoskelet Disord* 13: 218–242.
45 Hill AV, Long CHN, Lupton H (1924) Muscular exercise, lactic acid and the supply and utilisation of oxygen: parts VII–VIII. *Proc Royal Soc* 97: 155–76.
46 Mosso A (1915) *Fatigue*. London: Allen and Unwin Ltd.
47 Noakes TD (2012) Fatigue is a brain-derived emotion that regulates the exercise behaviour to ensure the protection of whole-body homeostasis. *Front Physiol* 3: 1–13.
48 Ulmer HV (1996) Concept of an extracellular regulation of muscular metabolic rate during heavy exercise in humans by psychophysiological feedback. *Experientia* 15: 416–20.
49 Lambert EV, St Clair Gibson A, Noakes TD (2005) Complex systems model of fatigue: integrative homeostatic control of peripheral physiological systems during exercise in humans. *Br J Sports Med* 39: 52–62.
50 Noakes TD (2000) Physiological models to understand exercise fatigue and the adaptations that predict or enhance athletic performance. *Scand J Med Sci Sports* 10: 123–45.
51 Noakes TD, Peltonen JE, Rusko HK (2001) Evidence that a central governor regulates exercise performance during acute hypoxia and hyperoxia. *J Exp Biol* 204: 3225–34.
52 Noakes TD, St Clair Gibson A, Lambert EV (2005) From catastrophe to complexity: a novel model of integrative central neural regulation of effort and fatigue during exercise in humans: summary and conclusions. *Br J Sports Med* 39: 120–4.
53 St Clair Gibson A, Noakes TD (2004) Evidence for complex system integration and dynamic neural regulation of skeletal muscle recruitment during exercise in humans. *Br J Sports Med* 38: 797–806.
54 Tucker R (2009) The anticipatory regulation of performance: the physiological basis for pacing strategies and the development of a perception-based model for exercise performance. *Br J Sports Med* 43: 392–400.
55 Crewe H, Tucker R, Noakes TD (2008) The rate of increase in rating of perceived exertion predicts the duration of exercise to fatigue at a fixed power output in different environmental conditions. *Eur J Appl Physiol* 103: 569–77.
56 Schabort EJ, Hawley JA, Hopkins WG, Mujika I, Noakes TD (1998) A new reliable laboratory test of endurance performance for road cyclists. *Med Sci Sports Exerc* 30: 1744–50.
57 Kay D, Marino FE, Cannon J, St Clair Gibson A, Lambert MI, Noakes TD (2001) Evidence for neuromuscular fatigue during high-intensity cycling in warm, humid conditions. *Eur J Appl Physiol* 84: 115–21.
58 St Clair Gibson A, Schabort EJ, Noakes TD (2001) Reduced neuromuscular activity and force generation during prolonged cycling. *Am J Physiol* 281: R187–96.

59 Marcora SM, Staiano W (2010) The limit to exercise tolerance in humans: mind over muscle? *Eur J Appl Physiol* 109: 763–70.
60 Wittekind AL, Micklewright D, Beneke R (2011) Teleoanticipation in all-out short duration cycling. *Br J Sports Med* 45: 114–9.
61 Edwards AM, Polman RCJ (2013) Pacing and awareness: brain regulation of physical activity. *Sports Med* 43(11): 1057–64.
62 Noakes TD (2011) Time to move beyond a brainless exercise physiology: the evidence for complex regulation of human exercise performance. *Appl Physiol Nutr Metab* 36: 23–35.
63 Paterson S, Marino FE (2004) Effect of deception of distance on prolonged cycling performance. *Percept Mot Skill* 98: 1017–26.
64 Dugas J, Oosthuizan U, Tucker R, Noakes TD (2009) Rates of fluid ingestion alter pacing but not thermoregulatory responses during prolonged exercise in hot and humid conditions with appropriate convective cooling. *Eur J Appl Physiol* 105: 69–80.
65 Marcora SM, Staiano W, Manning V (2009) Mental fatigue impairs physical performance in humans. *J Appl Physiol* 106: 857–64.
66 Rauch H, St Clair Gibson A, Lambert EV (2005) A signalling role for muscle glycogen in the regulation of pace during prolonged exercise. *Br J Sports Med* 39: 34–8.
67 Marino FE (2004) Anticipatory regulation and avoidance of catastrophe during exercise-induced hyperthermia. *Comp Biochem Physiol B Biochem Mol Biol* 139: 561–9.
68 Mauger AR, Jones AM, Williams CA (2009) Influence of feedback and prior experience on pacing during a 4-km cycle time trial. *Med Sci Sports Exerc* 41: 451–8.
69 Micklewright D, Papadopoulou E, Swart J, Noakes T (2010) Previous experience influences pacing during 20 km time trial cycling. *Br J Sports Med* 44: 952–60.
70 Saunders AG, Dugas JP, Tucker R, Lambert MI, Noakes TD (2005) The effects of different air velocities on heat storage and body temperature in humans cycling in a hot, humid environment. *Acta Physiol Scand* 183: 241–55.
71 Tucker R, Bester A, Lambert EV, Noakes TD, Vaughan CL, St Clair Gibson A (2006) Non-random fluctuations in power output during self-paced exercise. *Br J Sports Med* 40: 912–7.
72 Baden DA, McLean TL, Tucker R, Noakes TD, St Clair Gibson A (2005) Effect of anticipation during unknown or unexpected exercise duration on rating of perceived exertion, affect, and physiological function. *Br J Sports Med* 39: 742–6.
73 Eston R, Stansfield R, Westoby P, Parfitt G (2012) Effect of deception and expected exercise duration on psychological and physiological variables during treadmill running and cycling. *Psychophysiol* 49: 462–9.
74 Bolgar MA, Baker CE, Goss FL, Nagle E, Robertson RJ (2010) Effect of exercise intensity on differentiated and undifferentiated ratings of perceived exertion during cycling and treadmill exercise in recreationally active and trained women. *J Sports Sci Med* 9: 557–63.
75 Morton RH (2009) Deception by manipulating the clock calibration influences cycle ergometer endurance time in males. *J Sci Med Sport* 12: 332–7.
76 Faulkner J, Arnold T, Eston R (2011) Effect of accurate and inaccurate distance feedback on performance markers and pacing strategies during running. *Scand J Med Sci Sports* 21: e176–83.
77 Billaut F, Bishop DJ, Schaerz S, Noakes TD (2011) Influence of knowledge of sprint number on pacing during repeated-sprint exercise. *Med Sci Sports Exerc* 43: 665–72.

78 Swart J, Lindsay TR, Lambert MI, Brown JC, Noakes TD (2012) Perceptual cues in the regulation of exercise performance – physical sensations of exercise and awareness of effort interact as separate cues. *Br J Sports Med* 46: 42–8.
79 Presland JD, Dowson MN, Cairns SP (2005) Changes of motor drive, cortical arousal and perceived exertion following prolonged cycling to exhaustion. *Eur J Appl Physiol* 95: 42–51.
80 Tucker R, Marle T, Lambert EV, Noakes TD (2006) The rate of heat storage mediates an anticipatory reduction in exercise intensity during cycling at a fixed rating of perceived exertion. *J Physiol* 574: 905–15.
81 Noakes T (2008) Testing for maximum oxygen consumption has produced a brainless model of human exercise performance. *Br J Sports Med* 42: 551–5.
82 Noakes TD (2000) Physiological models to understand exercise fatigue and the adaptations that predict or enhance athletic performance. *Scand J Med Sci Sports* 10: 123–45.
83 Marcora SM (2008) Do we really need a central governor to explain brain regulation of exercise performance? *Eur J Appl Physiol* 104: 929–31.
84 Marcora S (2009) Perception of effort during exercise is independent of afferent feedback from skeletal muscles, heart, and lungs. *J Appl Physiol* 106: 2060–2.
85 Gallagher KM, Fadel PJ, Stromstad M, Ide K, Smith SA, Querry RG, Raven PB, Secher NH (2001) Effects of partial neuromuscular blockade on carotid baroreflex function during exercise in humans. *J Physiol* 533: 861–70.
86 Kjaer M, Hanel B, Worm L, Perko G, Lewis SF, Sahlin K, Galbo H, Secher NH (1999) Cardiovascular and neuroendocrine responses to exercise in hypoxia during impaired neural feedback from muscle. *Am J Physiol* 277: R76–85.
87 Smith SA, Querry RG, Fadel PJ, Gallagher KM, Stromstad M, Ide K, Raven PB, Secher NH (2003) Partial blockade of skeletal muscle somatosensory afferents attenuates baroreflex resetting during exercise in humans. *J Physiol* 551: 1013–21.
88 Myers J, Atwood JE, Sullivan M, Forbes S, Friis R, Pewen W, Froelicher V (1987) Perceived exertion and gas exchange after calcium and β-blockade in atrial fibrillation. *J Appl Physiol* 63: 97–104.
89 Braith RW, Wood CE, Limacher MC, Pollock ML, Lowenthal DT, Phillips MI, Staples ED (1992) Adnormal neuroendocrine responses during exercise in heart transplant recipients. *Circulation* 86: 1453–63.
90 Grazzini M, Stendardi L, Gigliotti F, Scano G (2005) Pathophysiology of exercise dyspnea in healthy subjects and in patients with chronic obstructive pulmonary disease (COPD). *Respir Med* 99: 1403–12.
91 Noakes TD, Tucker R (2008) Do we really need a central governor to explain brain regulation of exercise performance? A response to the letter of Dr Marcora. *Eur J Appl Physiol* 104: 933–5.
92 Smirmaul B (2012) Sense of effort and other unpleasant sensations during exercise: clarifying concepts and mechanisms. *Br J Sports Med* 46: 308–11.
93 Shephard RJ (2009) Is it time to retire the 'central governor'? *Sports Med* 39: 709–21.
94 Micklewright D, Parry D (2010) The central governor model cannot be adequately tested by observing its components in isolation. *Sports Med* 40: 91–4.

Part III

Fatigue

Is it the same for everyone?

Chapter 7

Factors influencing the causes of fatigue

7.1 Introduction

Part II discussed some primary candidates behind the development of fatigue during exercise. For clarity, the influence of factors that could modulate these candidates were not discussed. One of the primary modifiers of fatigue is the nature of exercise and the associated demands placed on the exercising individual. However, causes of fatigue can also be influenced by gender, training status, age, health, and more. The focus of this book prevents discussion of the role of age and health status in fatigue (these topics would require an entire book to themselves). However, exercise demand, gender, and training status will be discussed.

To address the issue of exercise demand on causes of fatigue, this chapter will be structured differently to those in Part II (Part II will be quite heavily referred to; therefore it is recommended that the reader addresses Part II before reading this chapter). The chapter will highlight types of exercise that have different physical requirements, and potential fatigue mechanisms from Part II will be linked to each exercise type. In this way, it will be possible to differentiate potential fatigue mechanisms based on exercise requirements, and emphasise sources of confusion or lack of knowledge regarding fatigue mechanisms during different types of exercise. Following the discussion of exercise demand, the issues of gender and training status will be overviewed, highlighting what is currently known about the modifying role of these two factors in exercise fatigue.

A few important points before reading this chapter: first, for ease of communication potential fatigue mechanisms will be presented almost in a 'stand-alone' fashion. Remember that physiological and biochemical function is extremely complex and highly integrated, and it is unlikely that just one of the mechanisms highlighted will be solely responsible for fatigue in any particular exercise situation. Second, as has been touched upon in previous chapters, the relative influence of a particular fatigue mechanism may depend in part on the environmental conditions in which exercise takes place. For example, exercising in a hot and humid environment is going to place greater emphasis on fatigue mechanisms associated with dehydration and hyperthermia compared to exercise in a cool environment. For clarity, this chapter will discuss exercise taking place in a thermoneutral environment, in a situation that is not excessively humid or subject to any other external factors that could influence fatigue processes (unless specifically stated). Third, only those mechanisms that are likely to contribute significantly to fatigue during particular exercise demands will be discussed. If a fatigue mechanism is not discussed, it is because existing research does not support it as a major source of fatigue during that form of exercise; however, it does not mean that the mechanism should be completely or permanently discounted (remember, knowledge on fatigue processes is ever changing). This point is of particular relevance to the central/anticipatory feedback model of performance that was discussed in Chapter 6. While this model of exercise regulation is very interesting, its complexity means that its existence is generally inferred from research findings that cannot be explained by other measured factors. As a result, it is not currently possible to state using clear research support that central/anticipatory regulation is a significant modifier of exercise performance across a variety of different exercises. Where focused literature does exist, this has been discussed. For other types of exercise, central/anticipatory feedback has been alluded to in summary figures as a potential factor that should not be overlooked, but requires further investigation.

7.2 The influence of exercise demand on fatigue mechanisms

7.2.1 Prolonged submaximal exercise

Prolonged submaximal exercise refers to exercise carried out at a moderate intensity for 30–180 minutes. The key performance requirements and associated fatigue mechanisms during endurance exercise are summarised in Figure 7.1. It is important to note that the focus of this chapter is not to provide a detailed breakdown of every physical variable that is important to the overall performance of each exercise (this would be more relevant in a discussion of talent identification and training). Instead, the focus is on identifying key body systems and processes that are important for performance, and how fatigue may impact these systems.

Prolonged submaximal exercise is dependent on cardiovascular function to transport oxygenated blood from the lungs, to the heart, and then into the systemic circulation for delivery to working tissues. Oxygen delivery is required to enable aerobic resynthesis of ATP using carbohydrate, fat, and lactate, which is by far the most important source of ATP resynthesis during prolonged submaximal exercise (energy from PCr breakdown is important during the first few minutes of prolonged submaximal exercise and if increases in exercise intensity are required, but after that carbohydrate and fat become

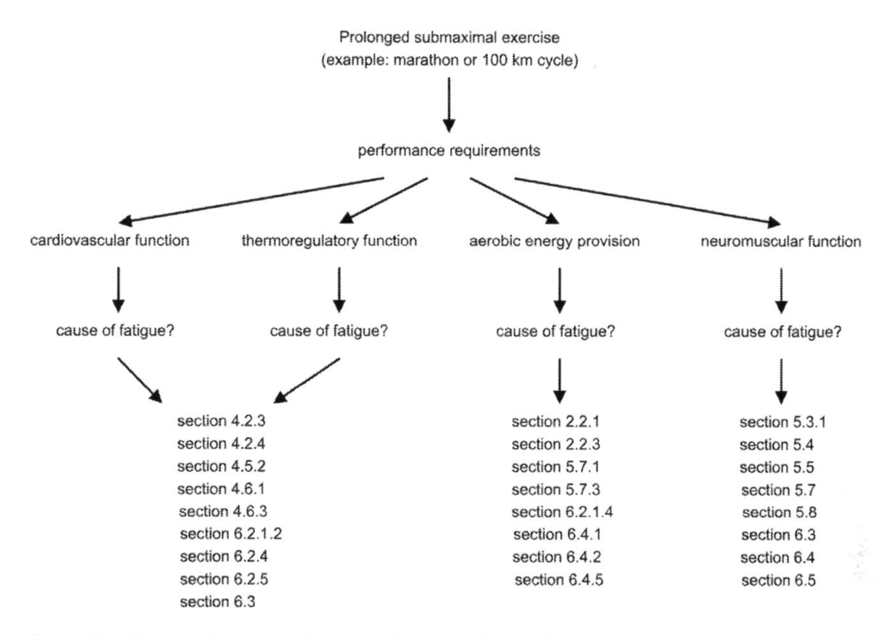

Figure 7.1 Potential causes of fatigue during prolonged submaximal exercise. Only those performance requirements that may play a direct, significant role in the fatigue process are highlighted. The section numbers refer to sections of this book that discuss the potential causes of fatigue associated with each of the identified performance requirements.

the principal fuels). Blood flow to working tissues also removes carbon dioxide (produced in greater amounts via aerobic metabolism), and aids hydrogen (H^+) removal from the muscle. Appropriate cardiovascular function is also required for regulation of body temperature, through the distribution of blood flow to both the working tissues and the skin for convective and evaporative body heat loss. Neuromuscular function is also crucial for maintenance of appropriate muscle activation and contractile function for the duration of the exercise bout.

7.2.1.1 What are the likely 'causes' of fatigue during prolonged submaximal exercise?

Prolonged submaximal exercise is reliant on the rate of aerobic metabolism of a limited energy store (i.e. carbohydrate) and the exercise intensity that can be maintained without development of hyperthermia or impaired neuromuscular function.[1] The movement economy of the exercising person (the energy cost, usually measured as VO_2, relative to the movement velocity) will also play a role in the ability to maintain a given intensity.[1] Therefore, it is logical to assume that potential causes of fatigue during prolonged submaximal exercise will relate to disturbances in energy metabolism, acid/base regulation, thermoregulation, and neuromuscular function.

7.2.1.1.1 CARDIOVASCULAR FUNCTION AND THERMOREGULATION

During prolonged submaximal exercise, fluid loss via sweating (among other avenues) may decrease blood plasma volume. Reduced plasma volume may reduce the volume of blood entering the heart in each cardiac cycle, which could reduce stroke volume and cardiac output, meaning that heart rate must increase to maintain the necessary oxygen delivery to working tissue (Section 4.2.3 and Figure 4.2). These alterations represent a reduction in cardiac efficiency, which could lead to impaired exercise performance.[2]

If body water loss continues, reduced plasma volume may generate a competition for blood flow between core organs, working tissues, and the skin. It is biologically imperative that core organs receive sufficient blood flow to maintain appropriate function, therefore skin blood flow may be reduced to the extent that evaporative heat loss is impaired, and core temperature subsequently increases. However, it is questionable whether the attainment of a 'critical' high core temperature is a direct cause of fatigue during exercise (Section 4.6.3). Instead, increases in skin temperature (which can occur due to reduced sweat rate and evaporative heat loss) may be more important than high core temperature in contributing to hyperthermia-induced fatigue. High skin temperatures require a higher skin blood flow, which may impair cardiac efficiency, reduce VO_{2max}, and increase the relative exercise intensity, causing the athlete to fatigue earlier (Section 4.6.3).

Key point

Increases in skin temperature may be a more important component of fatigue during prolonged submaximal exercise than increases in core temperature.

Despite equivocal evidence for the negative effect of a 'critical' core temperature, it seems likely that dehydration does negatively affect exercise performance, and that these effects are central rather than peripheral. Potential peripheral factors associated with hyperthermia (reduced blood and oxygen delivery to working muscles, increased muscle glycogen use) do not have good evidence as causes of fatigue, yet central alterations (increased brain temperature, reduced brain blood and oxygen delivery, impaired motor output) do appear to exert more of a negative influence on performance (Section 4.6.2).

Section 4.3 discussed that drinking to the dictates of thirst appears to be a useful strategy for ameliorating many of the potentially negative consequences of dehydration during prolonged submaximal exercise. Cyclists tend to consume higher volumes of fluid during exercise compared to runners,[3] probably due to the greater gastrointestinal distress that runners encounter when consuming fluid during their activity.[4] Lower fluid intake may place endurance runners at greater risk of fatigue related to dehydration than other endurance athletes. Finally, central fatigue appears to exert more of an effect on endurance running performance than endurance cycling performance of a similar duration.[5] This finding may suggest that endurance runners could be more disadvantaged by hyperthermia-induced central impairments than endurance cyclists.

7.2.1.1.2 AEROBIC ENERGY PROVISION

High-level marathon runners derive approximately two thirds of their energy requirement from carbohydrate, primarily muscle glycogen and to a lesser extent blood glucose.[1] Top marathon runners can run a marathon at an average intensity of more than 80% VO_{2max}, which cannot be maintained without sufficient carbohydrate stores.[1] Reductions in muscle glycogen therefore require a reduction in exercise intensity to a level that can be maintained by fat, blood glucose, and lactate metabolism.[1] Muscle glycogen depletion can occur after approximately 2 hours of exercise, although this is a broad timeframe that is influenced by exercise intensity, environmental conditions, pre-exercise muscle glycogen concentration, and athlete training status. Well-trained endurance athletes show an enhanced ability to metabolise fat at a given exercise intensity, which may allow them to 'spare' muscle glycogen and maintain a higher exercise intensity for longer. Interestingly, studies have not been completed that investigate the influence of training status on the degree to which carbohydrate depletion may cause fatigue during prolonged exercise.[1] While muscle glycogen depletion will impair the intensity at which prolonged submaximal exercise can be completed, the specific mechanisms behind this impairment are still debated (Section 2.2.3).

Key point

Well-trained endurance athletes oxidise more fat and less carbohydrate at a given relative exercise intensity. This may enable endurance athletes to spare glycogen stores and delay the onset of fatigue associated with glycogen depletion. However, it is becoming more likely that the role of glycogen depletion in muscle fatigue is dependent on the specific site of depletion.

Hypoglycaemia can occur during prolonged submaximal exercise, secondary to liver glycogen depletion. The extent of hypoglycaemia will depend on exercise duration and intensity (liver glucose release increases linearly with exercise intensity, and is also higher during long-duration exercise, when muscle glycogen stores become depleted), the pre-exercise energy status of the athlete (i.e. how much liver glycogen they begin exercise with), and whether or not the athlete consumes carbohydrate during exercise (which may spare liver glycogen and/or independently maintain blood glucose levels; Section 2.2.3.2.2). The development of hypoglycaemia can contribute to fatigue during prolonged submaximal exercise by limiting fuel supply to working muscles. The brain also has a limited glycogen store, and needs to take up blood glucose during exercise. Therefore, hypoglycaemia can also contribute to central fatigue during prolonged submaximal exercise; however, it should be remembered that the influence of hypoglycaemia on muscle carbohydrate oxidation, endurance capacity, and fatigue development is debated (Section 2.2.3.2.2).

Key point

Hypoglycaemia may contribute to the development of central fatigue during prolonged exercise. However, the role of hypoglycaemia in fatigue is inconsistent, and dependent on factors pre- and during exercise.

7.2.1.1.3 NEUROMUSCULAR FUNCTION

Significant impairments in sarcoplasmic reticulum (SR) calcium (Ca^{2+}) release and reuptake have been found following prolonged submaximal cycling exercise,[6] and these impairments have been linked to fatigue.[7] Section 5.7.1 discussed the potential importance of muscle glycogen on SR function, due to mechanisms related or unrelated to glycogens traditional role as a fuel source (the specific mechanisms are still debated).[7] Muscle glycogen depletion can occur during prolonged submaximal exercise (Section 7.2.1.1.2). Therefore, impairments in SR function may occur during prolonged submaximal exercise via muscle glycogen depletion. Whatever the specific mechanism, prolonged submaximal exercise is likely impaired/limited to some extent by SR dysregulation.

Most human studies investigating extracellular potassium (K^+) accumulation have used intense single leg bouts of exercise lasting no more than a few minutes (Section 5.3.1). Results from these studies suggest that extracellular K^+ can accumulate rapidly (within 1–3 minutes). However, this research does not indicate whether or not extracellular K^+ accumulation may occur during prolonged submaximal whole body exercise. McKenna *et al.*[8] showed significant increases in extracellular and interstitial K^+ concentration during cycling exercise lasting approximately 50 minutes. Furthermore, supplementing participants with N-acetylcysteine (an antioxidant compound) reduced extracellular K^+ accumulation and improved cycling duration, thereby associating improved K^+ regulation with greater exercise endurance. Pires *et al.*[9] also found notable increases in extracellular K^+ concentration during cycle exercise to exhaustion at an intensity above the second lactate threshold. Time to exhaustion at this intensity was only approximately 22 minutes, compared to about 45 minutes at an intensity equal to the second lactate threshold and about 94 minutes at an intensity equal to the first lactate threshold. Interestingly, extracellular K^+ concentration reached a plateau after about 40% of the exercise duration, regardless of exercise intensity. Therefore, Pires *et al.*[9] concluded that changes in variables such as extracellular K^+ did not correlate with time to exhaustion. Overgaard *et al.*[10] found significant increases in plasma K^+ concentration following a 100-km run. However, the authors only measured plasma K^+ concentration before and after the run. Therefore, a cause and effect relationship between plasma K^+ accumulation and performance could not be established.

Key point

Prolonged submaximal exercise is probably impaired by SR dysregulation and altered Ca^{2+} kinetics, but the mechanisms behind this have not been conclusively determined. Significant extracellular K^+ accumulation can occur during prolonged submaximal exercise, but its association with performance is inconclusive.

7.2.1.1.4 CENTRAL FATIGUE, AND CENTRAL/ANTICIPATORY REGULATION OF PERFORMANCE

Many of the central fatigue hypotheses discussed in Section 6.2 are more likely to play a performance limiting role during prolonged exercise. Changes in brain neurotransmitter production and metabolism (Section 6.2.1.2), brain ammonia accumulation (Section 6.2.1.3) and pro-inflammatory cytokine production (Section 6.2.1.4) have all been implicated in the development of central fatigue during prolonged submaximal exercise. Furthermore, the influence of some of these mechanisms may be dependent on certain peripheral and/or central alterations. For example, the role of brain neurotransmitters on prolonged exercise performance may be more important during exercise in the heat (Section 6.2.1.2), and increased pro-inflammatory cytokine production likely occurs due to significant energy depletion in skeletal muscle (Section 6.2.1.4). Prevalent central fatigue hypotheses should be considered when discussing fatigue during prolonged submaximal exercise, but the presence of potential modulating factors on these hypotheses should also be determined on a case-by-case basis.

The potential for a central/anticipatory regulation of exercise performance was introduced in Section 6.3. The observations highlighted in support for such performance regulation can also be related to prolonged submaximal exercise[11] (general absence of catastrophic homeostatic failure at exhaustion, significant increases in intensity in the final stages of exercise, and the employment of varied pacing strategies depending on exercise intensity, environmental conditions, and the expected difficulty of the exercise). Furthermore, there is not a clear and consistent link between any physiological/peripheral variable and fatigue during exercise (Section 6.4.5). While this may provide indirect support for a central/anticipatory regulation of prolonged submaximal exercise, it should be remembered that the very existence of such a regulatory system is still keenly debated (Section 6.5).

Key point

Many of the observations made to support a central/anticipatory regulation of exercise performance can be found during prolonged submaximal exercise, indicating that the model could apply to this type of exercise. However, the very existence of such a model is still keenly debated.

7.2.2 Field-based team games

This section focuses on field-based team games such as soccer, rugby, and field hockey. Low intensity work (standing, walking, jogging) is predominant in most field-based team games. However, the requirement to perform several hundred brief intense actions along with rapid, continuous changes of activity suggests a notable stress on both aerobic and anaerobic energy pathways. The requirement to rapidly and forcefully activate skeletal muscle for short periods of time is a crucial difference between team games exercise and prolonged submaximal exercise, and may influence the fatigue processes at work in team games.

Average heart rate during field-based team games is approximately 75–95% of maximum heart rate,[12–13] and the estimated mean VO_2 during a soccer match is 70–80% VO_{2max}.[14] Mean blood lactate concentration ranges from approximately 2.8–10 mmol/litre, with peak concentrations notably greater than these values.[12,14] Carbohydrate is the primary fuel source during team games, despite the predominance of low-intensity work. The extent of muscle glycogen depletion is variable, and likely affected by playing position, game intensity, environmental conditions, muscle fibre type recruitment, and pre-game glycogen concentrations.[15–16]

Team games appear to impose a similar average physiological stress to that observed in prolonged submaximal exercise. Aerobic metabolism is dominant, but anaerobic contribution is crucial to successful performance. However, the moment-to-moment demand of team games requires a notable high- and maximal-intensity component, making it significantly different to steady-state exercise.

7.2.2.1 What are the likely 'causes' of fatigue during field-based team games?

Research investigating the physical demand and determinants of fatigue during team games has discovered two 'forms' of fatigue during this type of activity. It appears that team games players experience temporary fatigue following periods of high-intensity activity; this is referred to as transient fatigue. A progressive fatigue also develops that results in less high-intensity activity, sprinting, and overall distance covered towards the end of a match.[17–19] This section will discuss potential causes of both 'forms' of fatigue.

Key point

There are two distinct 'forms' of fatigue during team games exercise. One is a temporary fatigue that occurs following high-intensity periods of a game (transient fatigue); the other is a progressive fatigue that impairs high-intensity exercise and distance covered towards the end of a match.

7.2.2.1.1 TRANSIENT FATIGUE

7.2.2.1.1.1 Muscle/blood lactate, and pH The performance requirements of field-based team games and the fatigue mechanisms associated with transient fatigue are in Figure 7.2. Notable blood lactate concentrations have been reported during team games, suggesting significant use of anaerobic glycolysis. Therefore, fatigue during team games may be associated with high muscle lactate concentrations and/or intramuscular acidosis.[16] This suggestion has some support from studies demonstrating significant increases in muscle lactate and acidosis, and weak but statistically significant correlations between muscle lactate concentration and decreased sprint performance, following intense periods of play.[20] However, muscle lactate concentrations during team games are much lower than those found at exhaustion following high-intensity exercise.[16] Furthermore, the absence of a causative role for lactate in fatigue, and the beneficial roles of lactate production during exercise, were discussed in Chapter 3.

If intramuscular lactate accumulation is not a likely cause of transient fatigue during team games, what about a reduction in muscle pH via accumulation of H^+? While H^+ accumulation has been put forward as a candidate for transient fatigue, decreases in muscle pH during soccer are only moderate,[14] and these changes have not been related to impaired performance.[14,21] Also, there is evidence to show that muscle pH levels 1 1/2 minutes before exhaustion during intense intermittent exercise were not different to those values seen at exhaustion.[22] It therefore appears that reduced muscle pH is not a likely cause of transient fatigue during team games.[14] It is possible that the lack of a role for H^+ accumulation in transient fatigue may be due to the seemingly minimal role of H^+ in muscle fatigue that was discussed in Section 3.3.2.

Key point

Neither high muscle lactate concentration nor reduced muscle pH appear to be a cause of transient fatigue during team games.

7.2.2.1.1.2 Low muscle phosphocreatine concentration Section 2.2.2.2 discussed the significant positive relationship between the ability to resynthesise phosphocreatine (PCr) and the recovery of power output during repeated sprinting. These studies show that the ability to perform repeated sprints is partly dependent on PCr availability. However, correlation studies between PCr recovery and repeated sprint performance also show that PCr recovery is associated with about 45–71% of the recovery of power output, suggesting that there are other factors that also contribute to intermittent exercise performance.

Following intense periods of activity during team games, the decrease in muscle PCr concentration is correlated with impaired sprinting ability.[16,21] However, muscle PCr depletion following high-intensity periods of team games activity appears to be moderate,[23] and other research has shown no changes in muscle PCr concentration towards the end of intermittent exercise tests designed to replicate the repeated sprint nature of team games.[22] The bulk of the available evidence appears to suggest that depletion of muscle PCr is not the cause of transient fatigue during team games.[14,16,23]

7.2.2.1.1.3 Muscle membrane excitability Dysregulation of the SR can occur during prolonged exercise (Section 5.7), and this may be linked to

Key point

Despite correlations between reduced muscle PCr and impaired sprinting performance, PCr depletion following high-intensity periods of team games activity is moderate, and research has reported no change in muscle PCr concentration during intermittent tests designed to replicate the repeated sprint nature of team games. Therefore, it is questionable whether PCr depletion is responsible for transient fatigue during team games.

accumulation of P_i (Section 7.2.2.1.1.2) and muscle glycogen depletion (Section 7.2.2.1.3.1). Therefore, it is plausible that SR dysregulation could contribute to fatigue during field-based team games exercise. However, data investigating this suggestion is currently lacking.

The potential role of reduced pH on extracellular K^+ accumulation, and the potential for exceeding the capacity of the Na+, K^+ pump during high-intensity exercise, indicates that extracellular K^+ accumulation may be greater during high-intensity exercise (Section 5.3 and 5.5). Therefore, extracellular K^+ accumulation may be implicated in transient fatigue during team games. However, Section 5.4 discusses the evidence against the role of extracellular K^+ accumulation on muscle fatigue. Furthermore, Section 5.5 suggests caution in accepting extracellular K^+ accumulation as a cause of muscle fatigue until more supportive *in vivo* research is produced. Given this information, what is known of the potential role of extracellular K^+ accumulation on transient fatigue during team games?

The answer to the above question is, not very much. While we know that intense short-term exercise causes sufficient extracellular K^+ accumulation to depolarise the muscle membrane potential and reduce force production, very little work has been done investigating K^+ turnover during team games.[16] For example, we know that blood K^+ levels are elevated during a soccer match,[20] but this study did not provide information on the accumulation of K^+ in the muscle interstitium. A more recent study found that caffeine ingestion improved the performance of intense intermittent exercise similar to that undertaken during team games, and that the caffeine caused a reduction in interstitial K^+ concentration.[24] These authors suggested that improved performance with caffeine ingestion indicates a role of interstitial K^+ accumulation in impairing performance during team games type exercise. However, the authors also note than other influences of caffeine ingestion, such as elevated catecholamine concentrations and/or a reduced central fatigue, may have contributed to improved performance, with reduced interstitial K^+ concentration a coincidental finding. This possibility is further supported by the finding that interstitial K^+ concentrations in the control trial were not high enough to contribute to fatigue.[24] As a result, it cannot be conclusively determined whether extracellular K^+ accumulation plays a role in transient fatigue during team games.

Key point

Blood K^+ levels are elevated during a soccer match, which may indicate a net loss of K^+ from the muscle and possible K^+ accumulation in the interstitium. However, this has not been measured in team games exercise. There is some indirect evidence that extracellular K^+ accumulation may play a role in transient during team games, but not enough to come to a conclusive decision.

7.2.2.1.2 SUMMARY

The specific cause(s) of transient fatigue during team games is currently unknown. While there are candidates, none of these has been consistently or clearly shown to cause transient fatigue. An interesting consideration is that, if physical/metabolic/biochemical factors cannot adequately explain transient fatigue, then perhaps the cause lies elsewhere. For example, transient fatigue may represent a form of pacing to enable the player to complete a full game without excessive performance loss or the requirement for a long recovery period, which is rarely available in field-based team games. The discussions in Chapter 6 focused on the concept of anticipatory regulation of exercise performance via real-time interpretation of exercise demands (Sections 6.3 and 6.4). Given that transient fatigue is often observed following high-intensity periods of activity, the concept of a continual regulation of exercise intensity based on existing exercise demands would appear to fit the nature of transient fatigue during team games. However, to date insufficient research has investigated the potential role of perceptual regulation in transient fatigue during team games.

7.2.2.1.3 PROGRESSIVE FATIGUE

In addition to transient fatigue, which can develop and 'dissipate' multiple times during team games, a more progressive fatigue also sets in as a game progresses. Unlike transient fatigue, progressive fatigue is not rectified before the end of the game.

7.2.2.1.3.1 Muscle glycogen depletion The extent of muscle glycogen depletion during team games is variable, and is likely affected by playing position, game intensity, environmental conditions, muscle fibre type

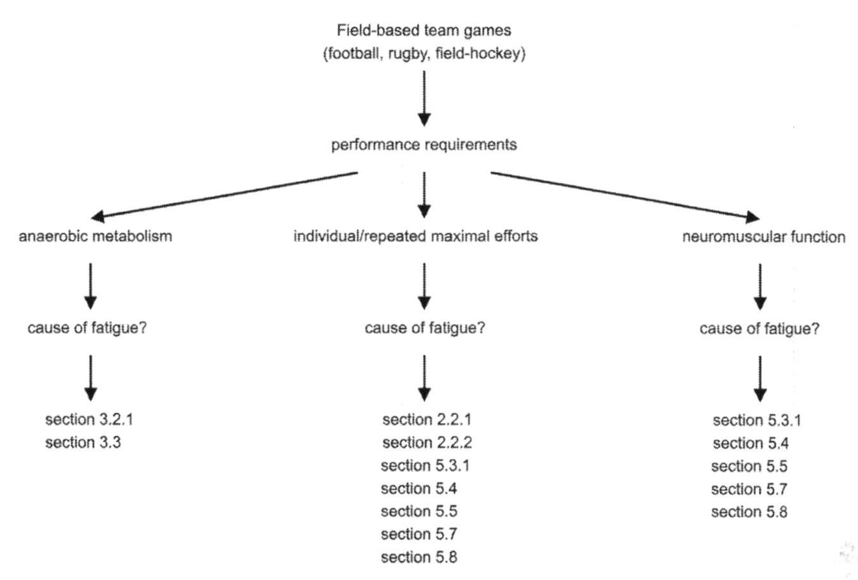

Figure 7.2 Potential causes of transient fatigue during field-based team games. Only those performance requirements that may play a direct significant role in the fatigue process are highlighted. The section numbers refer to sections of this book that discuss the potential causes of fatigue associated with each of the identified performance requirements.

recruitment, and pre-game muscle glycogen concentration.[15–16,25] However, it is generally accepted that muscle glycogen concentration during team games can fall to a level where performance, particularly in the latter stages of the game, might be impaired.[21] This suggestion is supported by the wealth of research documenting performance improvements and a delay in the onset of fatigue when carbohydrate supplements are used during team games exercise (Section 2.2.3.2.3). However, the critique of the carbohydrate supplementation literature (summarised in Table 2.1) should be considered.

Observation of progressive increases in blood free fatty acid concentrations during the second half of team games[20,25] suggests an increased reliance on fat as a fuel source, perhaps due to reduced glycogen availability.[14] When players start a soccer match with partial glycogen depletion, significant reductions occur by half-time and stores are almost fully depleted at the end of the game, in contrast to players who start with full glycogen stores.

While muscle glycogen concentrations can be significantly reduced during team games exercise, this does not necessarily imply a causative relationship between muscle glycogen depletion and progressive fatigue. Some studies have shown reductions in muscle glycogen during team games to levels that are insufficient to maintain maximal glycolytic rate (approximately 200 mmol/kg dry weight),[14] whereas other studies demonstrate much less muscle glycogen depletion. For example, Krustrup *et al.*[20] found that muscle glycogen concentrations at the end of a football game ranged from 150–350 mmol/kg dry weight. However, the authors looked more closely and found that about half of the type I and type II quadriceps muscle fibres were almost or completely depleted of muscle glycogen following the match. Findings such as this have led to the suggestion that fatigue towards the end of a game could be related to muscle glycogen depletion in individual muscle fibres. This relates back to the discussions in Section 2.2.3 and 5.7.1 that there is certainly a link between muscle glycogen depletion and fatigue, but that the nature of this link is not fully known. Section 5.7.1 discussed the potential for localised muscle glycogen depletion to contribute to impaired Ca^{2+} kinetics via reduced ATP concentrations in areas of the cell responsible for Ca^{2+} release and uptake, or by means unrelated to glycogen's role as an energy source. Therefore, localised muscle glycogen depletion in individual fibres could contribute to fatigue development during team games via these mechanisms. However, no research studies have specifically investigated this possibility. As a result, we are currently left with the conclusion that muscle glycogen depletion does likely play a role in progressive fatigue during team games, but the extent of this role and the exact mechanisms behind it are not yet known.

Development of hypoglycaemia to the extent where performance may be inhibited is uncommon in sport and exercise (Section 2.2.3.2.2). Furthermore, blood glucose concentrations do no reach critical values during soccer.[20] Therefore, development of hypoglycaemia as a prevalent cause of fatigue during team games can be discounted.

Key point

It is likely that muscle glycogen depletion plays some role(s) in progressive fatigue during team games exercise. The exact nature of this role is still under investigation, but may relate to depletion of glycogen in specific locations within individual muscle fibres. Under normal circumstances, hypoglycaemia is not a cause of fatigue during team games exercise.

7.2.2.1.3.2 Dehydration and thermoregulation During competitive field based team games in thermoneutral conditions, fluid losses of up to 3 litres have been reported, increasing to 4–5 litres in hot and humid environments.[26–8] Fluid losses during 90-mins soccer training equate to about 1.4–1.6% of pre-exercise body mass (BM),[26,28] with fluid deficits of 1–2% BM typical during competition across the majority of environmental conditions.[29]

As discussed in Section 4.3, a belief has existed for a long time that fluid losses of ≥ 2% BM can impair physiological and psychological function during exercise. This would suggest that team games players may be susceptible to dehydration-induced performance decrements. However, Section 4.3 discussed issues with the early research that was used to 'promote' this 2% threshold, and introduces more recent studies that appear to refute altogether the notion of the 2% threshold. Of course, it is likely that large volumes of fluid loss could impact negatively on team games performance. However, as mentioned above, typical fluid losses during team games training and competition, particularly soccer, are only 1–2% BM.

Key point

Typical fluid losses during team games training and competition amount to 1–2% body mass. This is unlikely to contribute to a significant reduction in performance.

Actual supporting evidence regarding dehydration and performance decrements in team games research is lacking. McGregor *et al.*[30] showed a 5% decrement in performance of a sprint-dribbling test following completion of a simulated team games exercise protocol with no fluid ingestion, which produced a fluid loss of approximately 2.4% BM. Mental concentration was unaffected. Edwards *et al.*[31] also found no change in concentration following 45 min of outdoor soccer match-play in the absence of fluid intake. Performance of a post-match sport-specific fitness test was impaired, and RPE, sensation of thirst, and core temperature were significantly greater compared with a fluid intake trial. Core temperature did not rise to a level that would be thought to contribute to fatigue.

Section 4.3 discussed how drinking according to the dictate of individual thirst may be the most effective approach to hydration during exercise. If this is the case, it poses a problem for team games players that may impact their performance. Team games players are confined to the rules of their sport. This means, for the majority of field based team games such as soccer, rugby, and hockey, that there are no scheduled breaks in play to consume fluid. Therefore, players are limited to consuming fluid at half-time and during any unforeseen breaks in play, for example to attend to an injured player. As a result, team games players may not be able to respond to their own thirst drive. This suggestion was put forward by Edwards and Noakes,[29] who proposed that rather than a direct cause of fatigue, dehydration is one in a number of dynamic markers within the central governor/anticipatory feedback model of exercise performance (Section 6.3 and 6.4). According to the authors, each player would begin a match with a 'pacing plan' that would enable them to reach the end of the game in a functioning state (Figures 6.4 and 6.5, Table 6.1). Conscious perception of a developing homeostatic disturbance, in this case loss of body water, triggers an increased perception of effort and behavioural changes, namely an increased desire to drink and a reduction in exercise intensity (voluntary fatigue), that prevents physiological system failure and failure to complete the match. In this hypothesis, the conscious perception of thirst may be more important to performance than actual fluid loss.[29,31] This self-pacing hypothesis is supported by observations of similar sweat rates across team games played in widely different environmental conditions; minimal to moderate fluid losses during games; no difference in core temperature between the first and second halves of games;[32] lack of attainment of a 'critical' core temperature during soccer matches (Section 4.6.3);[33] the ability of individuals of wide fitness levels to complete a full match; and that *ad libitum* drinking maximises exercise performance despite varying levels of dehydration.[34] To date, the influence of the thirst drive on team games performance, independent of changes in hydration status or thermoregulation, has not been closely investigated.

It appears that team games players (at least well-conditioned players) rarely reach a core temperature that could be considered 'critical' for performance impairment.[29] However, Section 4.6.3 mentioned that high skin temperatures can impair exercise performance, independently from changes in core temperature. Therefore, skin temperature response may play a role in the development of fatigue during team games. While there are studies that have shown improved exercise performance when increases in skin temperature are reduced or prevented,[35–6] there is currently not much data reporting the skin temperature responses to team games exercise, independent from changes in core temperature. Therefore, it is not possible to determine whether or not skin temperature is a potential cause of fatigue during team games, or whether strategies to reduce skin temperature would improve team games performance.

Key point

Drinking to the dictates of thirst may be the optimal strategy for exercise performance. If this is the case, team games players are hampered, as there are no scheduled breaks in play during most field-based team games where fluid could be routinely consumed. However, the relationship between the thirst drive and team games performance has not been closely investigated.

7.2.2.1.3.3 Central fatigue Section 4.6.2 discussed the link between hyperthermia, alterations in cerebral function, and impaired force of sustained voluntary muscle contractions. Hyperthermia-induced reduction in voluntary motor output requires elevated core and/or brain temperature, suggesting that this mechanism may only play a role in fatigue during team games played in high ambient temperatures (Section 7.2.2.1.3.2). However, research has reported reductions in electromyography (EMG; Section 1.3.2) activity of the quadriceps muscles during and after actual and simulated soccer exercise, and reductions in maximal voluntary contraction force (MVC; Section 1.2.1) immediately following soccer played in normal ambient temperatures.[37–9] These findings imply that a central aspect to fatigue during team games may be present even in normal ambient temperatures. However, implying a central component as the cause of reduced muscle EMG activity is speculative, as changes to EMG activity of a muscle do not necessarily signify altered central neural drive, and muscle EMG activity can change during and after exercise, but these changes do not necessarily alter muscle force production.[40] Despite this, evidence for reduced MVC during and after team games exercise does suggest a central component to the fatigue process in team games. The exact causes of this central fatigue component, particularly in the absence of hyperthermia, require further study.

Key point

There may be a central component to progressive fatigue during team games exercise. However, this requires more robust study, particularly regarding the nature of the possible central fatigue in the absence of hyperthermia.

7.2.2.1.3.4 Muscle/blood lactate and pH As mentioned in Section 7.2.2.1.1.1, increases in muscle or blood lactate concentration, or decreases in muscle or blood pH, do not appear to be a cause of transient fatigue during team games exercise. Therefore, it is highly unlikely that increases in lactate/decreases in pH would be a significant cause of the progressive fatigue found towards the end of a game, particularly as the frequency of high-intensity activities (which would be most likely to increase lactate levels/decrease pH) decreases in the second half.

7.2.3 Middle-distance exercise

Middle-distance exercise refers to exercise carried out for approximately 90 seconds to 5 minutes (equivalent to an approximate running distance of 800 or 1,500 metres). The key performance requirements and associated fatigue mechanisms during middle-distance exercise are in Figure 7.4.

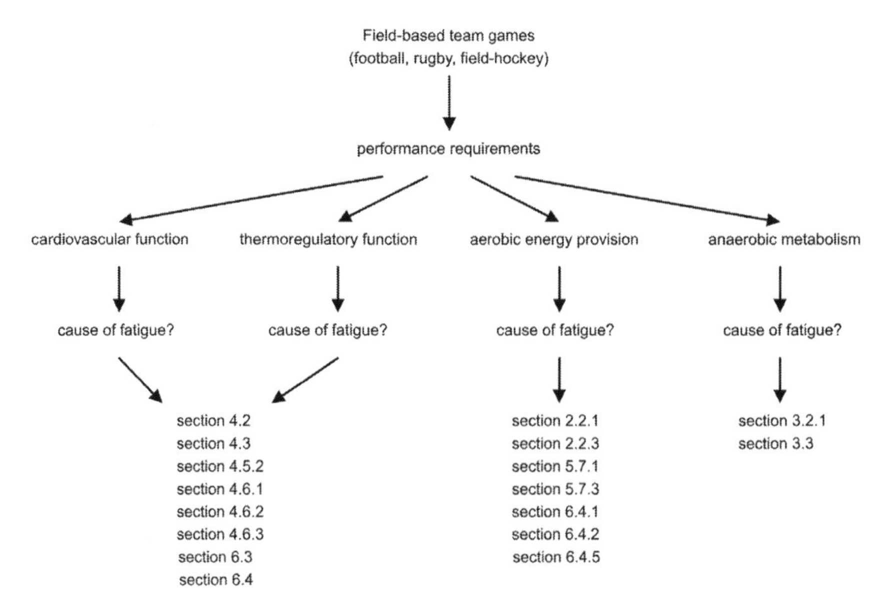

Figure 7.3 Potential causes of fatigue that develops towards the end of field-based team games. Only those performance requirements that may play a direct significant role in the fatigue process are highlighted. The section numbers refer to sections of this book that discuss the potential causes of fatigue associated with each of the identified performance requirements.

Peak muscle lactate concentrations occur following exercise that causes exhaustion in approximately 3–7 minutes. Therefore, it is not surprising that both an 800-metre and 1,500-metre run require notable contributions from the aerobic and anaerobic energy pathways. For an 800-metre run, the approximate percentage contribution of aerobic/anaerobic energy systems to total ATP resynthesis is 60–70/30–40%.[41–2] For the 1,500 metre run, the approximate aerobic/anaerobic contribution is 84/16%.[42] For both the 800- and 1,500-metre distance, the 'crossover' from a predominantly anaerobic to a predominantly aerobic ATP resynthesis occurs between 15 to 30 seconds into the run.[42] The importance of the anaerobic energy system diminishes as exercise duration increases.[43]

Research has identified the relationship between VO_{2max} and running economy, VO_2 at the second ventilatory threshold, and running speed at the second ventilatory threshold, as important indicators of middle-distance performance.[44–5] Measurement and interpretation of these variables appears to enable discrimination between an athlete's predisposition as either a middle or long distance runner.[45]

An often-overlooked factor that could impact the performance of middle distance runners is the adaptations gained from resistance training. Resistance

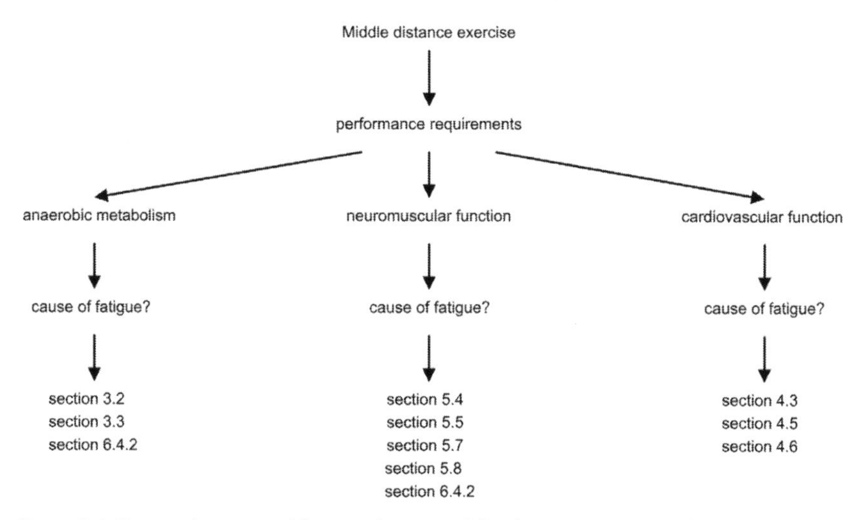

Figure 7.4 Potential causes of fatigue during middle-distance exercise. Only those performance requirements that may play a direct significant role in the fatigue process are highlighted. The section numbers refer to sections of this book that discuss the potential causes of fatigue associated with each of the identified performance requirements.

training using body weight and external resistance has been shown to improve running economy, either through changes in running mechanics or through factors associated with storage and return of elastic energy in the muscle.[46–7]

7.2.3.1 What are the likely 'causes' of fatigue during middle-distance exercise?

7.2.3.1.1 CARDIOVASCULAR FUNCTION

Section 7.2.3 identified aerobic metabolism as crucial for performance in middle-distance events. Therefore, factors that impair cardiovascular responses, and hence the ability to deliver oxygen to working muscles, could be a source of fatigue during middle-distance exercise.

The primary factors addressed in this book that could impair cardiovascular function during exercise are dehydration and hyperthermia. Both dehydration and hyperthermia are usually associated with longer duration activity, as it takes time for both of these conditions to develop (depending on the pre-exercise state of the athlete). It is highly unlikely that either dehydration or hyperthermia would negatively impact the cardiovascular response of athletes during an event lasting 90 seconds to 5 minutes. There may be some situations where either dehydration or hyperthermia could impact middle-distance performance, for example if an athlete began a run without appropriate preparation (i.e. significant pre-existing hypohydration), and/or if the event took part in extreme conditions (particularly regarding temperature and humidity). However, in the majority of situations it is unlikely that impaired function of the cardiovascular system would play a role in fatigue development during middle-distance exercise.

Key point

Under normal circumstances, it is unlikely that impairments to cardiovascular function are a cause of fatigue during middle-distance exercise.

7.2.3.1.2 MUSCLE/BLOOD LACTATE, AND PH

Section 7.2.3 confirms that middle-distance running requires significant contributions from the anaerobic energy pathways, which will lead to production of muscle lactate and H^+. The role of lactate in fatigue has already been considered in this chapter (Section 7.2.2.1.1.1), and will not be repeated here. Once again, the reader is referred to Sections 3.2 and 3.3 for a more focused discussion of lactate and fatigue.

Potentially of more relevance to middle distance exercise is H^+ production. During high-intensity exercise muscle pH can drop to below 6.5, which would indicate increased acidosis via H^+ production. As discussed in Section 3.3, at physiological temperatures and pH levels, metabolic acidosis has a smaller impact on SR Ca^{2+} release, muscle membrane excitability, and glycolytic rate than was originally thought. This information therefore argues against a significant role of intramuscular H^+ production in fatigue during middle-distance events. However, reductions in muscle pH can stimulate group III and IV muscle afferents, potentially increasing sensations of muscular pain/discomfort, and inhibiting central drive (via muscle afferent stimulation and/or arterial haemoglobin desaturation) and thereby contributing to the development of central fatigue (Section 3.3.1 and 3.3.2.5).

Many studies have shown an improvement in high-intensity exercise (including 800-metre and 1,500-metre running) performance following ingestion of sodium bicarbonate.[48–51] Sodium bicarbonate is a compound that makes the blood more alkaline. This increased alkalinity creates a greater pH gradient between the muscle and blood, allowing the blood to more readily 'accept' greater amounts of H^+ from the muscle, which would allow greater intramuscular H^+ production before any potentially fatiguing issues arise. The performance benefit seen with sodium bicarbonate ingestion is very similar to the performance decrement seen when ammonium chloride (a compound that increases the acidity of the blood) is ingested.[50] However, it is interesting that some studies which found performance improvements with sodium bicarbonate ingestion during high-intensity exercise also reported no difference in muscle pH at the end of exercise with or without sodium bicarbonate.[52] The lack of influence of sodium bicarbonate on muscle pH in the face of a performance improvement suggests that there may be other mechanisms by which sodium bicarbonate improves high-intensity exercise performance, for example by reducing central fatigue associated with extracellular acidosis (Section 3.3.2.5).[53–9]

Key point

The significant H^+ production, and associated muscle pH reduction, during middle-distance exercise may contribute to fatigue by alterations in Ca^{2+} kinetics, muscle membrane excitability, and glycolysis. However, the influence of pH on these factors in vivo is less than previously thought. Hydrogen production may induce central fatigue either via stimulation of type III and IV muscle afferents and/or causing arterial oxygen desaturation and cerebral hypoxia.

7.2.3.1.3 EXTRACELLULAR POTASSIUM ACCUMULATION

Section 7.2.1.1.3 stated that extracellular K^+ accumulation can occur within 1–3 minutes of intense exercise. However, limited data is available on the K^+ dynamics associated with intensive whole body exercise. The available data shows significant elevations in extracellular K^+ concentration after just one minute of exhaustive treadmill running.[60] This rate of accumulation suggests that any role of extracellular K^+ accumulation on fatigue may exert an effect within the timeframe of middle-distance exercise.

While extracellular K^+ accumulation can occur during middle-distance exercise, the degree to which this may contribute to fatigue should be considered. As discussed in Sections 5.4 and 5.5, the body has many mechanisms that work to prevent losses in muscle excitability (the main way in which extracellular K^+ accumulation is proposed to contribute to fatigue) during exercise. These mechanisms, combined with a lack of specific data on the K^+ dynamics of middle-distance exercise, mean that a consensus regarding the role of extracellular K^+ accumulation on fatigue during middle-distance exercise is not possible. However, the potential influence of elevated blood K^+ concentration on the central nervous system (CNS) via group III and IV afferent stimulation (Section 5.3.1), and therefore its potential association with development of central fatigue, is interesting, although further study is certainly required. Currently it is prudent to remember the statement from Section 5.5, that until more data is generated, we should be cautious about accepting extracellular K^+ accumulation as a cause of fatigue during middle-distance exercise.

Key point

Notable extracellular K^+ accumulation may occur during middle-distance exercise, which may impair muscle membrane excitability and muscle function. However, many mechanisms exist to reduce the effect of extracellular K^+ accumulation on muscle membrane excitability. Potassium accumulation may influence the CNS and contribute to central fatigue, however more research is needed before this can be confirmed.

7.2.3.1.4 CALCIUM KINETICS

Middle-distance running is characterised not only by the requirement for well-trained aerobic and anaerobic energy systems, but also for the maintenance of running economy at high movement speeds. Middle-distance runners show smaller declines in ground contact time with increasing speed compared with long-distance runners, which appears to reduce the metabolic cost for middle-distance runners of running at faster speeds.[61] The knowledge that running performance and running economy are related to the ability of the neuromuscular system to produce force[62] implies that alterations in this force producing ability could impair middle-distance exercise performance.

Section 5.7 discussed the possible role of changes in Ca^{2+} kinetics in exercise fatigue. Calcium kinetics can be impaired by glycogen depletion (Section 5.7.1). However, this is not likely to play a role during middle-distance exercise, as muscle glycogen availability is typically not a limiting factor during exercise of this duration. Similarly, the impact of metabolic acidosis on SR Ca^{2+} release and on the contractile process itself appears to be minimal (Section 3.3.2). Therefore, despite significant H^+ production during middle-distance exercise, this is unlikely to impair performance via changes to Ca^{2+} kinetics.

Accumulation of P_i during high-intensity exercise (from the breakdown of PCr and ATP) can reduce the sensitivity of the muscle contractile machinery to a given Ca^{2+} concentration (Section 5.7.2). This reduction in Ca^{2+} sensitivity appears to increase the closer muscle temperatures get to normal physiological temperature, suggesting that impaired Ca^{2+} sensitivity due to P_i accumulation may play an important role in muscle fatigue. Furthermore, P_i accumulation may contribute to reduced SR Ca^{2+} release by affecting the SR Ca^{2+} release mechanism and by precipitating with Ca^{2+} within the SR, reducing the amount of free Ca^{2+} that is available to be released into the muscle (Section 5.7.2). The potentially negative influence of P_i accumulation on Ca^{2+} kinetics could play a role in fatigue during middle-distance exercise, by reducing the force generating capability of the muscle. However, Section 5.7.2 warns about some of the limitations of the *in vitro* research that has been carried out into P_i and Ca^{2+} kinetics.

Reductions in ATP concentration near the SR pumps can result in less efficient removal of Ca^{2+} from the myoplasm. Furthermore, both reduced ATP and increased magnesium (Mg^{2+}) concentration impair SR Ca^{2+} release. Therefore, localised accumulation and/or depletion of specific metabolites within the muscle may impair Ca^{2+} kinetics, and hence muscle force production, during middle-distance exercise.

Altered Ca^{2+} kinetics may be a strong candidate for at least contributing to fatigue during middle-distance exercise. However, as mentioned in Section 5.8, our reliance on *in vitro* data regarding muscle Ca^{2+} kinetics means we should be aware of possible differences in responses *in vivo*, as some *in vitro* studies do not accurately reflect the complex environment of intact, contracting human muscle.

Key point

Impaired Ca^{2+} kinetics, possibly via P_i and Mg^{2+} accumulation and/or localised ATP depletion, may play a role in muscle fatigue during middle-distance exercise.

7.2.4 Long-distance sprints

The key performance requirements and associated fatigue mechanisms during long-distance sprinting are in Figure 7.5. Long-distance sprinting refers to maximal exercise lasting approximately 30–60 seconds, such as a 400-metre run. Notable fatigue occurs during this form of exercise, as evidenced by reductions in running speed of 20–40% by the end of a run.[63] Long-distance sprinting is dependent on high rates of anaerobic metabolism, a high VO_{2max}, and neuromuscular function to generate large muscle power.[43] It may be surprising to read that a high VO_{2max} has been associated with performance during long-distance sprinting; however, the aerobic/anaerobic energy contribution to a 400-metre sprint is approximately 35–45/55–65%.[41–2] Indeed, it is worth remembering that Spencer and Gastin[42] show the cross-over from predominantly anaerobic to predominantly aerobic energy supply occurs between 15–30 seconds into exercise. During a 400-metre run, PCr degradation is the predominant source of ATP resynthesis during the first 100 metres, followed by glycolysis from 100 to 300 metres, with almost no contribution from PCr in the final quarter of the run.[43,64–5] The notable

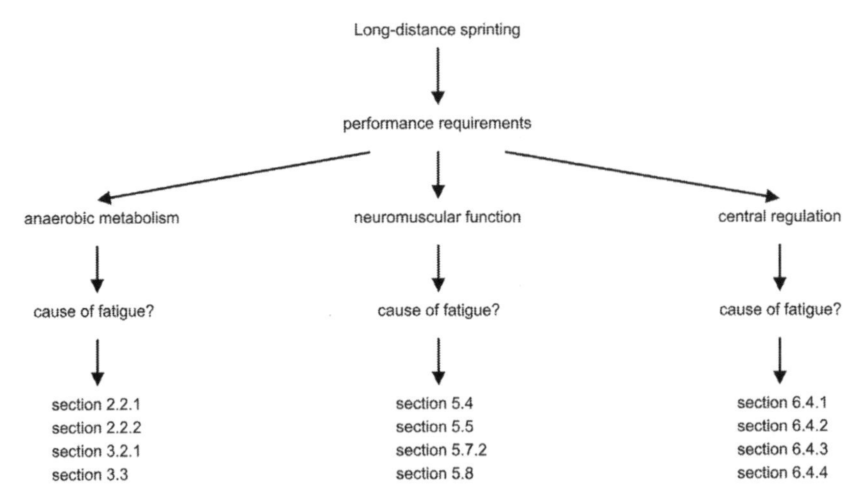

Figure 7.5 Potential causes of fatigue during long-distance sprinting. Only those performance requirements that may play a direct significant role in the fatigue process are highlighted. The section numbers refer to sections of this book that discuss the potential causes of fatigue associated with each of the identified performance requirements.

contribution of glycolysis to ATP resynthesis may explain why there is a strong correlation between 400-metre performance and both anaerobic energy contribution[41] and peak blood lactate concentration.[65] Peak running velocity occurs 50–100 metres into the run, following by a progressive decrease in velocity until 300 metres, and a notable reduction in velocity occurs in the final 100 metres.[66] This velocity pattern appears to be similar regardless of ability level, and in fact the greatest decrement in velocity during the final 100 metres is seen in world-class 400-metre runners.[66] The difference is that peak running velocity is greater in higher quality runners, and velocity remains significantly higher for at least the first half of the race.[66]

A high anaerobic capacity may relate to performance in long-distance sprinting by increasing power output and running velocity, as the rate at which ATP can be supplied anaerobically influences both of these factors.[41] This suggestion is supported by research showing that greater explosive strength, strength-endurance, and power leads to better 400-metre performance.[43,67]

7.2.4.1 What are the likely 'causes' of fatigue during long-distance sprints?

7.2.4.1.1 MUSCLE/BLOOD LACTATE, AND PH

The role of lactate production and pH changes on fatigue during long-distance sprinting is likely similar to that during middle distance running

(Section 7.2.3.1.2), so will only be discussed briefly. The importance of anaerobic metabolism to sprinting performance increases as sprint distance decreases, suggesting a relatively greater importance of anaerobic metabolism during 400-metre running compared with middle-distance running. However, as discussed in Section 3.3, reductions in muscle pH associated with H^+ production have a much smaller impact on muscle contractile function and metabolism in a normal *in vivo* environment than originally thought.

Section 7.2.3.1.2 also discussed how increases in muscle and blood H^+ concentration might stimulate group III and IV muscle afferents and desaturate arterial haemoglobin, respectively, potentially causing central fatigue. Research has shown notable reductions in MVC force immediately following a 400-metre run (Section 1.2.1);[63] however, notable reductions in muscle torque production via electrical stimulation of the muscle were also found (Section 1.2.1). It therefore appears that reductions in muscle force production following a 400-metre run are mainly due to peripheral causes, with central causes having less of an influence.[63] Possible peripheral causes of reduced muscle force are discussed below.

Key point

Reductions in muscle force production following long-distance sprinting are probably due to peripheral causes rather than central fatigue.

7.2.4.1.2 MUSCLE MEMBRANE EXCITABILITY

The rapid accumulation of extracellular K^+ during intense exercise (Section 7.2.3.1.3) means that K^+ accumulation in the interstitium or the t-tubules should be considered as a potential cause of fatigue during long-distance sprints. Studies have found that muscle membrane excitability appears to be preserved following a long-duration sprint.[63] Also, the time course of recovery of muscle torque (more than 30 minutes) is far longer than would be expected if reduced muscle membrane excitability due to extracellular K^+ accumulation was a significant cause of fatigue.[63,68] The apparent lack of a role for extracellular K^+ accumulation in fatigue development during long-duration sprints may be specific to this form of exercise, or may reflect the more general lack of influence of extracellular K^+ accumulation on muscle membrane excitability that was discussed in Sections 5.4 and 5.5.

7.2.4.1.3 CALCIUM KINETICS

While muscle membrane excitability may not be notably impaired during long-distance sprinting, alterations in intramuscular Ca^{2+} kinetics may play a more significant role in fatigue during this type of exercise. Following long-distance sprinting, peak muscle torque, maximal rate of force development, and relaxation are all impaired.[63,68] Findings such as this have led to the conclusion that fatigue during long-distance sprints is peripheral and likely related to alterations in excitation-contraction coupling.[68] More specifically, inhibition of SR Ca^{2+} release by P_i, and Ca^{2+}–P_i precipitation in the SR, are the most likely factors, rather than alterations at the contractile apparatus itself.[63,68–9] Impaired SR Ca^{2+} release may also be due to reductions in ATP and/or increases in myoplasmic Mg^{2+} (Sections 5.7.3 and 5.8).

Key point

Extracellular K^+ accumulation probably does not play a notable role in fatigue during long-distance sprints. However, Ca^{2+} kinetics may be impaired during this form of exercise.

7.2.4.1.4 ATP AND PHOSPHOCREATINE DEPLETION

As discussed in Section 2.2.1, significant whole-muscle ATP depletion is not seen during exercise at a variety of durations and intensities, including short-distance, high-intensity exercise.[70–1] Therefore, ATP depletion (at least at the whole-muscle level) would not be considered a direct cause of fatigue during long-distance sprinting.

While ATP depletion may not be a direct cause of fatigue, depletion of the sources of ATP resynthesis may be. Section 2.2.2.1 discussed how muscle PCr concentrations can be reduced by approximately 80% during a 30-second sprint, and that significant correlations exist between the recovery of PCr and subsequent power output. This indicates that single sprint performance is influenced by PCr depletion. However, it should be considered that athletes completing a 400-metre sprint do not begin running at their maximum speed, as this would result in an excessive reduction in speed towards the end of the race. Therefore, the energy system contributions modelled during all-out sprint efforts may not be the same as the responses during long sprint events, where a degree of pacing is involved that would influence the rate of ATP resynthesis, and hence the required energy system contribution (Section 7.2.4.1.5). As a result, PCr stores may last longer during a 400-metre run compared with the duration suggested by research using all-out long sprints.[72] This suggestion is supported by research showing that running velocity during a 400-metre run in world-class athletes does begin to decline until 11–13 seconds into the run,[66] which is longer than the time taken for velocity to drop during a short-distance sprint (Section 7.2.5). Nevertheless, a reduction in PCr concentration would reduce the rate at which ATP could be resynthesised, and would necessitate a slowing of running velocity. As a result, PCr depletion does likely contribute to the development of fatigue during long-distance sprinting, but as part of a combination of changes occurring in the muscle (Sections 7.2.4.1.1 and 7.2.4.1.3) and, potentially, the CNS (Section 7.2.4.1.5).[66]

Key point

Phosphocreatine depletion probably does contribute to fatigue during long-distance sprints, but as part of a combination of changes occurring in the periphery and, potentially, the central nervous system.

7.2.4.1.5 ANTICIPATORY REGULATION OF PERFORMANCE

Pacing strategies are arguably present in the majority of sporting events, whether as a conscious attempt to maximise performance or as a subconscious effort to prevent significant homeostatic disruption to body systems (Section 6.4.3). Specific research into the pacing strategies of 400-metre running, and the reasons driving these pacing strategies, is limited (Section 7.2.4). However, a pacing strategy is observed during all-out cycling lasting approximately 45 seconds.[73] This pacing strategy consists of a lower peak power output and initial mean power output (0–10 seconds of the test), and a reduced degree of fatigue in the first 15 seconds of the test, compared with 15 and 30-second all-out cycling bouts. Interestingly, there appears to be a relationship between RPE and blood lactate concentration during long all-out sprints, suggesting the possibility of lactate acting as an afferent signal that influences RPE and the pacing strategy employed.[73] If this were the case, it would indicate that anticipatory regulation might play a role in modulating long-distance sprint performance (Sections 6.4.1, 6.4.2, 6.4.3, 6.4.4). It has been shown that the contractile ability of the muscle begins to decline within 10 seconds of the beginning of a 400-metre run,[65] which may be indicative of some form of central, anticipatory regulation.

Key point

Observation of pacing strategies during all-out 45-second cycle sprints suggests that pacing is present during long-distance sprinting. Whether this is a conscious strategy or related to subconscious anticipatory performance regulation is unclear.

7.2.5 Short-distance sprints

The key performance requirements and associated fatigue mechanisms during short-distance sprinting are in Figure 7.6. Short-distance sprinting is defined as the equivalent of a 100–200-metre sprint (approximately 10–30 seconds of maximal effort). For optimal performance in short-distance sprinting, it is crucial for athletes to obtain and maintain their maximum or near-maximum velocity throughout the race.[43] However, decrements in velocity of about 8% and 20% occur during 100 and 200-metre races, respectively.[63] In 100-metre running, peak velocity is attained about 40–60 metres into the race, after which it begins to decline.[74] A similar pattern is seen in the 200-meter race, except peak velocity tends to be lower and the drop-off in velocity smaller but, of course, going on for longer.[75] This velocity trend helps to explain how Usain Bolt set the 100-metre world record of 9.58 seconds in 2009, as during that race Bolt was able to maintain his peak velocity from 50–80 metres before beginning to slow. This indicates that the person most likely to win a short-duration sprint is the person who slows down the least during the race.

The aerobic/anaerobic energy contribution to a 100-metre run is approximately 10–20/80–90%,[76] and for a 200-metre run approximately 30/70%.[42] Unsurprisingly, anaerobic metabolism is dominant, but the aerobic contribution of 10–30% suggests that the aerobic system should not be completely ignored when training for short-distance sprinting.[42] Despite this suggestion,

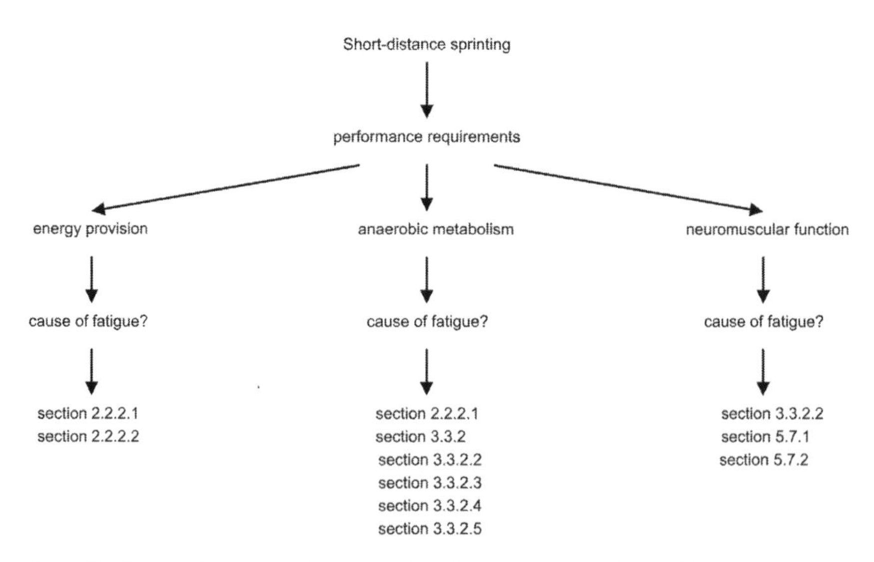

Figure 7.6 Potential causes of fatigue during short-distance sprinting. Only those performance requirements that may play a direct significant role in the fatigue process are highlighted. The section numbers refer to sections of this book that discuss the potential causes of fatigue associated with each of the identified performance requirements.

aerobic capacity does not appear to be related to performance in either the 100 or 200-metre run.[43] In contrast, performance in both distances is significantly related to anaerobic capacity.[43,76–7] Neuromuscular function and muscle power are also primary factors in performance during short-distance sprinting.[43]

7.2.5.1 What are the likely 'causes' of fatigue during short-distance sprints?

The short time to complete 100- and 200-metre sprints may give the perspective that there are fewer and, perhaps, less complex causes of fatigue in this type of activity compared to endurance-based exercise. However, it is almost certain that the causes of fatigue during short sprints are still multi-factorial.[72]

7.2.5.1.1 ADENOSINE TRIPHOSPHATE AND PHOSPHOCREATINE DEPLETION

Section 7.2.4.1.4 reiterated that significant whole-muscle ATP depletion is not seen during exercise at a variety of durations and intensities, including short duration, high-intensity exercise. This appears to preclude ATP depletion as a direct cause of fatigue during short-distance sprinting.

Phosphocreatine contributes approximately 50% of the ATP resynthesised during a 6 second sprint and 25% of the ATP during a 20 second sprint, with the remainder supplied by glycolysis and aerobic metabolism (Section 2.2.2.1 and Figure 2.2). The rapid reduction in PCr during sprinting may reduce the rate at which ATP can be resynthesised, thereby necessitating a reduction in running velocity. This suggestion is partly supported by research showing a significant increase in running velocity during a 100-metre sprint following a period of creatine supplementation, which can increase muscle PCr concentrations.[78] Greater PCr availability could improve sprint performance by maintaining ATP resynthesis via high energy phosphates for longer into the sprint.[78] However, creatine supplementation has shown mixed results regarding performance improvement (Section 2.2.2.2). Nevertheless, the association between PCr resynthesis and subsequent sprint performance (Section 2.2.2.2) indicates that PCr depletion does play a limiting role in short-distance sprint performance.

Key point

Phosphocreatine contributes a significant amount of the ATP required during short-distance sprints, and strong associations are present between PCr availability and short-duration sprint performance. Therefore, PCr depletion has a performance limiting role during short-distance sprinting.

7.2.5.1.2 MUSCLE/BLOOD LACTATE, AND PH

It was originally thought that anaerobic glycolysis was only activated once PCr stores were depleted; however, many studies have since documented significant increases in blood lactate concentration within 10-seconds of hard exercise.[79] Furthermore, anaerobic glycolysis contributes approximately 40–45% of the required ATP during a 10-second sprint, and 50% of the required ATP during a 20-second sprint (Section 2.2.2.1, Figure 2.2). Muscle and blood lactate begins to accumulate during sprints as short as 40 metres; however, the concentrations of muscle and blood lactate, and the reduction in blood pH, at the end of a 100-metre sprint are not sufficient to conclude that alterations in acid–base balance are a cause of fatigue during this event.[80–1]

While acidosis does not play a role in fatigue during the 100-metre sprint, in the 200-metre sprint athletes are required to continue running maximally for a further 10 seconds or so. Following 20-seconds of cycle sprinting, muscle pH falls significantly.[80] This reduction in pH may be sufficient to impair performance in at least two ways: 1: By reducing the activity of glycolysis, as has been shown at low muscle pH *in vitro*. However, pH-mediated impairment of glycolysis does not have clear support in the literature (Section 3.3.2.3); 2: By impairing the force output of actin and myosin when in their high-force state (Section 3.3.2.4). Type II muscle fibres show more pronounced reductions in muscle pH, and the depressive effect of low pH on muscle force is greater in this fibre type.[82–3] Sprinters will most likely have a greater percentage of type II muscle fibres, suggesting that any role of reduced pH on cross-bridge force production may be more prevalent in sprinters, and may be prevalent in the fatigue process during short-distance sprinting. However, as discussed in Section 3.3.2.4, many of the studies showing reductions in cross-bridge muscle force with reduced pH were conducted *in vitro* and at lower than normal physiological temperatures (the influence of temperature on pH-mediated changes in biochemical and physiological function is discussed elsewhere; see Section 3.3 and 3.3.2.4). Therefore, it is difficult to conclusively state the significance of reduced pH on cross-bridge force production in an exercising human.

Key point

The concentrations of muscle and blood lactate, and reduction in blood pH, following a 100 m sprint are not sufficient to be a cause of fatigue. Significant reductions in muscle pH following a 20-second cycle sprint suggest that reduced pH may contribute to fatigue during sprints of this duration. The exact nature of this contribution is still debated.

7.2.5.1.3 INORGANIC PHOSPHATE

Section 7.2.4.1.3 highlighted the possible role of alterations in intramuscular Ca^{2+} kinetics due to P_i accumulation in the myoplasm. Unfortunately, few (if any) data exist regarding Ca^{2+} cycling during short-distance sprints. However, significant increases in muscle P_i concentrations have been reported following 10- and 20-second sprints.[80] It has also been shown that peak power output is unaffected by the presence of high intramuscular P_i concentrations.[80] This finding casts doubt on the suggested role of high intramuscular P_i concentrations in the depression of maximal muscle force production (Section 5.7.2). It is also very difficult to establish the time-course of P_i accumulation *in vivo* during short-duration maximal sprinting. The extent of PCr breakdown has been shown to be very similar between a 40-metre and 100-metre sprint,[81] but it is still difficult to know whether a sufficient intramuscular accumulation of P_i would occur quickly enough to cause any disturbances in Ca^{2+} kinetics or cross-bridge force production during, for example, a 100-metre sprint (Section 5.7.2).

7.2.5.1.4 NEUROMUSCULAR FUNCTION

Impaired membrane excitability does not appear to be a cause of fatigue during long-distance sprinting (Section 7.2.4.1.2), and this also appears to be the case for short-distance sprints.[63] In fact, no significant correlations have been found between speed decrement and peripheral metabolic or neuromuscular changes during short-distance sprinting.[63]

Nevertheless, significant decreases in EMG activity of the leg muscles have been found following 100- and 200-metre sprints.[84] These changes may relate to sub-optimal output from the motor cortex (perhaps due to reduced motor neuron/muscle responsiveness, Section 6.5), peripheral fatigue (see the above sections), or decreased sensitivity of the stretch reflex following short-distance sprints, perhaps via stimulation of type III and IV muscle afferents (Section 3.3.1 and 7.2.3.1.2).[63,85] Reduced stretch reflex activity would impair the propulsive force of the athletes muscles, reducing muscle power and, hence, speed. The problem with testing hypotheses such as this is that specific muscles in the leg are affected by fatigue-induced changes during sprinting more than others. For example, the hamstring and calf muscles are affected more than the quadriceps muscles; and, the influence of fatigue on muscle function changes depending on the specific phase of the sprinting cycle[63] – more evidence for the complexity of studying fatigue in sport and exercise.

The relative importance of central fatigue to exercise performance becomes greater the longer that exercise continues. It would therefore be expected that central fatigue would have a minimal impact on short-distance sprinting. Indeed, Tomazin *et al.*[63] found little or no influence of central fatigue on isometric muscle contractions immediately following 100- and 200-metre sprints. However, the authors could not say for sure that central neural fatigue (particularly motor cortex output and reflex changes such as those discussed in the paragraph above) did not impact performance during the sprint. This is a particularly interesting line for further study, considering the apparent lack of association between speed decrement and peripheral changes during sprinting.

> **Key point**
>
> Central fatigue may develop and limit performance even during short-distance sprinting. However, the extent of central fatigue, and its causes, during short sprints are not clear. Further study would be interesting, considering the apparent lack of association between performance decrement and peripheral changes during sprinting.

7.2.6 Resistance exercise

Discussing fatigue mechanisms associated with resistance exercise requires a different approach to the previous sections. Resistance exercise is more of a training exercise as opposed to a competitive activity. Therefore, it is difficult to describe the performance requirements associated with success at resistance exercise, in contrast to highlighting the specific performance requirements of, say, prolonged submaximal exercise compared with long-distance sprinting. However, anyone who has tried resistance training will know that fatigue does occur during this form of exercise, usually manifesting in muscle pain/discomfort, a reduction in the speed at which the resistance can be moved, and perhaps even a complete inability to continue moving the resistance. Some proposed causes for these sensations are discussed below. Specific causes of fatigue may differ depending on the type of resistance training that is being done, but the current body of literature investigating fatigue processes during different forms of whole-body resistance training is smaller than that for other activities. Therefore, this section will focus on resistance training that would elicit maximal or near-maximal muscle contraction forces.

Recovery following maximal or near-maximal lifting (i.e. strength training) appears to occur more quickly than recovery following submaximal lifting to failure (i.e. endurance training).[86] This may appear paradoxical due to the possible perception that maximal lifting is 'tougher' than submaximal lifting. Importantly, though, it may indicate that fatigue processes in maximal strength training are different to those in submaximal endurance resistance training.

Maximal strength training is generally carried out at a low repetition range (usually 1–5), interspersed with long recovery durations (2–5 minutes).[86]

Key point

Recovery from maximal or near-maximal lifting is faster than recovery from submaximal lifting to failure. This suggests that fatigue processes in maximal lifting may be different to those during submaximal lifting.

Due to this work/rest pattern, a set of maximal strength training will generally take no longer than approximately 10 seconds, followed by substantial recovery. Despite a short work bout, a maximal effort is required, therefore it is likely that substantial PCr depletion is seen following a set of maximal strength lifts.[86–7] This PCr depletion would reduce the rate of ATP resynthesis, and could account at least partly for the decreased lifting velocity and reduced muscle torque seen following maximal or near-maximal muscle activation.[88–9] This could also explain the more rapid recovery of muscle strength; by the time the next set of lifting is required, a notable resynthesis of PCr will have occurred, which would enable the athlete to achieve maximal lifting loads.[87] Therefore, PCr kinetics could play a role in performance during maximal strength training. Significant correlations have also been found between reductions in muscle force and blood lactate concentration.[90] This correlation has led to the suggestion that fatigue during hypertrophy resistance training may be related to significant anaerobic glycolysis that produces H^+ and reduces muscle pH.[87] However, the issues with this hypothesis have been covered elsewhere (Section 3.3.2). A higher level of voluntary muscle activation (such as during maximal strength training) will lead to a more rapid energy depletion and metabolite accumulation.[88] In the case of maximal strength training, one of the key metabolites to accumulate could be P_i, via PCr breakdown. Accumulation of P_i may impair SR Ca^{2+} release, reducing muscle contractile force (Section 5.7.2).[88,91] However, direct measurements of such effects during maximal strength training are lacking. Furthermore, many studies have used electrical stimulation techniques on individual muscle groups as a model for the study of fatigue during maximal muscle contractions, and findings from such studies should be interpreted with this in mind.

Key point

Phosphocreatine depletion may contribute to reductions in lifting velocity and muscle torque during following maximal and near-maximal lifting. Inorganic phosphate accumulation and associated dysregulation of Ca^{2+} kinetics may also play a role, but this requires further study.

Both central and peripheral fatigue have been documented during maximal voluntary muscle contractions.[92] During a maximal isometric voluntary contraction, muscle force production begins to fall almost immediately, and the force increase induced by electrical stimulation increases, indicating the presence of central fatigue (Section 1.2.1).[93–4] A slowing of motor unit firing rates has been shown during sustained and repeated maximal muscle contractions,[95] and the mechanisms behind this are crucial for the understanding of central fatigue development during maximal muscle activation.[94] The potential mechanisms are quite complex; however, slowing of motor unit firing rate likely relates to one or more of the following: 1. A decrease in excitatory input through the motor neurons; 2. An increase in inhibitory input to the motor neurons; 3. A decrease in the responsiveness of the motor neurons themselves to stimulation.[94] Evidence suggests that the slowing of motor unit firing rates is most likely due to a combination of decreased responsiveness of the motor neurons and inhibition of motor neuron firing (perhaps via type III and IV afferent stimulation and reduced muscle spindle activity, see Sections 3.3.1 and 7.2.5.1.4).[96–7] Excitatory input may not decrease, but may become suboptimal by failing to compensate for changes to motor neuron function caused by reduced responsiveness and increased inhibition.[94]

Key point

Central fatigue may develop during maximal and near-maximal lifting via a number of potential changes in excitatory or inhibitory inputs to the motor neurons and/or decreased motor neuron responsiveness.

Some studies have reported a lack of central fatigue during resistance training, implying an importance of peripheral fatigue.[90] However, the extent of peripheral fatigue may depend on muscle fibre type, with type II fibres potentially more affected by peripheral fatigue,[98] and the degree of central fatigue may depend on training status, with more highly resistance-trained individuals capable of 'generating' more central fatigue.[90] Yet more evidence for the complexity of studying fatigue and drawing conclusions.

Key point

The relative influence of central and peripheral fatigue processes during resistance training may depend on factors such as muscle fibre type, resistance load, and training status.

7.3 The influence of gender on fatigue mechanisms

As you can hopefully appreciate from studying the chapters in this book, the causes of fatigue during exercise are specific to the demands of the task. This task specificity can vary between men and women because of gender differences in physiological responses to exercise.[99–100] Much is yet to be discovered about the gender differences in fatigue during dynamic, whole-body exercise.[100] This section will provide a concise overview of current knowledge on this topic.

7.3.1 How does fatigue differ between males and females?

During sustained or intermittent isometric contractions at the same relative intensity, females appear to be less fatigable than males.[99,101] Interestingly, fatigability between genders seems to be influenced by muscle group, with less fatigability seen in females for the elbow flexors, back extensors, knee extensors, and respiratory muscles,[100–3] less of a gender difference for the dorsiflexors,[104] and no gender difference for the elbow extensors.[105] The effect of gender on fatigability in specific muscle groups may depend on the neural, metabolic, and contractile make-up of each muscle group (discussed below). Gender differences in fatigability during isometric contractions are also greatly diminished as the intensity of the muscle contraction increases,[100–6] or when males and females are matched for muscle strength.

A similar pattern is seen during concentric muscle contractions, with females showing less fatigability than males, although the extent of the gender difference is smaller than for isometric contractions.[100] For concentric contractions, gender differences in fatigability can be lessened by independently increasing the intensity and speed of contraction.[107–8] For eccentric contractions, a slightly different picture is seen. Muscle force reduction after repeated eccentric contractions is either similar between genders[109] or is actually greater in females compared to males.[110]

Investigating the fatigue responses to specific contraction types in isolated muscle groups is interesting, but perhaps not the most relevant to sport and exercise contexts. A more externally valid model of research has investigated the fatigue response of males and females to repeated cycle sprints. This work has found that females are generally less fatigable (i.e. they show less of a reduction in power output) than males.[111] However, this is not a universal finding as some work shows no significant difference between genders,[112] particularly when males and females are matched for initial power output.[112] Females also seem to recover from repeated cycle sprints more quickly than males.[113]

Key point

During sustained and intermittent isometric contractions, concentric contractions, and repeated sprints, females are less fatigable than males. However, less fatigability in females is dependent on the muscle group tested, and is greatly reduced as the intensity of the contraction increases, or when genders are matched for muscle strength.

7.3.2 What might explain gender differences in exercise fatigue?

From a physiological standpoint, numerous potential explanations exist for gender differences in fatigability. These will be summarised in the following text, and in Figure 7.7. Interested readers are also encouraged to access the excellent review by Hunter[100] for further detail.

In Section 7.3.1, it was mentioned that when males and females are matched for strength or power output, gender differences in fatigability are greatly reduced or even negated. In fact, there are minimal gender differences in strength per unit of muscle.[100] Therefore, it seems that a potential cause of gender differences in fatigability relates to absolute strength differences between men and women. The larger muscle mass and greater force exerted by males can generate mechanical and metabolic consequences that could exacerbate fatigue compared with females.[100]

A reduction in blood flow to working muscle could exacerbate fatigue via changes in intramuscular metabolic and contractile conditions. Females have better muscle perfusion than males during low- to moderate-intensity isometric contractions (at least for some muscle groups).[103] Better perfusion in females may be due to less contraction-induced compression of the arteries supplying the muscle with blood. The difference in arterial compression between genders occurs because males are generally stronger than females, and exert more pressure on intramuscular arterial blood routes during contractions.[114] Alterations in muscle perfusion between genders may also help to explain why gender differences in fatigability are reduced when the intensity of muscle contraction increases and when genders are matched for strength. During high-intensity contractions, blood flow will be occluded to a similar level for both genders,[106] as it would be if contraction strength was similar. However, females also have a greater ability to dilate the arteries that supply muscles with blood[115] and have greater capillarisation of certain muscle groups (particularly those with more type I fibres), which may also help them to perfuse their muscles better than males. Importantly, greater vasodilation in females is independent of strength.[100]

It is well known that males and females differ in terms of muscle fibre type, size, number, metabolism and contractile properties. Any one of these differences could influence fatigability. Females have greater amounts of type I muscle fibres than males in many muscles involved in locomotion and functional movements.[116] Type I muscle fibres are more fatigue resistant than type II fibres. Specifically, type I fibres show slower Ca^{2+} kinetics than type II fibres.[117] In line with this, females have been shown to have slower rates of SR Ca^{2+} reuptake than males,[118] which would contribute to a slower rate of muscle relaxation. Less muscle fatigue in females has been correlated with slower muscle contractile properties.[119] It therefore seems that females possess a slower, more fatigue resistant muscle profile than males.[100] However, the influence of muscle fibre type on Ca^{2+} kinetics and rate of contraction indicates that the effect of these mechanisms on gender differences in fatigability will be muscle specific.[100]

Gender differences in muscle fibre type and contractile properties are also suggestive of differences in muscle metabolism during exercise. Indeed, it has been shown that females utilise glycolysis to a lesser extent than males during high-intensity isometric contractions,[120] and produce less blood lactate and a smaller reduction in ATP during sprinting, probably due to greater type I fibre content.[121] Conversely, no gender difference is seen for PCr or oxidative metabolism.[120] It is also well known that females oxidise more fat and less carbohydrate than males during exercise at the same relative intensity.[116] Again, this may relate in part to the greater type I fibre content of females, as type I fibres are more suited to aerobically oxidising lipid. Taken together, the metabolic response of females to exercise may be indicative of a more fatigue-resistant state, due to less production of potentially fatigue inducing metabolites from anaerobic glycolysis and a lesser reliance on finite glycogen and blood glucose as an energy source (Section 2.2.3 and 3.3).

Investigation of gender differences in voluntary muscle activation suggests that gender differences in fatigability may reside more in the periphery. There seem to be minimal gender differences in voluntary activation during brief maximal contractions of upper body muscles,[122] and no gender difference in the extent of central fatigue following low- and high-intensity isometric contractions of upper body muscles.[100] However, it does seem that males show a greater reduction than females in the ability to voluntarily activate lower limb muscles during maximal contractions.[123] A speculative suggestion for this upper-lower body gender difference is that males may generate greater peripheral afferent feedback from group III and IV muscle afferents in the lower limbs than females, perhaps due to the differences in muscle perfusion and metabolism discussed earlier in this section.[100]

Finally, it is appropriate to address the potential influence of the female menstrual cycle on fatigability during exercise. Currently, there is no clear evidence that fatigability is influenced by stages of the menstrual cycle,[124] at least during exercise in normal environmental conditions. However, menstrual cycle stage may influence physiological and perceptual responses to prolonged submaximal exercise in hot and humid conditions.[125]

Key point

Females may be less fatigable than males due to differences in muscle perfusion, type I muscle fibre content, muscle energy metabolism and metabolite production, and, potentially, differences in voluntary muscle activation (at least of lower limb muscles).

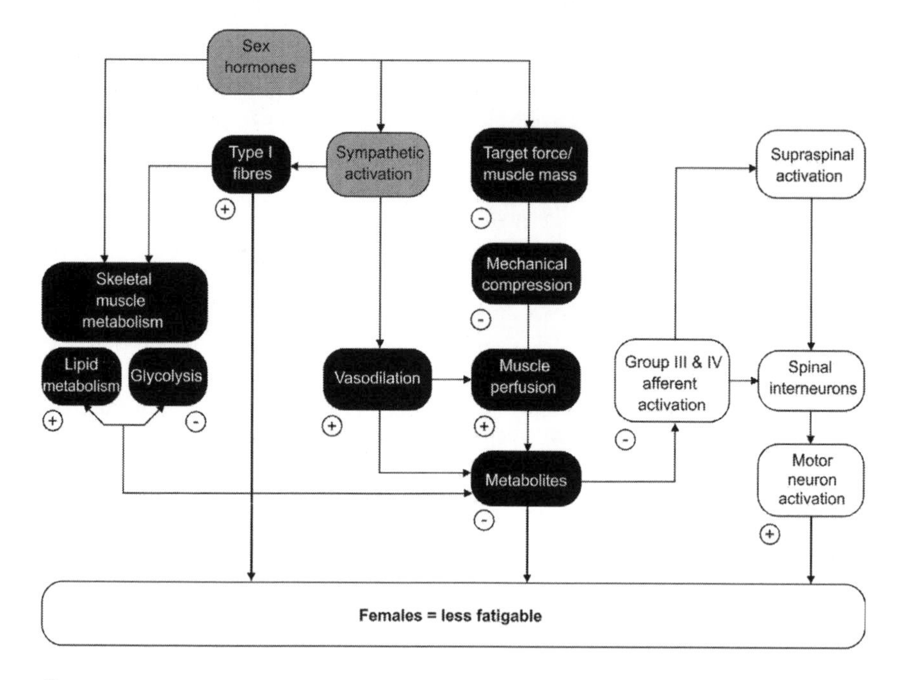

Figure 7.7 Potential physiological mechanisms behind the gender differences in muscle fatigability during exercise. The relative impact of specific mechanisms will depend on the exercise task (particularly type and intensity/strength of contraction, and muscle group(s) used). Black boxes = intramuscular processes; white boxes = nervous system processes; grey boxes = hormonal and sympathetic processes. Figure reproduced from Hunter.[100]

7.4 The influence of training status on fatigue mechanisms

Different types of training can generate different and often quite specific physiological adaptations. Of course, training also increases the physical capacity of the body to perform exercise. If different types of training yield different physiological adaptations, than it stands to reason that training *per se*, and specific types of training, may influence the fatigue mechanisms that can impair exercise performance. This section will provide an overview of how training status may impact fatigue mechanisms during exercise. For ease of reference, the section will specifically address the potential fatigue mechanisms discussed in Part II of this book, and does not provide an all-encompassing overview of the myriad potential influences of training status on exercise performance.

7.4.1 Energy metabolism

Classic adaptations to endurance exercise training include increased muscle mitochondrial density, aerobic enzyme concentration and activity, and muscle capillarisation and perfusion that together improve the ability of the muscles to aerobically resynthesise ATP. Endurance training also increases the expression and activity of intramuscular fatty acid transport proteins and metabolic enzymes. Collectively, these adaptations enable an endurance trained individual to oxidise more fat and less carbohydrate at a given relative exercise intensity.[126–7]

Increased fat and reduced carbohydrate oxidation suggest that endurance trained individuals may be able to reduce the rate at which they deplete endogenous glycogen stores during exercise, and thereby be less affected by potential fatigue mechanisms associated with glycogen depletion (Section 2.2.3). For instance, one of the ways in which muscle glycogen depletion is thought to impair exercise performance is by reducing SR Ca^{2+} release due to depletion of intramyofibrillar glycogen and an associated impairment of ATP resynthesis near the muscle triads (Section 2.2.3.2.1). Type I muscle fibres contain more subsarcolemmal and intramyofibrillar glycogen than type II fibres.[128] As endurance trained athletes will likely have a greater proportion of type I muscle fibres, this may confer an advantage by increasing the amount of time before intramyofibrillar glycogen is depleted. The subcellular localisation of glycogen is influenced by training status,[129] with subsarcolemmal glycogen accumulating most rapidly through training.[128] However, while subsarcolemmal and intermyofibrillar glycogen can be increased after several weeks of endurance training, intramyofibrillar glycogen concentration may only increase after long-term training, or in highly trained athletes.[128] Highly endurance trained athletes do still show impairment in SR Ca^{2+} release that is associated with low intramyofibrillar glycogen content,[130] however the association between low muscle glycogen and fatigue is less pronounced in more highly trained people.[130] While endurance training may not increase intramyofibrillar glycogen concentrations, it could be speculated that it may attenuate the rate of intramyofibrillar glycogen depletion, thereby delaying the onset of potential dysregulation of SR Ca^{2+} kinetics. While some authors have implicated differences in training status as a reason for different study findings,[130] more specific research is required that compares subcellular glycogen use and associated SR dysfunction in people of differing training states.

Performance during repeated-sprint exercise is related to the ability to break down PCr during the sprint, and replenish it during the subsequent recovery period (Section 2.2.2.2). Sprint trained athletes have the highest PCr degradation rates,[81] probably due in part to greater activity of creatine kinase in type II muscle fibres,[131] of which sprint-trained athletes will likely have a greater proportion. Conversely, endurance trained athletes have the greatest PCr resynthesis rates.[132] Replenishment of PCr stores is reliant on the aerobic resynthesis of ATP, and strong positive correlations have been found between submaximal measures of endurance performance, VO_{2max}, and PCr resynthesis rates.[133–4] The relationship between aerobic fitness and PCr resynthesis rates suggests that during repeated-sprint exercise, more aerobically fit individuals would begin each sprint with higher PCr concentrations, which may attenuate reductions in sprint performance attributed to PCr depletion. Indeed, it has been shown that endurance trained people maintain power output significant better than team games players during ten 6-second sprints interspersed with 30 seconds recovery.[135] The greater rate of PCr depletion in sprint/power trained people, and greater rate of resynthesis of PCr in endurance trained people, suggests that sprint/power athletes may be more susceptible to any fatiguing effects of PCr depletion, particularly during repeated-sprint exercise (Section 2.2.2.1 and 2.2.2.2). These findings also suggest that, from a training perspective, it is important for team games players to develop aerobic fitness as well as sprint speed/power, as this may improve PCr resynthesis rate and enable better high-intensity performance throughout a match. This suggestion is supported by research showing improvements in sprint number and overall match intensity following 8 weeks of aerobic interval training in soccer players.[136] However, it is not possible to conclusively attribute this improved performance to mechanisms associated with PCr kinetics (Section 7.2.2.1.1.2).[137]

Key point

Endurance trained people oxidise more fat and less carbohydrate at a given relative exercise intensity, which may reduce, or delay, the influence of fatigue mechanisms associated with glycogen depletion. Endurance training may also increase the rate of PCr resynthesis, enabling better maintenance of performance during repeated sprint exercise.

7.4.2 Metabolic acidosis

Team games athletes have a greater muscle H^+ buffering capacity than endurance trained or untrained people.[138] Greater muscle buffer capacity may enable greater performance during high-intensity exercise, particularly involving repeated sprints. This suggestion is supported by work showing a correlation between muscle buffer capacity and work completed during repeated sprints, meaning that the greater the muscle buffer capacity, the more work could be completed.[52] The greater muscle buffer capacity of team games players may be an adaptation to the type of training they carry out, which would involve repeated bouts of high-intensity exercise that may stimulate adaptations to buffering processes.[138]

Sprint trained athletes tend to have a higher prevalence of type II muscle fibres. These muscle fibres contain high concentrations of glycogen and anaerobic enzymes, and are therefore able to generate energy via anaerobic glycolysis more effectively than type I fibres. Anaerobic glycolysis produces lactate and H^+ (Section 3.3), and it appears to be important for optimal function to remove particularly H^+ from the muscle. Type II muscle fibres contain a much larger concentration of monocarboxylate transporter 4 (MCT4) protein than type I fibres.[139] These transporters function to remove lactate and H^+ from the muscle cells and move it either into the blood or into adjacent muscle cells for use in aerobic ATP resynthesis (Sections 3.3 and 3.3.1).[140] Therefore, individuals with a greater type II fibre profile may be more effective at removing lactate and H^+ from working muscle.

While sprint trained athletes may have specific mechanisms for buffering and transporting lactate and H^+, it appears that endurance training also causes adaptations that may influence lactate and H^+ production and removal. First, endurance athletes tend to have greater proportions of type I muscle fibres, which are more suited to oxidative rather than anaerobic metabolism. As a result, endurance trained athletes produce less muscle lactate at a given exercise intensity than non-endurance trained athletes.[141–2] Second, endurance training is designed to potentiate the aerobic capacity of these muscle fibres. The ability to remove blood lactate has been strongly correlated with muscle oxidative capacity.[143] This may relate to the finding that the expression of monocarboxylate transporter 1 (MCT1) is greater in type I muscle fibres and that aerobic training increases the expression of MCT1 protein in the sarcolemma and mitochondria of skeletal muscle.[140,144] Sarcolemmal MCT1 may contribute to lactate and H^+ uptake into type I fibres from the blood, and removal to other muscle fibres in the cell-cell lactate shuttle, and mitochondrial MCT1 could facilitate intracellular transport of lactate and H^+ into the mitochondria to take part in oxidative ATP resynthesis.[140,145–6]

The nature of lactate and H^+ movement into and out of the blood and skeletal muscle is complex, influenced by muscle morphology and the exercise demand, and is still being investigated. However, the fundamental role of training status is that sprint trained and team games athletes have more effective muscle lactate/H^+ buffering and removal processes than endurance trained athletes, and in turn endurance trained athletes are more effective at transporting lactate and H^+ into adjacent muscle fibres for use in aerobic ATP resynthesis, and have muscle fibre profiles that produce less lactate and H^+ at a given relative exercise intensity.

Key point

Team games athletes have a greater muscle H^+ buffering capacity than endurance or sprint trained athletes. Sprint-trained athletes are able to move lactate and H^+ out of the muscle very effectively. Endurance-trained athletes produce less lactate and H^+ at a given relative exercise intensity, and have an enhanced ability to move lactate and H^+ into muscle mitochondria for use in the aerobic resynthesis of ATP.

7.4.3 Thermoregulation

There is some suggestion that people with greater aerobic fitness are better able to tolerate exercise in high ambient temperatures than less aerobically fit people. More aerobically fit people begin exercise in hot conditions with a lower core temperature, are able to continue exercising for significantly longer, and end exercise with a significantly higher core temperate than less fit people.[147] If aerobic fitness is able to offset some of the negative influences of hyperthermia (Sections 4.5.2 and 4.6), it may be of benefit to performance, particularly of prolonged exercise. Neuroendocrine markers of central fatigue appear to follow a temperature-dependent increase and be similarly present in trained and untrained people at exhaustion during exercise in the heat.[148]

Unsurprisingly, the ability of more aerobically fit people to better tolerate exercise in the heat has been attributed to the regular exercise and physical activity that is likely undertaken by fitter people. More specifically, aerobically fitter people are able to tolerate a higher core temperature during exercise, suggesting that a given core temperature increase generates a greater relative thermal strain in less-fit individuals.[148] Reasons why aerobically fitter people are able to tolerate higher core temperatures are still debated. Aerobically fitter people encounter a lower circulatory strain at a given core temperature during exercise in the heat due to their greater blood volume and stroke volume.[149] However, cardiovascular responses of trained and untrained people during exercise in the heat do not support the suggestion that less cardiovascular strain enables fitter people to better tolerate exercise in the heat.[150] The perception of physiological strain during exercise in the heat is also lower for more aerobically trained individuals.[148] This finding again suggests that trained people are able to tolerate higher core temperatures during exercise due to the familiarity of regular increases in core temperature during training.[150] Intriguingly, this suggestion links greater exercise tolerance of aerobically fit people to the anticipatory model of exercise regulation, particularly the use of prior exercise experience in developing a perception of the exercise bout to come (Section 6.3.2, Figure 6.4 and Table 6.1). It is also possible that lower body fat levels enable a greater tolerance to exercise in the heat, as fat has a greater capacity for heat storage than lean tissue.[150] However, the influence of body fat on tolerance to exercise in the heat may also be independent of aerobic fitness.[150]

As is generally the case with the intricate and interrelated human physiological responses to exercise, it is likely that the mechanisms behind aerobically fitter people's ability to better tolerate exercise in the heat are multifaceted. It must also be considered that not all research supports the influence of aerobic fitness on greater tolerance to exercise in the heat.[151]

Key point

Aerobically-trained people have a greater ability to tolerate exercise in high temperatures, which is linked to the ability to tolerate higher core temperatures. This ability may be related to lower cardiovascular strain, reduced perception of physical strain, or lower body fat levels.

7.4.4 Calcium and potassium kinetics

Type II muscle fibres have a faster Ca^{2+} release from, and uptake into, the SR, a greater rate of Ca^{2+} release per muscle action potential, and more Ca^{2+} binding sites on troponin C than type I fibres.[69,152] These differences contribute to the greater force production and faster contraction velocity of type II fibres, and demonstrate how the mechanics of a muscle fibre are suited to its function. However, type I muscle fibres have greater SR Ca^{2+} concentrations, which would better facilitate Ca^{2+} release by increasing the open probability of SR release channels.[153] The greater open probability of Ca^{2+} release channels may also make the SR of type I fibres less susceptible to potentially inhibiting effects of Mg^{2+} (Sections 5.7.2 and 5.7.3)[154] and less susceptible to fatigue.[152] Furthermore, type II muscle fibres show greater increases in P_i concentration than type I muscle fibres, due to their ability to break down ATP and PCr at faster rates.[82] A greater intramuscular P_i concentration in type II fibres may make them more susceptible to Ca^{2+}–P_i precipitation in the SR (Section 5.7.2).

Despite the potentially beneficial properties of type I muscle fibres with regard to Ca^{2+} kinetics, SR Ca^{2+} release and uptake is significantly reduced in endurance trained, resistance trained, and untrained individuals.[155] However, the decline in SR function is greater in untrained compared with endurance trained people. Furthermore, the extent of impairment in SR function is correlated with the percentage of type II fibres, suggesting a greater functional impairment in this fibre type.[155] Interestingly, short-term endurance training causes a reduction in the rate of SR Ca^{2+} release and uptake.[156] While at first glance this may be counter-intuitive and suggestive of a negative training adaptation, reduced Ca^{2+} kinetics may actually represent the beginning of functional changes geared towards improving the oxidative capacity of the muscle.[156] Indeed, longer duration endurance training increases levels of proteins involved in skeletal muscle Ca^{2+} handling,[157] and similar findings have also been reported in type II muscle fibres.[158]

As with most of the fatigue processes discussed in this book, there is debate as to the functional significance of *in vivo* extracellular K^+ accumulation on exercise fatigue (Sections 5.3 and 5.4). However, the lack of conclusive *in vivo* evidence (Section 5.5) suggests that extracellular K^+ accumulation should still be considered when discussing exercise fatigue, particularly when it is noted that training-induced changes in muscle K^+ kinetics are seen.

High-intensity intermittent training reduces extracellular K^+ accumulation during incremental single-leg exercise to exhaustion.[159] It appears that reduced extracellular K^+ accumulation following training is due to greater reuptake of K^+ into the muscle via increased activity of Na^+, K^+ pumps.[144,159] Density of skeletal muscle Na^+, K^+ pumps is increased by about 14–20% by endurance training, 16% by sprint training, and 10–18% by high-intensity intermittent and resistance training.[144,160–2] It therefore appears that individuals involved in most forms of training may be able to improve their ability to attenuate extracellular K^+ accumulation. However, this may be of most importance to sprint/power based athletes, as type II muscle fibres may be more susceptible to extracellular K^+ accumulation.[152]

Key point

The function of the SR of type I muscle fibres may be less impaired by Mg^{2+} and P_i accumulation than that of type II fibres. Indeed, the decline in SR function during exercise is related to type II fibre content. Endurance, resistance, and sprint training all increase Na^+, N^+ pump content, suggesting all forms of training may improve the ability to attenuate extracellular K^+ accumulation.

7.4.5 Central governor/anticipatory regulation of performance

Inferences about the potential influence of training status on central/anticipatory regulation of exercise performance are made largely using the information discussed in Sections 7.4.1–7.4.3. As mentioned in Section 6.5, central/anticipatory regulation of performance as proposed by existing models (Section 6.3.2 and Figure 6.4) is complex and very difficult to experimentally study. Therefore, perhaps unsurprisingly, the influence of training status on central/anticipatory regulation has not been sufficiently well isolated in a research setting.

The employment of a pacing strategy during exercise (Section 6.4.3) may provide support for central/anticipatory regulation of performance, as it is proposed that continual adjustment of exercise intensity occurs in line with a pre-developed template RPE, which is developed by peripheral afferent feedback, knowledge of expected exercise demands, and prior exercise experience (Figure 6.4). It has been shown that the ability to refine a pacing strategy in order to complete a given exercise task more quickly or efficiently is improved with training and experience (Section 6.4.3). If pacing strategies are indeed part of a central/anticipatory regulation of performance designed to enable exercise completion without significant physical damage, then training experience may be crucial to the success of this regulatory system.

Afferent peripheral feedback is also proposed to contribute to the generation of conscious RPE that is used as a regulator of exercise performance (Section 6.3.2, Figure 6.4). Sections 7.4.1–7.4.3 highlight that training, particularly high-intensity aerobic and more traditional endurance training, may attenuate the potential influence of exercise-induced peripheral metabolic, ionic, and thermoregulatory alterations on fatigue. Therefore, it could be suggested that individuals of a higher training status may generate less peripheral afferent feedback at a given exercise intensity, which could translate to a more favourable comparison between conscious and template RPE during exercise, and hence, better exercise performance. This suggestion is supported by research showing lower RPE at a given relative exercise intensity in aerobically fitter individuals compared to those of lower fitness levels.[163] However, more research is required here.

Key point

Training status and prior exercise experience improve the ability to pace during exercise. If pacing strategies are indicative of central/anticipatory regulation, then training experience may be beneficial in this process. People with greater training status may also generate less peripheral afferent feedback, potentially improving the comparison between conscious RPE and template RPE, and hence performance.

7.5 Summary

- During prolonged submaximal exercise, performance may be impaired by altered cardiovascular function, thermoregulation, and central function due to excessive fluid loss (under certain circumstances), glycogen depletion, impaired SR function, and extracellular K^+ accumulation.
- Observations made in support of the central/anticipatory regulation model of exercise performance can also be applied to prolonged submaximal exercise. However, the debate surrounding the existence of a central regulator of performance should be considered.
- During field-based team games, a transient fatigue occurs following high-intensity periods of activity, and a more progressive fatigue develops towards the end of a game.
- The cause of transient fatigue during team games is not known, and it appears that decreased muscle and blood pH, PCr depletion, and altered muscle membrane excitability are not strong causative factors. It is interesting to consider the possibility of transient fatigue as a form of pacing during team games, perhaps as part of a central/anticipatory regulation of performance. However, this suggestion needs to be investigated.
- Progressive fatigue during team games may be influenced by muscle glycogen depletion, limitations to fluid intake (but not necessarily actual fluid loss), and central fatigue.
- Middle-distance exercise performance could be impaired by H^+ production and reduced pH stimulating group III and IV afferents and/or desaturating arterial haemoglobin and inducing cerebral hypoxia, both of which would contribute to central fatigue. Significant extracellular K^+ accumulation can occur within the timeframe of middle-distance exercise, which may impair muscle function. Inorganic phosphate and Mg^{2+} accumulation in muscle may also impair Ca^{2+} kinetics.
- Long-distance sprinting performance may be impaired by altered excitation–contraction coupling, possibly via impaired SR function and Ca^{2+} kinetics, and PCr depletion. There may also be an aspect of anticipatory regulation of performance during long-distance sprinting, evidenced by a relationship between blood lactate concentration and RPE, and altered muscle contractile ability within 10 seconds of the onset of long-distance sprints.
- Short-distance sprinting is impaired by PCr depletion. Performance in 200-metre sprinting may be impaired by reductions in muscle pH, but this is not a cause of fatigue in the 100-metre sprint. More research is required to determine the potential influence of P_i accumulation and altered Ca^{2+} kinetics on short sprint performance. Short sprint performance can also be impaired by alterations in neuromuscular function, possibly mediated by changes to motor neuron responsiveness, peripheral fatigue, or decreased stretch reflex sensitivity.

- High-load resistance training may be impaired by PCr depletion and intramuscular metabolite accumulation. High-load resistance training may also be influenced by the development of central fatigue, although the relative influence of peripheral and central fatigue may depend on muscle fibre type and training status.
- Females appear less fatigable than males during sustained and intermittent isometric contractions, concentric contractions, and repeated sprinting. The better fatigability of females is greatly reduced or negated with increasing contraction intensity, or when genders are matched for strength.
- Reasons for the greater fatigability of females include better muscle perfusion, greater type I muscle fibre content, differences in metabolic responses to exercise, and better voluntary activation of the lower limb muscles.
- Endurance trained individuals oxidise more fat and less carbohydrate at a given relative exercise intensity, and are able to replenish PCr at a faster rate. This may negate, or at least delay, fatigue processes associated with glycogen depletion, and enable better maintenance of performance during repeated sprint exercise.
- Team games athletes have a greater ability to buffer muscle H^+ production than endurance trained or untrained people, which may enable greater repeated-sprint performance. Type II muscle fibres contain greater MCT4 content, which may allow sprint-trained athletes to move lactate and H^+ out of the muscle more effectively. Endurance trained athletes tend to have a muscle fibre profile that favours reduced lactate and H^+ production, but also have greater muscle MCT1 content, which may allow better transport of lactate and H^+ from cell to cell, and also transport into the mitochondria for use in aerobic ATP resynthesis.
- Individuals with a higher aerobic fitness can better tolerate exercise in high temperatures, seemingly due to a greater tolerance for high core temperatures and reduced perception of thermal strain.
- Type I muscle fibres have greater SR Ca^{2+} concentrations, which will facilitate Ca^{2+} release and make the SR less susceptible to inhibitory influences during exercise. Type II fibres show greater increases in P_i concentration, which may increase susceptibility to Ca^{2+}–P_i precipitation in the SR. All forms of training appear to induce adaptations that improve the ability to attenuate extracellular K^+ accumulation.
- Endurance-trained individuals report a lower RPE at a given relative exercise intensity, and demonstrate training adaptations that may attenuate potential afferent feedback from peripheral changes in metabolic, ionic, and thermoregulatory status. If central/anticipatory performance regulation is governed by afferent peripheral feedback and conscious RPE, it may mean that endurance-trained people are less 'held-back' by this performance-regulating system. However, this suggestion requires experimental study.

Test yourself

Answer the following questions to the best of your ability. Try to understand the information gained from answering these questions before you progress with the book.

1. Summarise the potential causes of fatigue during each of these exercise types: prolonged submaximal exercise, field-based team games, middle-distance exercise, long-distance sprinting, short-distance sprinting, resistance training.
2. List the potential reasons why females show greater fatigability than males during some forms of muscular exercise.
3. Why might the gender difference in fatigability be reduced, or even negated, with greater muscle contraction intensities or when genders are matched for strength?
4. How might endurance training reduce the impact of fatigue processes associated with glycogen depletion? How may it enable better maintenance of repeated sprint performance?
5. How might different types of training influence potential fatigue mechanisms associated with metabolic acidosis?
6. Summarise the influence of endurance training on the tolerance to exercise in the heat.
7. How are Ca^{2+} kinetics influenced by muscle fibre type? How does this relate to specific training statuses?
8. What is the influence of training status on extracellular K^+ accumulation?
9. How might training status be speculated to influence the potential role of central/anticipatory regulation of exercise performance?

References

1 Coyle EF (2007) Physiological regulation of marathon performance. *Sports Med* 37: 306–11.
2 Casa DJ, Armstrong LE, Hillman SK, Montain SJ, Reiff RV, Rich BSE, Roberts WO, Stone JA (2000) National Athletic Trainers Association position statement: fluid replacement for athletes. *J Athl Train* 35: 212–24.
3 Pfeiffer B, Stellingwerff T, Hodgson AB, Randell R, Pottgen L, Res P, Jeukendrup AE (2012) Nutritional intake and gastrointestinal problems during competitive endurance events. *Med Sci Sports Exerc* 44: 344–51.
4 Lambert GP, Lang J, Bull A, Eckerson J, Lanspa S, O'Brien J (2008) Fluid tolerance while running: effect of repeated trials. *Int J Sports Med* 29: 878–82.
5 Millet GP, Vleck VE, Bentley DJ (2009) Physiological differences between cycling and running: lessons from triathletes. *Sports Med* 39: 179–206.
6 Leppik JA, Aughey RJ, Medved I, Fairweather I, Carey MF, McKenna MJ (2004) Prolonged exercise to fatigue in humans impairs skeletal muscle Na^+-K^+ ATPase activity, sarcoplasmic reticulum Ca^{2+} release, and Ca^{2+} uptake. *J Appl Physiol* 97: 1414–23.
7 Wada M, Kuratani M, Kanzaki K (2013) Calcium kinetics of sarcoplasmic reticulum and muscle fatigue. *J Phys Fitness Sports Med* 2: 169–78.

8 McKenna MJ, Medved I, Goodman CA, Brown MJ, Bjorksten AR, Murphy KT, Petersen AC, Sostaric S, Gong X (2006) N-acetylcysteine attenuates the decline in muscle Na^+, K^+-pump activity and delays fatigue during prolonged exercise in humans. *J Physiol* 576: 279–88.
9 Pires FO, Noakes TD, Lima-Silva AE, Bertuzzi R, Ugrinowitsch C, Lira FS, Kiss MAPDM (2011) Cardiopulmonary, blood metabolite and rating of perceived exertion responses to constant exercises performed at different intensities until exhaustion. *Br J Sports Med* 45: 1119–25.
10 Overgaard K, Lindstrøm T, Ingemann-Hansen T, Clausen T (2002) Membrane leakage and increased content of Na^+-K^+ pumps and Ca^{2+} in human muscle after a 100-km run. *J Appl Physiol* 92: 1891–8.
11 Noakes TD (2007) The central governor model of exercise regulation applied to the marathon. *Sports Med* 37: 374–7.
12 Duthie G, Pyne D, Hooper S (2003) Applied physiology and game analysis of rugby union. *Sports Med* 33: 973–91.
13 Gabbett T, King T, Jenkins D (2008) Applied physiology of rugby league. *Sports Med* 38: 119–38.
14 Bangsbo J, Mohr M, Krustrup P (2006) Physical and metabolic demands of training and match-play in the elite football player. *J Sports Sci* 24: 665–74.
15 Abt G, Zhou S, Weatherby R (1998) The effect of a high-carbohydrate diet on the skill performance of midfield soccer players after intermittent treadmill exercise. *J Sci Med Sport* 1: 203–12.
16 Mohr M, Krustrup P, Bangsbo J (2005) Fatigue in soccer: a brief review. *J Sports Sci* 23: 593–9.
17 Bangsbo J, Nørregaard L, Thorsø F (1991) Activity profile of competition soccer. *Can J Sport Sci* 16: 110–6.
18 Bangsbo J, Mohr M (2005) Variations in running speed and recovery time after a sprint during top-class soccer matches. *Med Sci Sports Exerc* 37: S87.
19 Mohr M, Krustrup P, Bangsbo J (2003) Match performance of high-standard soccer players with special reference to development of fatigue. *J Sports Sci* 21: 519–28.
20 Krustrup P, Mohr M, Steensberg A, Bencke J, Kjaer M, Bangsbo J (2003) Muscle metabolites during a football match in relation to a decreased sprinting ability. Communication to the Fifth World Congress of Soccer and Science, Lisbon, Portugal.
21 Krustrup P, Mohr M, Steensberg A, Bencke J, Kjaer M, Bangsbo J (2006) Muscle and blood metabolites during a soccer game: implications for sprint performance. *Med Sci Sports Exerc* 38: 1165–74.
22 Krustrup P, Mohr M, Amstrup T, Rysgaard T, Johansen J, Steensberg A, Pedersen PK, Bangsbo J (2003) The Yo-Yo intermittent recovery test: physiological response, reliability and validity. *Med Sci Sports Exerc* 35: 695–705.
23 Bangsbo J, Iaia FM, Krustrup P (2007) Metabolic response and fatigue in soccer. *Int J Sports Physiol Perf* 2: 111–27.
24 Mohr M, Nielsen JJ, Bangsbo J (2011) Caffeine intake improves intense intermittent exercise performance and reduces muscle interstitial potassium accumulation. *J Appl Physiol* 111: 1372–9.
25 Balsom PD, Gaitanos GC, Söderlund K, Ekblom B (1999) High-intensity exercise and muscle glycogen availability in humans. *Acta Physiol Scand* 165: 337–45.
26 Maughan RJ, Shirreffs SM, Merson SJ, Horswill CA (2005) Fluid and electrolyte balance in elite male football (soccer) players training in a cool environment. *J Sports Sci* 23: 73–9.
27 Reilly T (1997) Energetics of high-intensity exercise (soccer) with particular reference to fatigue. *J Sports Sci* 15: 257–63.

28 Shirreffs SM, Aragon-Vargas LF, Chamorro M, Maughan RJ, Serratosa L, Zachwieja JJ (2005) The sweating response of elite professional soccer players to training in the heat. *Int J Sports Med* 26: 90–5.
29 Edwards AM, Noakes TD (2009) Dehydration: cause of fatigue or sign of pacing in elite soccer? *Sports Med* 39: 1–13.
30 McGregor SJ, Nicholas CW, Lakomy HKA, Williams C (1999) The influence of intermittent high-intensity shuttle running and fluid ingestion on the performance of a soccer skill. *J Sports Sci* 17: 895–903.
31 Edwards AM, Mann ME, Marfell-Jones MJ, Rankin DM, Noakes TD, Shillington DP (2007) Influence of moderate dehydration on soccer performance: physiological responses to 45 min of outdoor match-play and the immediate subsequent performance of sport-specific and mental concentration tests. *Br J Sports Med* 41: 385–91.
32 Edwards AM, Clark NA (2006) Thermoregulatory observations in soccer match play: professional and recreational level applications using an intestinal pill system to measure core temperature. *Br J Sports Med* 40: 133–8.
33 Aughey RJ, Goodman CA, McKenna MJ (2014) Greater chance of high core temperatures with modified pacing strategy during team sport in the heat. *J Sci Med Sport* 17: 113–8.
34 Robinson TA, Hawley JA, Palmer GS, Wilson GR, Gray DA, Noakes TD, Dennis SC (1995) Water ingestion does not improve 1-h cycling performance in moderate ambient temperatures. *Eur J Appl Physiol* 71: 153–60.
35 Schlader ZJ, Simmons SE, Stannard SR, Mündel T (2011) Skin temperature as a thermal controller of exercise intensity. *Eur J Appl Physol* 111: 1631–9.
36 Temfemo A, Carling C, Said A (2011) Relationship between power output, lactate, skin temperature, and muscle activity during brief repeated exercises with increasing intensity. *J Strength Cond Res* 25: 915–21.
37 Rahnama N, Lees A, Reilly T (2006) Electromyography of selected lower-limb muscles fatigued by exercise at the intensity of soccer match-play. *J Electromyogr Kinesiol* 16: 257–63.
38 Rampinini E, Bosio A, Ferraresi I, Petruolo A, Morelli A, Sassi A (2011) Match-related fatigue in soccer players. *Med Sci Sports Exerc* 43: 2161–70.
39 Robineau J, Jouaux T, Lacroix M, Babault N (2012) Neuromuscular fatigue induced by a 90-min soccer game modelling. *J Strength Cond Res* 26: 555–62.
40 Gandevia SC (2001) Spinal and supraspinal factors in human muscle fatigue. *Physiol Rev* 81: 1726–89.
41 Duffield R, Dawson B, Goodman C (2005) Energy system contribution to 400-metre and 800-metre track running. *J Sports Sci* 23: 299–307.
42 Spencer MR, Gastin PB (2001) Energy system contribution during 200- to 1500-m running in highly trained athletes. *Med Sci Sports Exerc* 33: 157–62.
43 Dal Pupo J, Arins FB, Guglielmo LGA, Da Silva R, Moro ARP, Dos Santos SG (2013) Physiological and neuromuscular indices associated with sprint running performance. *Res Sports Med* 21: 124–35.
44 Ingham SA, Whyte GP, Pedlar C, Bailey DM, Dunman N, Nevill AM (2008) Determinants of 800-m and 1500-m running performance using allometric models. *Med Sci Sports Exerc* 40: 345–50.
45 Rabadán M, Díaz V, Calderón FJ, Benito PJ, Peinado AB, Maffulli N (2011) Physiological determinants of speciality of elite middle- and long-distance runners. *J Sports Sci* 29: 975–82.
46 Jung AP (2003) The impact of resistance training on distance running performance. *Sports Med* 33: 539–52.
47 Saunders PU, Telford RD, Pyne DB, Peltola EM, Cunningham RB, Gore CJ, Hawley JA (2006) Short-term plyometric training improves running economy in highly trained middle and long distance runners. *J Strength Cond Res* 20: 947–54.

48 Bird SR, Wiles J, Robbins J (1995) The effect of sodium bicarbonate ingestion on 1500-m racing time. *J Sports Sci* 13: 399–403.
49 Carr AJ, Gore CJ, Hopkins WG (2011) Effects of acute alkalosis and acidosis on performance: a meta-analysis. *Sports Med* 41: 801–14.
50 McNaughton LR, Siegler J, Midgley A (2008) Ergogenic effects of sodium bicarbonate. *Curr Sports Med Rep* 7: 230–6.
51 Wilkes D, Gledhill N, Smyth R (1983) Effect of acute induced metabolic alkalosis on 800-m racing time. *Med Sci Sports Exerc* 15: 277–80.
52 Bishop D, Edge J, Davis C, Goodman C (2004) Induced metabolic alkalosis affects muscle metabolism and repeated-sprint ability. *Med Sci Sports Exerc* 36: 807–13.
53 Cairns SP (2006) Lactic acid and exercise performance: culprit or friend? *Sports Med* 36: 279–91.
54 Knicker AJ, Renshaw I, Oldham ARH, Cairns SP (2011) Interactive processes link the multiple symptoms of fatigue in sport competition. *Sports Med* 41: 307–28.
55 Nybo L, Secher NH (2004) Cerebral perturbations provoked by prolonged exercise. *Prog Neurobiol* 72: 223–61.
56 Amann M, Calbert JAL (2008) Convective oxygen transport and fatigue. *J Appl Physiol* 104: 861–70.
57 Gandevia SC, Allen GM, Butler JE, Taylor JL (1996) Supraspinal factors in human muscle fatigue: evidence for suboptimal output from the motor cortex. *J Physiol* 490: 529–36.
58 Nielsen HB, Bredmose PR, Strømstad M, Volianitis S, Quistorff B, Secher NH (2002) Bicarbonate attenuates arterial desaturation during maximal exercise in humans. *J Appl Physiol* 93: 724–31.
59 Swank A, Robertson RJ (1989) Effect of induced alkalosis on perception of exertion during intermittent exercise. *J Appl Physiol* 67: 1862–7.
60 Medbø JI, Sejersted OM (1990) Plasma K^+ changes with high intensity exercise. *J Physiol* 421: 105–22.
61 Chapman R, Laymon AS, Wilhite DP, McKenzie JM, Tanner DA, Stager JM (2012) Ground contact time as an indicator of metabolic cost in elite distance runners. *Med Sci Sports Exerc* 44: 917–25.
62 Nummela AT, Paavolainen LM, Sharwood KA, Lambert MI, Noakes TD, Rusko HK (2006) Neuromuscular factors determining 5 km running performance and running economy in well-trained athletes. *Eur J Appl Physiol* 97: 1–8.
63 Tomazin K, Morin JB, Strojnik V, Podpecan A, Millet GY (2012) Fatigue after short (100-m), medium (200-m) and long (400-m) treadmill sprints. *Eur J Appl Physiol* 112(3): 1027–36.
64 Hirvonen J, Numella A, Rusko H, Rehunen M, Härkönen M (1992) Fatigue and changes of ATP, creatine phosphate and lactate during the 400 m sprint. *Can J Sport Sci* 17: 477–83.
65 Nummela A, Vuorima T, Rusko H (1992) Changes in force production, blood lactate and EMG activity in the 400m sprint. *J Sports Sci* 10: 217–28.
66 Hanon C, Gajer B (2009) Velocity and stride parameters of world-class 400-meter athletes compared with less experienced runners. *J Strength Cond Res* 23: 524–31.
67 Miguel PJ, Reis VM (2004) Speed strength endurance and 400m performance. *New Stud Athlet* 19: 39–45.
68 Lattier G, Millett GY, Martin A, Martin V (2004) Fatigue and recovery after high-intensity exercise part I: neuromuscular fatigue. *Int J Sports Med* 25: 450–6.
69 Allen DG, Lamb GD, Westerblad H (2008) Skeletal muscle fatigue: cellular mechanisms. *Physiol Rev* 88: 287–332.
70 Cheetham ME, Boobis LH, Brooks S, Williams C (1986) Human muscle metabolism during sprint running. *J Appl Physiol* 61: 54–60.
71 Gaitanos GC, Williams C, Boobis LH, Brooks S (1993) Human muscle metabolism during intermittent maximal exercise. *J Appl Physiol* 75: 712–9.

72 Maughan R, Gleeson M (2004) *The Biochemical Basis of Sports Performance*. Oxford: Oxford University Press.
73 Wittekind AL, Micklewright D, Beneke R (2011) Teleoanticipation in all-out short-duration cycling. *Br J Sports Med* 45: 114–9.
74 Mackala K (2007) Optimisation of performance through kinematic analysis of the different phases of the 100 metres. *New Studies in Athletics* 22: 7–16.
75 Mureika JR (2003) Modelling wind and altitude effects in the 200 m sprint. *Can J Phys* 81: 895–910.
76 Duffield R, Dawson B, Goodman C (2004) Energy system contribution to 100-m and 200-m track running events. *J Sci Med Sport* 7: 302–13.
77 Nevill AM, Ramsbottom R, Nevill ME, Newport S, Williams C (2008) The relative contributions of anaerobic and aerobic energy supply during track 100-, 400- and 800-m performance. *J Sports Med Phys Fitness* 48: 138–42.
78 Skare OC, Skadberg Ø, Wisnes AR (2001) Creatine supplementation improves sprint performance in male sprinters. *Scand J Med Sci Spor* 11: 96–102.
79 Spencer M, Bishop D, Dawson B, Goodman C (2005) Physiological and metabolic responses of repeated-sprint activities specific to field-based team sports. *Sports Med* 35: 1025–44.
80 Bogdanis GC, Nevill ME, Lakomy HKA, Boobis LH (1998) Power output and muscle metabolism during and following recovery from 10 and 20 s of maximal sprint exercise in humans. *Acta Physiol Scand* 163: 261–72.
81 Hirvonen J, Rehunen S, Rusko H, Härkönen M (1987) Breakdown of high-energy phosphate compounds and lactate accumulation during short supramaximal exercise. *Eur J Appl Physiol* 56: 253–9.
82 Fitts RH (2008) The cross-bridge cycle and skeletal muscle fatigue. *J Appl Physiol* 104: 551–8.
83 Metzger JM, Moss RL (1987) Greater hydrogen ion-induced depression of tension and velocity in skinned single fibres of rate fast than slow muscles. *J Physiol* 393: 727–42.
84 Mero A, Peltola E (1989) Neural activation fatigued and non-fatigued conditions of short and long sprint running. *Biol Sport* 6: 43–58.
85 Ross A, Leveritt M, Riek S (2001) Neural influences on sprint running: training adaptations and acute responses. *Sports Med* 31: 409–25.
86 Willardson JM (2006) A brief review: factors affecting the length of the rest interval between resistance exercise sets. *J Strength Cond Res* 20: 978–84.
87 Sahlin K, Ren JM (1989) Relationship of contraction capacity to metabolic changes during recovery from a fatiguing contraction. *J Appl Physiol* 67: 648–54.
88 Nordlund MM, Thorstensson A, Cresswell AG (2004) Central and peripheral contributions to fatigue in relation to level of activation during repeated maximal voluntary isometric plantar flexions. *J Appl Physiol* 96: 218–25.
89 van den Tillaar R, Saeterbakken A (2014) Effect of fatigue upon performance and electromyographic activity in 6-RM bench press. *J Hum Kinet* 40: 57–65.
90 Ahtiainen JP, Hakkinen K (2009) Strength athletes are capable to produce greater muscle activation and neural fatigue during high-intensity resistance exercise than nonathetes. *J Strength Cond Res* 23: 1129–34.
91 Westerblad H, Allen DG (2002) Recent advances in the understanding of skeletal muscle fatigue. *Curr Opin Rheumatol* 14: 648–52.
92 Taylor JL, Allen GM, Butler JE, Gandevia SC (2000) Supraspinal fatigue during intermittent maximal voluntary contractions of the human elbow flexors. *J Appl Physiol* 89: 305–13.
93 Gandevia SC, Allen GM, Butler JE, Taylor JL (1996) Supraspinal factors in human muscle fatigue: evidence for suboptimal output from the motor cortex. *J Physiol* 490: 529–36.

94 Taylor JL, Gandevia SC (2008) A comparison of central aspects of fatigue in submaximal and maximal voluntary contractions. *J Appl Physiol* 104: 542–50.
95 Rubinstein S, Kamen G (2005) Decreases in motor unit firing rate during sustained maximal-effort contractions in young and older adults. *J Electromyogr Kinesiol* 15: 536–43.
96 Andersen B, Westlund B, Krarup C (2003) Failure of activation of spinal motoneurons after muscle fatigue in healthy subjects studied by transcranial magnetic stimulation. *J Physiol* 551: 345–56.
97 Butler JE, Taylor JL, Gandevia SC (2003) Responses of human motoneurons to corticospinal stimulation during maximal voluntary contractions and ischemia. *J Neurosci* 23: 10224–30.
98 Boerio D, Jubeau M, Zory R, Maffiuletti NA (2005) Central and peripheral fatigue after electrostimulation-induced resistance exercise. *Med Sci Sports Exerc* 37: 973–8.
99 Hunter SK (2009) Sex differences and mechanisms of task-specific muscle fatigue. *Exerc Sport Sci Rev* 37: 113–22.
100 Hunter SK (2014) Sex differences in human fatigability: mechanisms and insight into physiological responses. *Acta Physiol* 210: 768–89.
101 Guenette JA, Romer LM, Querido JS, Chua R, Eves ND, Road JD, McKenzie DC, Sheel AW (2010) Sex differences in exercise-induced diaphragmatic fatigue in endurance-trained athletes. *J Appl Physiol* 109: 35–46.
102 Fulco CS, Rock PB, Muza SR, Lammi E, Cymerman A, Butterfield G, Moore LG, Braun B, Lewis SF (1999) Slower fatigue and faster recovery of the adductort pollicis muscle in women matched for strength with men. *Acta Physiol Scand* 167: 233–9.
103 Hunter SK, Enoka RM (2001) Sex differences in the fatigability of arm muscles depends on absolute force during isometric contractions. *J Appl Physiol* 91: 2686–94.
104 Avin KG, Naughton MR, Ford BW, Moore HE, Monitto-Webber MN, Stark AM, Gentile AJ, Law LA (2010) Sex differences in fatigue resistance are muscle group dependent. *Med Sci Sports Exerc* 42: 1943–50.
105 Dearth DJ, Umbel J, Hoffman RL, Russ DW, Wilson TE, Clark BC (2010) Men and women exhibit a similar time to task failure for a sustained, submaximal elbow extensor contraction. *Eur J Appl Physiol* 108: 1089–98.
106 Yoon T, Schlinder Delap B, Griffith EE, Hunter SK (2007) Mechanisms of fatigue differ after low- and high-force fatiguing contractions in men and women. *Muscle Nerve* 36: 512–24.
107 Maughan RJ, Harmon M, Leiper JB, Sale D, Delman A (1986) Endurance capacity of untrained males and females in isometric and dynamic muscular contractions. *Eur J Appl Physiol* 55: 395–400.
108 Senefeld J, Yoon T, Bement MH, Hunter SK (2013) Fatigue and recovery from dynamic contractions in men and women differ for arm and leg muscles. *Muscle Nerve* 48: 436–9.
109 Power Ga, Dalton BH, Rice CL, Vandervoort AA (2010) Delayed recovery of velocity-dependent power loss following eccentric actions of the ankle dorsiflexors. *J Appl Physiol* 109: 669–76.
110 Sewright KA, Hubal MJ, Kearns A, Holbrook MT, Clarkson PM (2008) Sex differences in response to maximal eccentric exercise. *Med Sci Sports Exerc* 40: 242–51.
111 Billaut F, Bishop D (2012) Mechanical work accounts for sex differences in fatigue during repeated sprints. *Eur J Appl Physiol* 112: 1429–36.
112 Smith KJ, Billaut F (2012) Tissue oxygenation in men and women during repeated-sprint exercise. *Int J Sports Physiol Perf* 7: 59–67.

113 Laurent CM, Green JM, Bishop PA, Sjokvist J, Schumacker RE, Richardson MT, Curtner-Smith M (2012) Effect of gender on fatigue and recovery following maximal intensity repeated sprint performance. *J Sports Med Phys Fitness* 50: 243–53.
114 Hunter SK, Griffith EE, Schlachter KM, Kufahl TD (2009) Sex differences in time to task failure and blood flow for an intermittent isometric fatiguing contraction. *Muscle Nerve* 39: 42–53.
115 Parker BA, Smithmyer SL, Pelberg JA, Mishkin AD, Herr MD, Proctor DN (2007) Sex differences in leg vasodilation during graded knee extensor exercise in young adults. *J Appl Physiol* 103: 1583–91.
116 Roepstorff C, Thiele M, Hillih T, Pilegaard H, Richter EA, Wojtaszewski JF, Kiens B (2006) Higher skeletal muscle alpha2AMPK activation and lower energy charge and fat oxidation in men than in women during submaximal exercise. *J Physiol* 574: 125–38.
117 Li JL, Wang XN, Fraser SF, Carey MF, Wrigley TV, McKenna MJ (2002) Effects of fatigue and training on sarcoplasmic reticulum Ca^{2+} regulation in human skeletal muscle. *J Appl Physiol* 92: 912–22.
118 Harmer AR, Ruell PA, Hunter SK, McKenna MJ, Thom JM, Chisholm DJ, Flack JR (2014) Effects of type 1 diabetes, sprint training and sex on skeletal muscle sarcoplasmic reticulum Ca^{2+} uptake and Ca^{2+}-ATPase activity. *J Physiol* 592: 523–35.
119 Wust RC, Morse CI, de Haan A, Jones DA, Degens H (2008) Sex differences in contractile properties and fatigue resistance of human skeletal muscle. *Exp Physiol* 93: 843–50.
120 Russ DW, Lanza IR, Rothman D, Kent-Braun JA (2005) Sex differences in glycolysis during brief, intense isometric contractions. *Muscle Nerve* 32: 647–55.
121 Esbjornsson M, Sylven C, Holm I, Jansson E (1993) Fast twitch fibres may predict anaerobic performance in both females and males. *Int J Sports Med* 14: 257–63.
122 Keller ML, Pruse J, Yoon T, Schlinder-Delap B, Harkins A, Hunter SK (2011) Supraspinal fatigue is similar in men and women for a low-force fatiguing contraction. *Med Sci Sports Exerc* 43: 1873–83.
123 Martin PG, Rattey J (2007) Central fatigue explains sex differences in muscle fatigue and contralateral cross-over effects of maximal contractions. *Pflugers Arch* 454: 957–69.
124 Janse de Jonge, XA (2003) Effects of the menstrual cycle on exercise performance. *Sports Med* 33: 833–51.
125 Janse DEJXA, Thompson MW, Chuter VH, Silk LN, Thom JM (2012) Exercise performance over the menstrual cycle in temperate and hot, humid conditions. *Med Sci Sports Exerc* 44: 2190–8.
126 Phillips SM, Green HJ, Tarnopolsky MA, Heigenhauser GJF, Hill RE, Grant SM (1996) Effects of training duration on substrate turnover and oxidation during exercise. *J Appl Physiol* 81: 2182–91.
127 Venables MC, Achten J, Jeukendrup AE (2005) Determinants of fat oxidation during exercise in healthy men and women: a cross-sectional study. *J Appl Physiol* 98: 160–7.
128 Nielsen J, Holmberg H, Schroder HD, Saltin B, Ortenblad N (2011) Human skeletal muscle glycogen utilization in exhaustive exercise: role of subcellular localization and fibre type. *J Physiol* 589: 2871–85.
129 Nielsen J, Ortenblad N (2013) Physiological aspects of the subcellular localization of glycogen in skeletal muscle. *Appl Physiol Nutr Metab* 38: 91–9.
130 Ortenblad N, Nielsen J, Saltin B, *et al.* (2011) Role of glycogen availability in sarcoplasmic reticulum Ca^{2+} kinetics in human skeletal muscle. *J Physiol* 589 (3): 711–25.

131 Yamashita K, Yoshioka T (1991) Profiles of creatine kinase isoenzyme compositions in single muscle fibres of different types. *J Muscle Res Cell Motil* 12: 37–44.
132 Takahashi H, Inaki M, Fujimoto K, Katsuta S, Izumi A, Nutsu M, Itai Y (1995) Control of the rate of phosphocreatine resynthesis after exercise in trained and untrained human quadriceps muscles. *Eur J Appl Physiol* 71: 396–404.
133 Bogdanis GC, Nevill ME, Boobis LH, Lakomy HK, Nevill AM (1995) Recovery of power output and muscle metabolites following 30 s of maximal sprint cycling in man. *J Physiol* 482: 467–80.
134 Yoshida T, Watari H (1993) Metabolic consequences of repeated exercise in long distance runners. *Eur J Appl Physiol* 67: 261–5.
135 Hamilton AL, Nevill ME, Brooks S, Williams C (1991) Physiological responses to maximal intermittent exercise: differences between endurance-trained runners and team games players. *J Sports Sci* 9: 371–82.
136 Helgerud J, Engen LC, Wisløff U, Hoff J (2001) Aerobic endurance training improves soccer performance. *Med Sci Sports Exerc* 33: 1925–31.
137 Glaister M (2005) Multiple sprint work: physiological responses, mechanisms of fatigue and the influence of aerobic fitness. *Sports Med* 35: 757–77.
138 Edge J, Bishop D, Hill-Haas S, Dawson B, Goodman C (2006) Comparison of muscle buffer capacity and repeated-sprint ability of untrained, endurance-trained and team-sport athletes. *Eur J Appl Physiol* 96: 225–34.
139 Juel C, Halestrap AP (1999) Lactate transport in skeletal muscle – role and regulation of the monocarboxylate transporter. *J Physiol* 517: 633–42.
140 Dubouchaud H, Butterfield GE, Wolfel EE, Bergman BC, Brooks GA (2000) Endurance training, expression, and physiology of LDH, MCT1 and MCT4 in human skeletal muscle. *Am J Physiol* 278: E571–9.
141 Berg K (2003) Endurance training and performance in runners. *Sports Med* 33: 59–73.
142 Holloszy JO, Coyle EF (1984) Adaptations of skeletal muscle to endurance exercise and their metabolic consequences. *J Appl Physiol* 56: 831–8.
143 Thomas C, Sirvent P, Perrey S, Raynaud E, Mercier J (2004) Relationships between maximal muscle oxidative capacity and blood lactate removal after supramaximal exercise and fatigue indexes in humans. *J Appl Physiol* 97: 2132–8.
144 Juel C (2006) Training-induced changes in membrane transport proteins of human skeletal muscle. *Eur J Appl Physiol* 96: 627–35.
145 Gladden LB (2004) Lactate metabolism: a new paradigm for the third millennium. *J Physiol* 558: 5–30.
146 Thomas C, Perrey S, Lambert K, Hugon G, Mornet D, Mercier J (2005) Monocarboxylate transporters, blood lactate removal after supramaximal exercise, and fatigue indexes in humans. *J Appl Physiol* 98: 804–9.
147 Cheung SS, McLellan TM (1998) Heat acclimation, aerobic fitness, and hydration effects on tolerance during uncompensable heat stress. *J Appl Physiol* 84: 1731–9.
148 Wright HE, Selkirk GA, Rhind SG, McLellan TM (2012) Peripheral markers of central fatigue in trained and untrained during uncompensable heat stress. *Eur J Appl Physiol* 112: 1047–57.
149 Hopper MK, Coggan AC, and Coyle EF (1988) Exercise stroke volume relative to plasma volume expansion. *J Appl Physiol* 64: 404–8.
150 Selkirk GA, McLellan TM (2001) Influence of aerobic fitness and body fatness on tolerance to uncompensable heat stress. *J Appl Physiol* 91: 2055–63.
151 Mora-Rodriguez R (2012) Influence of aerobic fitness on thermoregulation during exercise in the heat. *Exerc Sport Sci Rev* 40: 79–87.

152 Stephenson DG, Lamb GD, Stephenson GMM (1998) Events of the excitation-contraction-relaxation (E-C-R) cycle in fast- and slow-twitch mammalian muscle fibres relevant to muscle fatigue. *Acta Physiol Scand* 162: 229–45.
153 Sitsapesan R, Williams AJ (1995) The gating of the sheep skeletal sarcoplasmic reticulum Ca^{2+}-release channel is regulated by luminal Ca^{2+}. *J Membr Biol* 146: 133–44.
154 Fryer MW, Stephenson DG (1996) Total and sarcoplasmic reticulum calcium contents of skinned fibres from rat skeletal muscle. *J Physiol (Lond)* 493: 357–70.
155 Li JL, Wang XN, Fraser SF, Carey MF, Wrigley TV, McKenna MJ (2002) Effects of fatigue and training on sarcoplasmic reticulum Ca^{2+} regulation in human skeletal muscle. *J Appl Physiol* 92: 912–22.
156 Green H, Burnett M, Kollias H, Jing O, Smith I, Tupling S (2011) Malleability of human skeletal muscle sarcoplasmic reticulum to short-term training. *Appl Physiol Nutr Metab* 36: 904–13.
157 Ferreira JC, Bacurau AV, Bueno CR, Cunha TC, Tanaka LY, Jardim MA, Ramires PR, Brum PC (2010) Aerobic exercise training improves Ca^{2+} handling and redox status of skeletal muscle in mice. *Exp Biol Med* 235: 497–505.
158 Morissette MP, Susser SE, Stammers AN, O'Hara KA, Gardiner PF, Sheppard P, Moffatt TL, Duhamel TA (2014) Differential regulation of the fiber type specific gene expression of the sarcoplasmic reticulum Ca^{2+}-ATPase (SERCA) isoforms induced by exercise training. *J Appl Physiol* 117(5): 544–55.
159 Nielsen JJ, Mohr M, Klarskov C, Kristensen M, Krustrup P, Juel C, Bangsbo J (2004) Effects of high-intensity intermittent training on potassium kinetics and performance in human skeletal muscle. *J Physiol* 554: 857–70.
160 Fraser SF, Li JL, Carey MF, Wang XN, Sangkabutra T, Sostaric S, Selig SE, Kjeldsen K, McKenna MJ (2002) Fatigue depresses maximal in vitro skeletal muscle Na(+)-K(+)-ATPase activity in untrained and trained individuals. *J Appl Physiol* 93: 1650–9.
161 McKenna MJ, Schmidt TA, Hargreaves M, Cameron L, Skinner SL, Kjeldsen K (1993) Sprint training increases human skeletal muscle Na^+-K^+-ATPase concentration and improves K+ regulation. *J Appl Physiol* 75: 173–80.
162 Green H, Dahly A, Shoemaker K, Goreham C, Bombardier E, Ball-Burnett M (1999) Serial effects of high-resistance and prolonged endurance training on Na^+–K^+ pump concentration and enzymatic activities in human vastus lateralis. *Acta Physiol Scand* 165: 177–84.
163 Travlos AK, Marisi DQ (1996) Perceived exertion during physical exercise among individuals high and low in fitness. *Percept Motor Skill* 82: 419–24.

Part IV

Summary

Where next?

Chapter 8

Conclusion

8.1 Where next?

Chapter 1 introduced some of the main ways in which fatigue can be measured and quantified. The importance of ensuring that measured variables actually reflect potentially fatigue-causing mechanisms, and the difficulty in measuring some potential modulators of fatigue, was discussed. New and emerging technology that is being implemented in the study of fatigue in sport and exercise was also introduced. Technological advances and the development of new measurement procedures enable access to new avenues of study and a greater understanding and appreciation of an area of research, and such advances have driven many of the recent developments into the study of the physiological regulation of sport and exercise.

Technological developments usually move at quite a rapid pace. Therefore, future research into fatigue in sport and exercise should, and almost certainly will, make use of these developments. It would be futile to suggest which specific mechanisms, organs, or variables should be focused on, as often the technological advance leads us to the next fatigue candidate, as opposed to the candidate necessitating the technological development. Therefore, the targets of fatigue research in the coming years may not have even been identified yet. However, there is certainly scope for further investigation into potential mechanisms of fatigue that have already been identified. For example, how we perceive the sensation of effort during exercise, the sensing of various peripheral biochemical and metabolic changes, how these signals may be integrated and contribute to the development of fatigue, and the role of the brain in fatigue (dependent and independent of peripheral signalling and effort perception) all require better understanding and a clearer application to the fatigue process. This is just one example of ongoing study that needs to be developed and explored further, as it may lead us in new directions of investigation.

Throughout this book, it has been stated that fatigue in almost all situations is likely to be an integrated, complex, and multi-faceted occurrence. This is reinforced by the failure of any single physiological variable to consistently and accurately predict or explain fatigue. Traditional experimental research involves manipulating a single variable and measuring the effect of that change on a specific outcome measure, while carefully controlling for any other factors that could also influence the outcome measure. While this level of control is beneficial for producing valid results regarding the effect of the manipulated variable, it is not reflective of the way the body functions during exercise. The human response to exercise is complex and highly integrated (particularly as exercise influences almost every body organ and system). Therefore, it is important that research attempts to reflect this complexity as much as possible, as changing or focusing on only one variable at a time will not give the full picture of the influence of that change, but also the 'knock-on' influence of the change on other variables/organs/body systems. An example of this is the association between lactate/lactic acid production and the development of fatigue (both lactate and lactic acid are referred to on purpose; see Section 3.3). Isolated measurement of high rates of lactate/lactic acid production at the point of fatigue led to the conclusion that lactate/lactic acid production causes fatigue. However, wider investigation into the dynamics of anaerobic glycolysis and the fate of intramuscular lactate has completely reshaped our understanding of the role of lactate/lactic acid in the fatigue process (Chapter 3). This change in thinking may have also encouraged the development of other lines of enquiry into fatigue development, as we could no longer fall back on the traditional explanation of lactate/lactic acid as the fatigue-inducing culprit.

There are examples in the literature of studies that attempt to 're-create' the integrated human exercise response, and the authors of such studies should be commended. The reason why this is not routinely done is that it is extremely difficult to retain the experimental control necessary for the results to have meaning. However, if fatigue research is to truly understand its subject, and provide answers as well as more questions, then new technologies and measurement tools must be utilised to maximise our ability to study the development of a multi-faceted phenomenon in the most appropriate way possible.

While specific research designs should try to utilise an integrative approach, so should fatigue researchers themselves. One of the hindrances when trying to assimilate fatigue research on a particular topic is the different procedures and measurements used by different research groups, even when those groups are studying a very similar topic. If someone reads two articles on a particular aspect of fatigue that appear to contradict one another, can that person be assured that the contrasting results represent genuine conflict about the topic, or could it simply be due to the different protocols used in the two studies? It is, of course, inappropriate to state that every research study on a particular topic should use the exact same methodology. However, it would be useful for research into fatigue in sport and exercise to be more collaborative, so that different research groups could confer on the best ways in which to study a particular topic, and then conduct those studies in a way that generates data which can be compared and contrasted with greater meaning about the specific fatigue mechanism, as opposed to study findings being compared on the basis of differences in the research approach. This may further knowledge in a more economical and time-efficient manner. It must be said that research groups in most areas of research would be happy to collaborate more with colleagues, but logistical issues (finance/funding, time, institutional restrictions etc) often get in the way. Therefore, this suggestion is made from an 'ideal world' perspective. Nevertheless, if it could happen, it may significantly benefit the study of fatigue in sport and exercise.

8.2 A word of caution

The preface of this book mentioned that it was not possible to encompass the full scope of sport and exercise fatigue research into a single undergraduate text, and that the focus was on some of the most prevalent fatigue hypotheses that have produced significant research interest and/or have entered public consciousness, and some contemporary issues in fatigue research. It is important that readers remember this, and do not see the book as the final word on all possible causes of sport and exercise fatigue. The book is a good place to start, but further study and exploration is encouraged (see Section 8.3).

The book has also focused almost exclusively on physiological causes of fatigue, or causes that at least have a physiological component in their hypothesis/model. Doubtless, there are potential contributions to fatigue in sport and exercise from psychological, nutritional (beyond energy availability), and biomechanical variables, in addition to the interesting perspective on sport and exercise fatigue brought by aspects of pathophysiology and other pathologies. Hopefully, this book may act as a stimulus for other authors to address such variables in a similar way.

8.3 Staying informed

Our understanding of fatigue in sport and exercise has expanded and deepened exponentially in the last few decades, due in part to the development of new technologies and research methodologies as mentioned in Section 8.1. There is no reason to believe that this rate of knowledge development will stop; In fact, it is more likely to increase. The rapidly evolving landscape of fatigue research reinforces the need to keep your knowledge up to date. Doing so will allow you to share the correct knowledge with colleagues/clients/students/athletes, and will help to prevent the perpetuation of outdated concepts.

It is easy to say that knowledge should remain up to date, but it is another thing to achieve it (particularly in the wide-ranging and conflicting world of sport and exercise fatigue research). This section will provide some hints and tips for maintaining a contemporary knowledge base in sport and exercise fatigue, as well as some things to be aware of to ensure that knowledge is being gained from the most appropriate and trusted sources. The following is not an exhaustive list; it is more a core strategy that can be employed to assist you in staying informed. Use the advice as you see fit, and also explore other ways of keeping informed that work for you.

8.3.1 Ways to stay informed

8.3.1.1 Access the primary literature

While this strategy may be the most obvious one, it is also the most important. Simply put, 'access the primary literature' means 'read the research'! More specifically, it means read original research that conducted a study designed to address a focused research question related to fatigue in sport and exercise. Undeniably, this is a useful strategy, but it is also deceptively difficult, particularly in a topic that covers as many bases as fatigue research. Accessing the primary literature in this topic will be likely to throw up some tricky questions and scenarios, such as: *do I need to look back at the historical research in order to better understand the contemporary studies?*; *if I should look at the historical work, how far back should I go?*; *what are the 'seminal' studies in each particular field of fatigue research?*; *there is so much potentially relevant original work in each field of fatigue research, I feel lost before I even begin.*

Some of the potential stumbling blocks that may be encountered when trying to develop and maintain a knowledge base of fatigue in sport and exercise may be alleviated by initially accessing a recent review of research on the topic. A literature review can come in at least two forms. A descriptive review is where the author collates a comprehensive number of studies that are related to the topic of the review, and describes the studies with a particular focus on methodological approach, key results, and the interpretation of those results by the original authors. Descriptive reviews are therefore overviews of a topic, with the collation of the studies not driven by a regimented protocol of selection (thereby precluding replication) and potentially open to author bias. Systematic reviews try to overcome these limitations. Systematic reviews attempt to review a body of evidence with the aim of addressing a particular question. For example, with regard to fatigue research, a systematic review could address the question: *does attainment of a critical core temperature cause fatigue during exercise in the heat in highly trained marathon runners?* The authors of the review would then set about searching for all available literature related to this question, using multiple methods of study retrieval (online databases, searching of study reference lists, etc). Importantly, the authors would need to access all literature on the topic, regardless of the study findings, as a systematic review must be unbiased in its presentation of current knowledge on the topic. Each study is then assessed for eligibility against pre-defined criteria, and included or excluded from the review. Selected studies are then evaluated in terms of their methodological approach, and poorly conducted studies discarded. For each of the remaining studies, key findings are summarised and combined to provide an 'answer' to the original question, and to provide evidence-based recommendations for further study that may be needed. Sometimes, a systematic review will include statistical analysis, such as in meta-analyses where a standardised effect size is calculated for the effect of the intervention in each individual study, and these effect sizes can be compared and/or combined to gain a clearer view of the magnitude of effect of a particular intervention. Importantly, the authors of a systematic review will publish their study retrieval and assessment protocol in full detail along with their review, so that it could be replicated (much in the same way as authors of original studies publish their methodology). If the systematic review procedure was sufficiently rigorous and unbiased, replication of the process should lead to the same conclusions.

While review articles are a useful tool for gaining an overarching insight into a topic area, they are still a summary of the area, and are not a substitute for reading the primary literature. Therefore, reviews should be used as a starting point in understanding a topic, and as a way of identifying key early and more contemporary primary literature.

8.3.1.2 Identify the 'key players'

Keeping your knowledge of fatigue in sport and exercise up to date may prove challenging due to the large amount of existing research, the rate of new publications, and the breadth of the field. It may help to streamline your literature searches by identifying the names of key authors or research groups (i.e. key players) that have a track-record of publications in particular areas of sport and exercise fatigue. Online research databases incorporate an advanced search facility, where keyword-based searches can be focused by the addition of, among other selections, publication date ranges (e.g. only retrieving articles with the chosen keywords that were published between 2008–2013) and the names of authors. Using these tools may enable you to track down relevant historical and contemporary papers in a more efficient way.

While it is critical to the development and maintenance of your knowledge to search databases of peer-reviewed research publications, other avenues of information should not be discounted. For example, many academics and researchers produce expert statements, guest articles, and other contributions for popular sport, health, fitness, and medical publications such as magazines, websites, and books for the general reader. One of the main reasons many academics/researchers may do this is to improve communication between producers of science and potential consumers of that science, and thereby demonstrate real-world impact of their research findings. This is particularly important for academics, as sometimes it is difficult to implement research findings in a real world setting. If key players involved in researching fatigue in sport and exercise are making the effort to achieve greater real-world impact, then students of sport and exercise fatigue should make the most of such opportunities. Other ways to engage with academics and researchers who 'reach out' are discussed in the next section.

8.3.1.3 Social media

In the section above, it was mentioned that many academics and researchers write occasional pieces for mainstream publications in order to demonstrate engagement and impact with the general public and the end-users of research findings. Other ways in which academics/researchers achieve this is via the use of social media. In recent years, a large number of researchers have developed a presence on social media and professional networking sites such as Research Gate, Twitter, and Linkedin, among others. These sites are freely available to the public, only requiring registration to create a user profile. Once registered, users can 'follow' other users, and gain access to the information they share.

Sites such as Research Gate encourage users to post research publication lists and conference presentations, allowing followers to see the track-record, as well as the latest work, of authors whose work they are interested in. These sites often have the facility to post questions on particular topics, which other users who have interest/expertise in the area of the question can answer. Sites such as Linkedin also allow users to post research publications, as well as such information as employment history and research interests. Such sites may also allow users to 'advertise' their skills and services, thereby encouraging professional networking. Finally, sites such as Twitter allow users to post short comments/observations about any topic they wish, links to other websites/articles/publications, and allow users to enter into conversation with one another.

It is increasingly common for academics/researchers to use social media to increase awareness of research being carried out by themselves and/or research groups in which they are a member. This is often done by simply discussing ongoing research, seeking advice/collaborations on a proposed research study, or providing 'sneak-peeks' of new research data, pre-publication. Many researchers also provide links to contemporary research of others that they find interesting or relevant, thereby providing another avenue for discovering new research. Academics may also enter into discussions and debates with one another, which sometimes provides a unique opportunity to gain access to the combined knowledge and perspectives of a researcher and his/her professional network.

Social media can be a powerful tool in gaining a greater understanding of current knowledge in a particular area of research, the key people who are developing this knowledge, emerging developments in the field, and providing communication access to the key players in ways that may not otherwise be possible. However, it is important to carefully cultivate a social media presence. Things to consider include which individuals/groups to follow, what information you may wish to share with users, and that any communication with fellow users should be carried out in a professional and formal fashion. Finally, even though you may be engaging on social media with professional academics and researchers, it should be remembered that much of the comments and information shared may be based on personal opinion or perspective, and will not necessarily have gone through any formal vetting/review process. Therefore, be wary of taking all social media communications at face value, and consider doing additional research or asking further questions as required.

8.3.1.4 Professional memberships

Several large sport and exercise science governing bodies/organisations exist, whose purpose includes acting as professional registers and support structures for those working in various aspects of the sport and exercise science industry, and working to raise and maintain the professional standards of sport and exercise science. Examples of such bodies (there are many others) include the British Association of Sport and Exercise Sciences (BASES), the European College of Sport Science (ECSS), and the American College of Sports Medicine (ACSM). Many of these organisations offer membership to those working in different roles within sport and exercise science, and to students studying the discipline.

Some governing bodies, particularly BASES and the ACSM, periodically publish position statements written by experts in the field. These position statements represent the most up to date viewpoint on a particular topic, and may also include recommendations and guidelines as appropriate. For example, a periodic position statement regarding fluid intake in sport and exercise is published by the ACSM. This position statement provides a review of the literature related to dehydration, rehydration, and fluid intake strategies in sport and exercise, makes inferences regarding the strength of existing evidence within each of these aspects, and provides recommendations for fluid intake practices. Governing bodies and organisations also organise special working groups, comprised of academics from specific fields, which work to develop research strategies and foster collaborative research opportunities. An annual student conference is held by BASES, and is open to all undergraduate and postgraduate sport and exercise science students, who can submit to present their research at the conference. The conference also features talks and other presentations by established academics and researchers, as well as networking opportunities and career advice. Most governing bodies/organisations also regularly publish their own members magazine, containing news from across the sport and exercise sciences, expert letters and articles, and opportunities to write in with questions about various aspects of sport and exercise science. Finally, many governing bodies/organisations hold short workshops on a variety of topics and issues in sport and exercise science, where attendees can address the issues and debate the latest findings.

Becoming a member of one or more of these governing bodies/associations can provide access to the above facilities. Such access provides another way of keeping up to date with the goings-on in sport and exercise science in general, and possibly with research into fatigue in sport and exercise.

8.3.2 Potential problems when trying to stay informed

8.3.2.1 The mainstream media

It is important to pay attention to the reporting of science in the media (newspapers, online news websites, television/radio). Doing so provides an insight into which scientific topics are making their way into the mainstream press, and which are not. However, it is very important to be able to address the mainstream media reporting of scientific findings from a critical perspective. This is because reporting in the mainstream media can be subject to misinterpretation (of study findings, researcher interviews/comments etc), misunderstanding (for example, by the reporter or editor), reporter/publisher bias (a particular 'spin' placed on a study finding to reflect the agenda of the publication), and sensationalism (dramatically overstating or overreaching the study findings to make the implications significantly more positive, negative, or impactful than was the researchers intentions). Such reporting can contribute to inaccurate perceptions of scientific concepts by the lay-person, and to the persistent belief in incorrect information that has been alluded to at various points throughout this book. As a student of the sciences, it is important that you are able to identify such reporting issues (perhaps using some of the strategies discussed in Section 8.3.1, and others you develop yourself), and pass this on to others who may not have the same background knowledge to do this for themselves (see Section 8.4). By doing this, you will contribute to the more accurate viewing of science as a gradual development in knowledge over many small steps, rather than large leaps and sweeping generalisations. You may also help to prevent the development of 'incorrect truths' arising from misrepresented scientific research.

8.3.2.2 Who is making the claims?

Section 8.3.1.3 discussed how social media can be a very useful tool for accessing the latest news, views, and research findings in a given topic. However, the section also cautioned that even though social media interactions may be with key-players in the field (see Section 8.3.1.2), many of the views shared might be based on personal perspectives, and may not have been formally vetted/reviewed for accuracy or substantiation. The same applies to individuals making claims/statements about scientific findings via all forms of media. It is important to consider who is making the statements/claims in order to evaluate their veracity. Key questions that may help you to do this include: *what is the professional background of the individual? Is the individual involved in the research on which the claims are based, or is the research being used 'second hand'? What companies/organisations does the individual work for? Does the individual have any financial/commercial/professional affiliations that could present a conflict of interest or potentially bias the statements they are making?* A healthy dose of scepticism is a good thing as it motivates you to look a little deeper, and not passively accept all that you see or hear.

8.4 A final word

Writing this book has at times been quite challenging. One of the reasons for this is because it can be daunting (and sometimes disheartening) to delve into the huge body of literature into fatigue in sport and exercise in an attempt to answer questions, challenge misconceptions, or simply provide more insight into any of the myriad topics in this area. My role as an academic and researcher has afforded me experience of sifting through research studies and collating findings in an attempt to reach a consensus about current knowledge in a particular topic. Nevertheless, it was at times exasperating to go through this process with the fatigue literature, due to the volume of disparate and contradictory research findings that have been published over the years, and continue to be published today. Going through this process has given me a clearer appreciation (and sympathy!) for students of the sport, health, and exercise sciences, and any other interested individuals, who try to do the same thing in order to further their knowledge. My experiences have also reinforced the importance of one of the key aims of the book: to collate current thinking on some key hypotheses/theories in sport and exercise fatigue in a clear, easy to understand way.

I hope that this aim has been achieved. I hope that you, the reader, feel able to use this book as a starting point or a guide for your studies into fatigue in sport and exercise. I also hope that you have been provided with an informative and thought-provoking insight into some of the current thinking in this field. Finally, I hope that you feel motivated and inspired to utilise the knowledge and insights gained from reading the book in whatever ways are appropriate to you both personally and professionally, and to spread this new knowledge and insight to friends and colleagues. In the preface, I mentioned that the reader should not read this book expecting that at the end, they would know precisely what causes fatigue in sport and exercise, as the majority of the answers to this question have not yet been found. You probably now understand the accuracy of this statement! However, even if you are motivated simply to spread the word on all that we *don't* yet know regarding fatigue in sport and exercise, this would be useful as well as accurate. In the process of communicating the complexity of fatigue and the limitations to our knowledge, you will also communicate that many of the long-held beliefs regarding what causes fatigue are limited in their ability to actually explain fatigue, or have even been disregarded as causes of fatigue in sport and exercise. The message is that regardless of what you say, it is beneficial to the topic to talk about sport and exercise fatigue.

Index

Note: page numbers in *italic* type refer to figures; those in **bold** type refer to tables.